Evidence-based Psychopharmacology

This book summarizes the recent advances in evidence-based pharmacological treatment of psychiatric disorders. There have been some significant developments in our understanding of the methods for systematically reviewing the literature, assessing clinical trials, and optimizing decision-making. This volume examines these issues with reference to the major psychiatric conditions and addresses issues such as selecting the best first-line psychopharmacological intervention for a particular disorder, for how long a particular intervention should be continued, and identifying the next-best treatment strategy should the first agent fail. The conditions covered include, amongst others, depression, schizophrenia, panic, posttraumatic stress disorder, obsessive-compulsive disorder, attention-deficit hyperactivity disorder, and eating disorders. There is also a chapter on the potential for complications as a result of adverse interactions between drugs. These issues lie at the heart of clinical psychopharmacology and the book will therefore appeal to all practicing clinicians, whether in a primary care or a specialist mental health setting.

Evidence-based Psychopharmacology

Dan J. Stein
University of Cape Town, South Africa

Bernard Lerer
Hadassah-Hebrew Medical Center, Israel

Stephen Stahl
University of California San Diego, USA

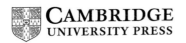

CAMBRIDGE
UNIVERSITY PRESS

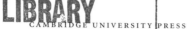
CAMBRIDGE UNIVERSITY PRESS

Cambridge, New York, Melbourne, Madrid, Cape Town, Singapore, São Paulo

Cambridge University Press

The Edinburgh Building, Cambridge CB2 2RU, UK

Published in the United States of America by Cambridge University Press, New York

www.cambridge.org
Information on this title: www.cambridge.org/9780521824818

© Cambridge University Press 2005

First published 2005

Printed in the United Kingdom at the University Press, Cambridge

A catalog record for this book is available from the British Library

Library of Congress Cataloging in Publication data

ISBN-13 978-0-521-82481-8 hardback
ISBN-10 0-521-82481-8 hardback

ISBN-13 978-0-521-53188-8 paperback
ISBN-10 0-521-53188-8 paperback

Cambridge University Press has no responsibility for the persistence or accuracy of URLs for external or third-party internet websites referred to in this book, and does not guarantee that any content on such websites is, or will remain, accurate or appropriate.

Every effort has been made in preparing this book to provide accurate and up-to-date information that is in accord with accepted standards and practice at the time of publication. Nevertheless, the authors, editors, and publisher can make no warranties that the information contained herein is totally free from error, not least because clinical standards are constantly changing through research and regulation. The authors, editors, and publisher therefore disclaim all liability for direct or consequential damages resulting from the use of material contained in this book. Readers are strongly advised to pay careful attention to information provided by the manufacturer of any drugs or equipment that they plan to use.

Contents

Contributors

Abraham Bakker, MD
National Centre for Eating Disorders
Robert Fleury Stichting
Leidschendam
The Netherlands

David S. Baldwin, MD
Department of Psychiatry
University of Southampton
Southampton
UK

Joseph Biederman, MD
Massachusetts General Hospital and
Harvard University
Boston MA
USA

Jacqueline Birks
Cochrane Dementia and Cognitive
Improvement Group
University of Oxford
Oxford
UK

Carlos Blanco, MD
Department of Psychiatry
Columbia College of Physicians
and Surgeons
New York NY
USA

C. Lindsay DeVane, PharmD
Department of Psychiatry and Behavioral
Sciences
Medical University of South Carolina
Charleston SC
USA

Robin Emsley, MB ChB, MMed, PhD
Department of Psychiatry
University of Stellenbosch
Stellenbosch
South Africa

John Grimley Evans
Cochrane Dementia and Cognitive
Impairment Group
University of Oxford
Oxford
UK

Naomi A. Fineberg, MA, MBBS, MRCPsych
Queen Elizabeth II Hospital
Welwyn Garden City
Herts
UK

Martine F. Flament, MD, PhD
University of Ottawa Institute of Mental
Health Resource
Royal Ottawa Hospital
Ottawa ON
Canada

Claudia Furino, BA
University of Ottawa Institute of Mental
Health Resource
Royal Ottawa Hospital
Ottawa ON
Canada

Tim M. Gale, PhD
Department of Psychology
University of Hertfordshire
Hatfield
Herts
UK

S. Nassir Ghaemi, MD
Cambridge Hospital and Harvard University
Cambridge MA
USA

Nathalie Godart, MD, PhD
Department of Psychiatry
Institut Mutualiste Montsouris
Paris
France

Douglas J. Hsu, BS
Cambridge Hospital and Harvard University
Cambridge MA
USA

Jeffrey Huffman, MD
Massachusetts General Hospital
and Harvard University
Boston MA
USA

Michael R. Liebowitz, MD
Department of Psychiatry
Columbia College of Physicians and
Surgeons
New York NY
USA

Andrew A. Nierenberg, MD
Massachusetts General Hospital
and Harvard University
Boston MA
USA

Piet Oosthuizen, MB ChB, MMed, PhD
Department of Psychiatry
University of Stellenbosch
Stellenbosch
South Africa

Michael J. Ostacher, MD, MPH
Massachusetts General Hospital
and Harvard University
Boston MA
USA

Roy Perlis, MD
Massachusetts General Hospital
and Harvard University
Boston MA
USA

Claire Polkinghorn, MD
Department of Psychiatry
Royal South Hants Hospital
Southampton
UK

C. Barbara Portier, MD
Department of Psychiatry
Sint Lucas Andreas Hospital
Amsterdam
The Netherlands

Muhammad S. Raza, MD
Department of Psychiatry
Columbia College of Physicians
and Surgeons
New York NY
USA

Franklin R. Schneier, MD
Department of Psychiatry
Columbia College of Physicians
and Surgeons
New York NY
USA

Thomas Spencer, MD
Massachusetts General Hospital
and Harvard University
Boston MA 02114
USA

Dan J. Stein, MD
Department of Psychiatry
University of Cape Town
Cape Town
South Africa

Anton J. L. M. van Balkom, MD
Department of Psychiatry
Vrije Universiteit
Amsterdam
The Netherlands

Gordon Wilcock
Department of Care of the Elderly
University of Bristol
Bristol
UK

Timothy Wilens, MD
Massachusetts General
Hospital and Harvard University
Boston MA
USA

Preface

The pioneers of modern psychopharmacology prided themselves on the empirical nature of their work, and the rigor of their clinical data. Evidence-based medicine emphasizes the importance of searching for relevant studies and making decisions in the light of the data (Sackett *et al.*, 1996), and therefore has immediate appeal for psychopharmacology. This volume attempts to summarize recent advances in the evidence-based medication treatment of psychiatric disorders.

Clinical decisions are only as good as the existing evidence, and critics have rightly pointed out the necessity for good clinical judgment and for further research when the data are poor (Klein, 1993; Wells, 1999; Rush, 2001). Nevertheless, there has been a steady growth in methods for systematically reviewing the literature, assessing the clinical trials database, and optimizing clinical decision-making (Chalmers and Altman, 1995; Eddy, 1996; Fawcett *et al.*, 1999). We therefore felt that it was timely to publish a collection of evidence-based articles in psychopharmacology.

This volume comprises articles on each of the major psychiatric disorders, and addresses questions such as: (1) what is the best first-line psychopharmacological intervention for a particular disorder? (2) how long should such an intervention be continued? and (3) what is the next best strategy should the first-line psychopharmacological agent fail? These questions lie at the heart of clinical psychopharmacology, and we are hopeful that the volume will therefore appeal to practicing clinicians, whether they work in a primary or specialty setting.

REFERENCES

Chalmers, I. and Altman, D. G. (1995). *Systematic Reviews*. London: BMJ Publishing Group.

Eddy, D. M. (1996). *Clinical Decision-Making: From Theory to Practice*. Sudbury, MA: Jones and Bartless.

Fawcett, J., Stein, D. J., and Jobson, K. O. (1999). *Textbook of Treatment Algorithms in Psychopharmacology*. Chichester: John Wiley.

Klein, D. F. (1993). Clinical psychopharmacological practice: the need for a developing research base. *Archives of General Psychiatry*, **50**, 491–4.

Rush, A. J. (2001). Clinical practice guidelines: good news, bad news, or no news? *Archives of General Psychiatry*, **50**, 483–90.

Sackett, D. L., Rosenberg, W. M. C., Muir Gray, J. A., *et al.* (1996). Evidence-based medicine: what it is and what it isn't. *British Medical Journal*, **312**, 71–2.

Wells, K. B. (1999). Treatment research at the crossroads: the scientific interface of clinical trials and effectiveness research. *American Journal of Psychiatry*, **156**, 5–10.

Introduction

Dan J. Stein

University of Cape Town, South Africa

This volume is based on the assumption that the concepts and methods of evidence-based medicine can make an important contribution to clinical psychopharmacology. In this introductory chapter, a brief background to evidence-based medicine is provided. The chapter outlines a definition of evidence-based medicine, considers some of the limitations of evidence-based medicine, discusses the growing emphasis on evidence-based guidelines and algorithms, and notes some of the evidence for evidence-based medicine.

What is evidence-based medicine?

There has been a significant growth in attention to evidence-based medicine in the past two decades. A search of the internet database PubMed reveals two citations on evidence-based medicine in 1992, but 3037 in 2004. Articles on evidence-based psychiatry first began appearing in the mid-1990s, and have similarly demonstrated an exponential increase. An immediate question is whether evidence-based medicine is merely old wine in a new bottle, or whether it represents a novel conceptual approach, along with new methodologies.

Sackett, a seminal author in the emergence of this new focus, has written that evidence-based medicine is the "conscientious, explicit, and judicious use of current best evidence in making decisions about the care of individual patients" (Sackett *et al.*, 1996). Evidence-based medicine addresses the question of how best to search the literature, how best to rate the quality of the relevant studies, and how best to synthesize the existing data (for example, using meta-analysis) (Guyatt and Rennie, 2002). Involvement of the patient in decision-making is also key.

The practice of evidence-based medicine involves, however, a good deal more than just the academic exercise of searching for and examining the existing research. In particular, evidence-based medicine involves "integrating individual clinical expertise with the best available external clinical evidence from systematic research" (Sackett *et al.*, 1996). Without clinical expertise, practice risks being tyrannized by evidence. Conversely, without current best evidence, practice risks becoming out-dated (Cochrane, 1972). Thus, evidence-based medicine should not be equated with "cookbook" medicine.

An immediate objection to the prominence claimed by evidence-based medicine is that it has long been recommended that medicine be based on scientific principles, and that its interventions therefore lie on a solid empirical base (Flexner, 1910). Nevertheless, it should be remembered that randomized controlled trials (RCTs), the gold standard of evidence, are a relatively new development in medicine and psychiatry, as are the large electronic databases that provide ready access to such work. Certainly, RCTs are now so numerous that clinicians often do not read (Loke and Derry, 2003) or apply (Bruce et al., 2003) them; appropriate theories and methods for synthesizing and applying the data at hand are therefore needed.

Even so, the limitations of the research base on which evidence-based medicine lies must be acknowledged. First, there may be few RCTs, or indeed, any studies, available to address any particular clinical question. The value of sequential and combined regimens is particularly difficult to address (Saver and Kalafut, 2001). Of course, absence of evidence of efficacy is not the same as absence of efficacy, so that while skepticism is crucial, it should also be tempered by clinical judgment. Similarly, a focus on measurable factors lies at the heart of evidence-based medicine, but in clinical psychopharmacology there are areas of practice where research measures are arguably insufficiently precise to match clinical phenomena (Williams and Garner, 2002). Certainly, despite the precedence given to RCTs, observational studies can provide accurate information (Concato et al., 2000).

Second, even when RCTs exist, these may have significant limitations. The majority of the large controlled trials undertaken in psychopharmacology today are sponsored by the pharmaceutical industry, and aim to demonstrate to regulatory authorities the efficacy of medication over placebo. There are far fewer trials demonstrating the effectiveness of medication in the clinical context, where patient samples are much more heterogeneous than those who enter registration trials (Wells, 1999). Current clinical trials have other important limitations, including large numbers of subjects who respond to both medication and placebo (Parker et al., 2003).

Third, meta-analysis of multiple available RCTs should be undertaken with due caution. Negative studies are often filed away in drawers rather than published, so that the published literature may be positively biased in favor of particular interventions (Melander et al., 2003). Available studies may employ widely different methods, so that formal comparison is inappropriate. In an incisive criticism of a meta-analysis comparing pharmacotherapy and psychotherapy trials, for example, Klein (2000) argued that "Meta-analyses compared effect sizes from disparate studies that were not uniformly blind, random, controlled, or high quality." Thus clinically useful distinctions can be obscured by using the supposed common metric of a single effect size.

Fourth, the conclusions of evidence-based medicine can be translated into inappropriately restricted policy. On the basis of the "evidence," crucial variables affecting the operation of health systems may be overlooked (Birch, 1997), and there may be undue rationing of psychiatric medication and treatment. Interestingly, the use of untested non-conventional treatments may have increased after widespread introduction of evidence-based medicine into the UK (Williams and Garner, 2002). At the end of the day, if we are going to emphasize the importance of evidence, we will need to address the evidence for evidence-based medicine. We return to this question below.

Guidelines and algorithms

Together with the growth of evidence-based medicine there has been the publication of a growing number of guidelines and algorithms, including those in the area of psychiatry and psychopharmacology. There is an increasing emphasis on "best practice" by clinicians, consumers, and health managers (in both public and private sectors); and guidelines are systematically developed statements designed to help practitioners and patients make decisions about appropriate health care for specific circumstances (Jackson and Feder, 1998), while algorithms attempt to clarify and present the inputs, sequences, and outputs involved in rule-based decision-making (Fawcett et al., 1999).

Guidelines and algorithms are particularly useful insofar as they summarize the evidence (including data on efficacy, on effectiveness, and on cost-effectiveness), and point out areas where there are insufficient data and so where further research is needed (Patel et al., 2001). They have the potential for helping to ensure that rigorous clinical standards are maintained, and for directing research to addressing gaps in the evidence base (Rush, 2001). Nevertheless, the proliferation of guidelines and algorithms does not necessarily translate into their being read, or into better clinical care, whether because of poor quality (Littlejohns et al., 1999; Shaneyfelt et al., 1999), or because of barriers to implementation (Cabana et al., 1999).

A good guideline should: (1) identify the key decisions (e.g., diagnosis, assessment strategy, treatment choice); (2) review the relevant, valid evidence on the benefits, risks, and costs of alternative decisions; and (3) present recommendations in a concise, accessible, updated format (Woolf, 1992; Jackson and Feder, 1998). Guidelines should give an indication of the level of evidence used and consequent level of certainty of advice (there is a need to make decisions when there is no evidence). Guidelines must be time-stamped and regularly updated – evidence changes rapidly over time and updating may require multidisciplinary feedback.

One area in which guidelines must show flexibility is in establishing a balance between specificity and generality (Klein, 1993). A useful guideline must walk a fine line between excessive specificity and excessive generality. Excessive specificity cannot be evidence-based, and by ignoring critical individual differences may be dangerous. Excessive generality, on the other hand, may provide insufficiently specific guidance for any particular decision.

Why don't physicians and consumers follow guidelines and algorithms (Haynes and Haines, 1998; Cabana *et al.*, 1999)? First, as noted above, the guidelines may be poor; they may not be user-friendly, relevant, or accurate. Second, there may be lack of effective dissemination and consequent poor access to recommendations. Third, there may be a lack of effective implementation and reinforcement. It may be crucial to target guidelines and algorithms in particular ways for particular users and purposes (Stein *et al.*, 2002).

Furthermore, important inherent limitations of guidelines and algorithms must be acknowledged. First, guidelines are only as good as the evidence base on which they rest; if this is poor, then the guideline may simply not provide an answer to any particular clinical question. Second, guidelines are no substitute for clinical expertise and judgment; they can't, for example, ensure an accurate diagnosis. The more complex the case, and the greater the specification of individual contributing clinical variables, arguably the less useful any particular guideline will be.

This volume is not specifically devoted to the development of guidelines and algorithms for clinical psychopharmacology. While guidelines are ideally evidence-based, many of those involved in the practice and teaching of evidence-based medicine focus rather on helping individual practitioners to address specific questions raised by patients. Here we focus on three key questions throughout: (1) What is the first-line pharmacotherapy? (2) For how long should this be maintained? and (3) What is the optimal approach to those who fail to respond to first-line pharmacotherapy?

What is the evidence for evidence-based medicine?

Given the emphasis of evidence-based medicine, an immediate question for those interested in its promulgation is whether there is any evidence that supports such a move. A small but growing literature has addressed this point, and the data are to some extent reassuring (Sackett *et al.*, 1996).

First, there are a number of positive controlled trials of teaching critical appraisal to medical students. Second, there is some evidence that educational outreach can modify health professional behavior, although not all data are consistent (Thomson-O'Brien *et al.*, 2000; Gilbody *et al.*, 2003). Third, there are a number of positive outcomes studies showing the benefit to patients of receiving effective therapies. Fourth, there are a number of positive controlled trials of the effects of guidelines and algorithms on clinical outcome, including work that has focused specifically on clinical psychopharmacology (Trivedi *et al.*, 2004).

On the other hand, although it has been argued that computerized decision support systems can promote adherence to guidelines and algorithms, RCTs have not demonstrated high rates of use or beneficial effects on the process or outcome of care (Rousseau *et al.*, 2003). Furthermore, there is some evidence that access to specialist services has been more beneficial than guideline implementations for the management of depression (Peveler & Kendrick, 2001). Thus, even while adhering to the principles of evidence-based medicine, there is a need for additional work to optimize evidence-based policy (Macintyre *et al.*, 2001).

While evidence-based medicine can be criticized for being insufficient, there are in reality few valid alternatives. We are continuously faced with the problem of dissociating researchers' therapy allegiances and their interpretation of treatment outcomes (Luborsky *et al.*, 2004). A tongue-in-cheek publication lists possible alternatives to evidence-based medicine as eminence-based medicine, vehemence-based medicine, eloquence-based medicine, providence-based medicine, diffidence-based medicine, nervousness-based medicine, and confidence-based medicine (Isaacs and Fitzgerald, 1999). All of these have obvious and significant disadvantages.

Evidence-based medicine is undoubtedly here to stay. Practitioners will increasingly need to feel comfortable with methodologies involving the assessment of the evidence. Despite the current limitations of the field, there are good reasons for accepting that this will ultimately benefit the practice of clinical psychopharmacology. The present volume rests on this assumption, and addresses the evidence-based psychopharmacology of each of the major psychiatric disorders.

REFERENCES

Birch, S. (1997). As a matter of fact: evidence-based decision-making unplugged. *Health Economics*, **6**, 547–59.

Bruce, S. E., Vasile, R. G., Goisman, R. M., *et al.* (2003). Are benzodiazepines still the medication of choice for patients with panic disorder with or without agoraphobia? *American Journal of Psychiatry*, **160**, 1432–8.

Cabana, M. D., Rand, C. S., Powe, N. R., *et al.* (1999). Why don't physicians follow clinical practice guidelines? A framework for improvement. *Journal of the American Medical Association*, **282**, 1458–65.

Cochrane, A. L. (1972). *Effectiveness and Efficiency: Random Reflections on Health Services*. London, UK: Nuffield Provincial Hospitals Trust.

Concato, J., Shah, N., and Horwitz, R. I. (2000). Randomized, controlled trials, observational studies, and the hierarchy of research designs. *New England Journal of Medicine*, **342**, 1887–92.

Fawcett, J., Stein, D. J., and Jobson, K. O. (1999). *Textbook of Treatment Algorithms in Psychopharmacology*. Chichester, UK: John Wiley.

Flexner, A. (1910). *Medical Education in the United States and Canada: A Report to the Carnegie Foundation for the Advancement of Teaching*. Bulletin no. 4. New York, NY: Carnegie Foundation for the Advancement of Teaching.

Gilbody, S., Whitty, P., Grimshaw, J., and Thomas, R. (2003). Educational and organizational interventions to improve the management of depression in primary care: a systematic review. *Journal of the American Medical Association*, **289**, 3145–51.

Guyatt, G. and Rennie, D. (2002). *Users' Guides to the Medical Literature: A Manual for Evidence-Based Clinical Practice*. Chicago, IL: AMA Press.

Haynes, B. and Haines, A. (1998). Barriers and bridges to evidence based clinical practice. *British Medical Journal*, **317**, 273–6.

Isaacs, D. and Fitzgerald, D. (1999). Seven alternatives to evidence based medicine. *British Medical Journal*, **319**, 1618.

Jackson, R. and Feder, G. (1998). Guidelines for clinical guidelines. *British Medical Journal*, **317**, 427–8.

Klein, D. F. (1993). Clinical psychopharmacological practice: the need for a developing research base. *Archives of General Psychiatry*, **50**, 491–4.

Klein, D. F. (2000). Flawed meta-analyses comparing psychotherapy with pharmacotherapy. *American Journal of Psychiatry*, **157**, 1204–11.

Littlejohns, P., Cluzeau, F., Bale, R., *et al.* (1999). The quantity and quality of clinical practice guidelines for the management of depression in primary care in the UK. *British Journal of General Practice*, **49**, 205–10.

Loke, Y. K. and Derry, S. (2003). Does anybody read "evidence-based" articles? *BMC Medical Research Methodology*, **3**, 14.

Luborsky, L., Diguer, L., Seligman, D. A., *et al.* (2004). The researcher's own therapy allegiances: a "wild card" in comparisons of treatment efficacy. *Clinical Psychology: Science and Practice*, **6**, 95–132.

Macintyre, S., Chalmers, I., Horton, R., and Smith, R. (2001). Using evidence to inform health policy: case study. *British Medical Journal*, **322**, 222–5.

Melander, H., Ahlqvist-Rastad, J., Meijer, G., and Beermann, B. (2003). Evidence b(i)ased medicine – selective reporting from studies sponsored by pharmaceutical industry: review of studies in new drug applications. *British Medical Journal*, **326**, 1171–3.

Parker, G., Anderson, I. M., and Haddad, P. (2003). Clinical trials of antidepressants are producing meaningless results. *British Journal of Psychiatry*, **183**, 102–4.

Patel, V. L., Arocha, J. F., Diermeier, M., How, J., and Mottur-Pilson, C. (2001). Cognitive psychological studies of representation and use of clinical practice guidelines. *International Journal of Medical Information*, **63**, 147–67.

Peveler, R. and Kendrick, T. (2001). Treatment delivery and guidelines in primary care. *British Medical Bulletin*, **57**, 193–206.

Rousseau, N., McColl, E., Newton, J., Grimshaw, J., and Eccles, M. (2003). Practice based, longitudinal, qualitative interview study of computerised evidence based guidelines in primary care. *British Medical Journal*, **326**, 314.

Rush, A. J. (2001). Clinical practice guidelines: good news, bad news, or no news? *Archives of General Psychiatry*, **50**, 483–90.

Sackett, D. L., Rosenberg, W. M. C., Muir Gray, J. A., and Richards, W. S. (1996). Evidence-based medicine: what it is and what it isn't. *British Medical Journal*, **312**, 71–2.

Saver, J. L. and Kalafut, M. (2001). Combination therapies and the theoretical limits of evidence-based medicine. *Neuroepidemiology*, **20**, 57–64.

Shaneyfelt, T. M., Mayo-Smith, M. F., and Rothwangl, J. (1999). Are guidelines following guidelines? The methodological quality of clinical practice guidelines in the peer-reviewed medical literature. *Journal of the American Medical Association*, **281**, 1900–5.

Stein, D. J., Xin, Y., Osser, D., Li, X., and Jobson, K. (2002). Clinical psychopharmacology guidelines: different strokes for different folks. *World Journal of Biological Psychiatry*, **3**, 64–7.

Thomson-O'Brien, M. A., Oxman, A. D., Davis, D. A., *et al.* (2000). Educational outreach visits: effects on professional practice and health care outcomes. *Cochrane Database Systematic Review* 2. CD000409.

Trivedi, M. H., Rush, J. A., Crismon, M. L., *et al.* (2004). Clinical results for patients with major depressive disorder in the Texas Medication Algorithm Project. *Archives of General Psychiatry*, **61**, 669–80.

Wells, K. B. (1999). Treatment research at the crossroads: the scientific interface of clinical trials and effectiveness research. *American Journal of Psychiatry*, **156**, 5–10.

Williams, D. D. R. and Garner, J. (2002). The case against 'the evidence': a different perspective on evidence-based medicine. *British Journal of Psychiatry*, **180**, 8–12.

Woolf, S. H. (1992). Practice guidelines, a new reality in medicine: II. Methods of developing guidelines. *Archives of Internal Medicine*, **152**, 946–52.

Evidence-based pharmacotherapy of major depressive disorder

Michael J. Ostacher, Jeffrey Huffman, Roy Perlis, and Andrew A. Nierenberg

Massachusetts General Hospital and Harvard University, Boston, MA, USA

Major depressive disorder (MDD) is estimated by the World Health Organization to be the fourth leading cause of loss of disability-adjusted life years. In the National Comorbidity Survey, MDD is the most common mental illness and is one of the most common and disabling of all illnesses (Kessler *et al.*, 1994). The lifetime risk for MDD is 10–25% in women and 5–12% in men, and at any point its prevalence is 5–9% in women and 2–3% in men. Given the widespread and disabling nature of the illness, MDD is of great public health concern.

The first useful antidepressants, imipramine and isoniazid, were serendipitously found to have antidepressant properties in the 1950s. These discoveries – coupled with the observation that reserpine, which depletes monoamines, induced depression – led to the development of the monoamine hypothesis of depression. This led to the rational development of drugs which affect central nervous system monoamines, primarily norepinephrine (noradrenaline), serotonin (5-HT), and dopamine.

The tricyclic antidepressants (TCAs) and monoamine oxidase inhibitors (MAOIs) formed the foundation for several decades of pharmacologic treatments for depression, although their side-effects (including lethality in overdose in the case of TCAs, and strict dietary restriction to avoid hypertensive crises in the case of MAOIs) limited their utility and tolerability. Pharmaceutical research focused on the development of drugs with improved tolerability and safety. Next-generation drugs such as trazodone, a 5-HT_2-receptor antagonist, were an incremental improvement, but not until the arrival to the market in 1988 of the first selective serotonin reuptake inhibitor (SSRI), fluoxetine (Prozac), did the use of antidepressants markedly change. Several other SSRIs followed, including paroxetine (Paxil), sertraline (Zoloft), fluvoxamine (Luvox), citalopram (Celexa), and escitalopram (Lexapro).

Antidepressants are not effective for all patients. In clinical practice, 40–50% of episodes do not completely respond to initial antidepressant drug therapy. Response to antidepressant medication is also delayed, with weeks to months until remission for those who do respond. Many patients are only partially responsive to treatment, and residual symptoms are responsible for significant morbidity and loss of function. A further generation of antidepressants was developed with effects on multiple neurotransmitter systems in the hope that drugs with effects on multiple neurotransmitter sites would be effective for a higher percentage of patients or have a more rapid onset of response. These so-called dual-action and triple-action antidepressants include venlafaxine (Effexor), nefazodone (Serzone), mirtazapine (Remeron), duloxetine, and bupropion (Wellbutrin). Reversible monoamine oxidase inhibitors (RIMAs) such as moclobemide and brofaromine were also developed, and may have an improved safety profile compared to earlier-generation non-reversible MAOIs. Conflicting data exist regarding the success of these latest-generation drugs in improving depression treatment beyond existing drugs.

For the purposes of this chapter, we searched MEDLINE and PsychLit for all controlled trials published in English between January 1981 and January 2004 in which adults with MDD were randomly assigned to receive medication, placebo, or active comparator drugs, and all meta-analyses of psychopharmacotherapy for MDD. The number of published randomized controlled trials (RCTs) of antidepressants for the acute treatment of MDD is too vast to allow for discussion of each study individually.

In order to recommend first-line treatment for MDD, we examined meta-analyses of RCTs of antidepressant drugs for MDD as a statistical means of weighing the relative efficacy of antidepressants that have not been compared directly. This was done both to evaluate the acute effectiveness of multiple antidepressant agents in MDD and to determine what recommendations are to be made for continuation and maintenance treatment of MDD with antidepressants. Meta-analysis increases the power to show a difference between treatment groups, in effect by increasing the sample size. This can reduce type II error; that is, the failure to find a difference when one actually exists. Because placebo response rates in antidepressant trials tend to be very high – thus causing many positive trials of active drugs to have small effect sizes – meta-analysis of multiple trials may be used to determine whether drug–placebo differences are meaningful.

The literature on evidence-based treatment for first-line antidepressant treatment failures is, to this date, quite limited. Few randomized, parallel-group trials of such treatments have been published; limited evidence from open trials will be reviewed.

What is the first-line pharmacotherapy of MDD?

All marketed antidepressants are effective in the treatment of depression. In determining which of these antidepressants can be recommended as first-line treatment for major depression, however, several factors are important. Does an antidepressant have demonstrable response and remission rates? Is the time to remission and recovery more rapid for a given antidepressant or class of antidepressant? Does superiority in terms of adverse events lead fewer patients to discontinue their medications, and thus lead to a greater percentage of responders at endpoint? To what extent should the safety of a drug – in overdose or due to side-effects – have an impact on prescribing? Do drugs differ in the response rates for different subtypes of depression (e.g., melancholic or psychotic) or in patients with comorbid conditions (e.g., anxiety disorders, substance abuse), or who differ in sex or age?

Randomized controlled efficacy trials generally use a straightforward, simple design to answer a basic question. As these studies tend to exclude patients with significant medical or psychiatric comorbidity, however, they offer only incomplete information about a drug's effectiveness in an unselected clinical population. Many studies exclude patients with active or recent substance abuse, even though the rate of comorbid substance abuse in mood disorders is substantial, thus limiting how generalizable the results are to actual clinical practice.

An essential task in recommending first-line treatment is to determine whether an individual antidepressant or class of antidepressant has superior efficacy compared to others. Meta-analyses of multiple antidepressant trials can improve the ability to distinguish between the relative equivalences of different antidepressants or classes of antidepressants. The methodology of the meta-analysis is important in interpreting the results, as the results can only be as good as the criteria for deciding which studies are analyzed. Only double-blind, parallel-group studies ought to be included. All available studies that meet criteria for data quality must be included, and not merely those with favorable results. Dosages of the medications in an individual study, for example, must be adequate (and comparable, in a comparator trial) or the results will not be interpretable.

SSRIs in MDD

The most widely prescribed antidepressants are the SSRIs. Most, though certainly not all, SSRI trials have shown superiority of active drug over placebo in the treatment of MDD. These studies generally fail to demonstrate a clear dose–response curve, suggesting that increasing SSRI dose beyond what is minimally effective does not increase response (although in some cases dropout rates are greater with higher dosages), although a meta-analysis of fixed- versus variable-dose trials of SSRIs found a 7–10% increased response rate for increased dosages (Baker *et al.*, 2003). It also appears that higher doses of SSRIs may have higher effect sizes, suggesting again that some dose–response relationship does exist for SSRIs (Khan *et al.*, 2003).

A Cochrane Collaboration meta-analysis identified 98 trials comparing SSRIs to other antidepressants, with a total of 5044 SSRI-treated patients, and failed to detect any clinically significant difference in efficacy between drugs (Geddes *et al.*, 2003). SSRIs also demonstrate efficacy for depression, without clear evidence of superiority over older drugs when studied in particular patient subgroups. A smaller meta-analysis including 365 SSRI-treated geriatric depressed patients found SSRIs and TCAs to be equally efficacious (Wilson *et al.*, 2003). Similarly, a meta-analysis which included 18 antidepressant studies, including six with SSRIs, in medically ill patients noted efficacy for multiple classes, but did not find one to be superior (Gill and Hatcher, 1999, 2003).

A well-designed meta-analysis funded by Eli Lilly compared fluoxetine to TCAs. Thirty trials (16 USA and 14 non-USA) and 4120 patients (3447 USA and 673 non-USA) were included in the study. The criteria for study inclusion in the analysis included adequate TCA and fluoxetine dosing, double-blind design, and the first 17 items of the Hamilton Rating Scale for Depression (HAM-D). Analyses were performed separately for studies conducted in the USA versus elsewhere. The effect size (−0.30) for fluoxetine compared to placebo was small for the main outcome measure, 50% decrease in HAM-D. There was not a statistically significant difference favoring fluoxetine versus TCAs overall. The European trials, comparing fluoxetine to newer TCAs, showed a non-significant trend in favor of the TCAs, while the US trials, comparing fluoxetine to older TCAs, showed a non-significant trend in favor of fluoxetine.

One recent study attempted to assess the effectiveness, rather than the efficacy, of SSRIs in clinical practice. The A R T I S T trial showed a non-significant trend in favor of the randomized 573 depressed patients in a primary care practice to open-label treatment with one of three SSRIs (paroxetine, fluoxetine, and sertraline). Over the 9-month trial, patients in all three groups improved, but the three groups did not differ statistically in degree of improvement. This supports the findings of a Cochrane Collaboration meta-analysis of individual trials of SSRIs (Geddes *et al.*, 2002).

One area where SSRIs may demonstrate benefit over older medications is in tolerability. A Cochrane Collaboration review that identified 136 randomized trials in which SSRIs and tricyclic antidepressants were compared among depressed patients found a modest but significant difference favoring SSRIs in terms of dropouts (Barbui *et al.*, 2003). Accordingly, the SSRIs have advantages in terms of safety and tolerability compared to many newer and older agents, and their place as a primary treatment choice for major depression is not disputed.

Dual- and triple-action agents and RIMAs in MDD

The most recent generation of antidepressants (which includes bupropion, mirtazapine, and venlafaxine) has proved effective for major depression in both outpatient and inpatient settings in placebo-controlled and comparator trials. Whether these newer-generation dual-action agents improve response compared to SSRIs is unclear, although there are some interesting data suggesting that this might be the case.

An early meta-analysis of double-blind, placebo-controlled trials of imipramine, bupropion, trazodone, and fluoxetine published between 1980 and 1990 found no difference in effect size for any of the antidepressants, suggesting equivalence between these antidepressants (Workman and Short, 1993). Although the criteria for study interpretability, however, did not include minimum dosages, the results are consistent with other analyses.

A meta-analysis funded by Wyeth, the manufacturer of venlafaxine, pooled eight trials of venlafaxine compared to SSRIs or SSRIs and placebo. After treatment with venlafaxine ($n = 851$), SSRIs (fluoxetine, paroxetine, fluvoxamine; $n = 748$) or placebo (four studies; $n = 446$), the study found remission rates (defined as HAM-D17 < 7) of 45% (382/851) for venlafaxine, 35% (260/748) for SSRIs, and 25% (110/446) for placebo ($P < 0.001$). The odds ratio for remission was 1.50 (1.3–1.9), favoring venlafaxine versus SSRIs (Thase *et al.*, 2001). Venlafaxine separated from placebo at week 2, while this only occurred at week 4 for SSRIs.

The study has several important limitations. First, previous non-responders to SSRIs were not excluded from any of the studies; as previous non-response to an SSRI would likely have predicted non-response to the study SSRI, this would have been an important exclusion criterion. Second, the difference in response was only true for venlafaxine doses greater than 150 mg/day; at 75 mg/day there was no difference in remission rates with venlafaxine compared to SSRIs. Third, two studies were 6 weeks in duration and the remainder 8 weeks. Whether the ultimate response rates over a longer period would have been more similar cannot be known.

Overall, no clear benefit for dual- and triple-action agents or RIMAs can be found in larger meta-analyses (Freemantle *et al.*, 2000). A meta-analysis using a modified intent-to-treat design compared older, newer, and alternative treatments for multiple depressive disorders (including major depression), and found equivalent benefit for older and newer antidepressants (Williams *et al.*, 2000). For MDD, there was equivalent effectiveness between the newer agents (SSRIs, serotonin norepinephrine reuptake inhibitors, RIMA, norepinephrine reuptake inhibitors,

5-HT$_2$-receptor antagonists, and dopamine reuptake inhibitors) and older agents (first-generation TCAs, tetracyclic antidepressants, second-generation TCAs, trazodone, and non-reversible MAOIs). Fifty-four percent of the patients randomly assigned to receive a newer antidepressant and 54% of those assigned to receive an older antidepressant experienced at least a 50% improvement in depressive symptoms (relative benefit, 1.0: confidence interval (CI) 0.97–1.06). The authors found an overall dropout rate of 30% across these studies, suggesting that actual clinical care must address the tendency of patients to stop their antidepressants. They rightfully point out that large "effectiveness" trials in actual clinical practice will be necessary to determine whether there are meaningful differences between drugs.

There have been several notable attempts to examine effectiveness in clinical practice. The Texas Medication Algorithm Project (TMAP) compared the use of expert consensus guidelines for the treatment of multiple psychiatric disorders, including MDD (Crismon *et al.*, 1999). There were several methodological problems in the design of the studies. Most significantly, there was no randomization to treatment. Instead different sites (primarily outpatient treatment centers) implemented the guideline algorithms with treatment-as-usual at control sites. The study is also limited in that it was implemented in a public sector, primarily indigent population; this aspect of the design may underestimate the effectiveness of all treatments.

A large National Institute of Mental Health (NIMH)-funded effectiveness study, the Sequenced Treatment Alternatives to Relieve Depression (STAR*D) trial, will attempt to clarify what differences there are between treatments in clinical practice. STAR*D will enroll up to 4000 depressed outpatients in open treatment with citalopram; those who fail to respond will then be randomized to various "next-step" interventions. STAR*D will provide data which will examine SSRI and second-line treatment efficacy in MDD, and attempt to fill gaps in information guiding current treatment (Fava *et al.*, 2003).

Depressive subtypes, comorbidity, and demographics

It has been suggested that certain antidepressants are more effective than others in different subpopulations of patients. If this is indeed the case, then recommendations for first-line treatment should bear this in mind. We examined the published data regarding the differential effects of different antidepressants on medical comorbidity, *Diagnostic and Statistical Manual of Mental Disorders*, 4th edition (DSM-IV) axis I and II comorbidity (including anxiety disorders), subtypes of depression (e.g., atypical, melancholic), and demographics such as sex and age. There have been no robust predictors of response in MDD; studies that suggest that one treatment may be preferable to another for given populations of patients are too small and underpowered to dictate treatment recommendations.

Medical comorbidity

Significant medical comorbidity often excludes patients from participating in randomized trials of antidepressants for MDD. When the medical risk of the drugs themselves was considered high, as it was with TCAs, general recommendations were to avoid using antidepressants in the medically ill (Koenig *et al.*, 1989). Newer drugs are expected to be safer for use in this population; analysis of randomized trials suggests benefit for all antidepressants for the treatment of MDD in this subgroup of patients (Gill and Hatcher, 2003).

A retrospective review of TCA treatment of medically ill patients with TCAs by a psychiatric consultation service found poor tolerability of the drug (30% dropouts due to side-effects) and limited response (40% responded) (Popkin *et al.*, 1985). Even though this was only a retrospective chart review, the study reinforced the impression that TCAs were not useful in medically ill patients.

A Cochrane Collaboration meta-analysis of the antidepressant treatment of medically ill patients, however, comes to a different conclusion (Gill and Hatcher, 2003). The study examined 18 RCTs of antidepressants in medically ill subjects (six of SSRIs, three of atypical antidepressants, and nine of tricyclics). There was substantial benefit to antidepressant treatment, with 52% responding to antidepressant overall compared to 30% responding to placebo (13 studies, odds ratio (OR) 0.37, 95% CI 0.27–0.51). There was a small but statistically significant increase in dropout rates for drug compared to placebo for TCAs and SSRIs (OR 1.66, 95% CI 1.14–2.40); for one study of mianserin there were fewer dropouts in the treatment group. The authors noted that there was a small increased treatment effect of TCAs over SSRIs, but that TCAs had a somewhat increased dropout rate.

A limitation of the Cochrane meta-analysis is that none of the studies analyzed included patients without significant medical illness as a comparator group. A naturalistic study which included both medically ill and healthy patients examined the effects of axis III comorbidity in the treatment of treatment-resistant depression with nortriptyline, and concluded that medical illness did not have an impact on the effectiveness of the drug compared to subjects without medical illness (Papakostas *et al.*, 2003).

Although the data suggest that response to antidepressants may not be impeded by the presence of medical illness, drug safety and tolerability are still concerns in treating MDD in the medically ill. It is worth avoiding orthostatic hypotension in the frail elderly, for instance, and drugs with these prominent side-effects should be avoided. It is also the case that large-scale trials comparing antidepressants in the medically ill population are lacking, so one antidepressant cannot be recommended over any other because of effectiveness.

Axis II comorbidity

A large study found that axis II personality disorder comorbidity had no effect on therapeutic outcome in the antidepressant treatment of acute MDD. A total of 635 patients with major depression and dysthymia were treated blindly with imipramine or sertraline (Russell *et al.*, 2003). The prevalence of axis II disorders was 46%; there was no clear impairment in the percentage of responders (>50% drop in HAM-D scores, HAM-D score <15, and Clinical Global Impression (CGI) improvement score of 1 or 2) or remitters (HAM-D score <7 and CGI improvement score of 1 or 2) compared to the subjects without any axis II disorder. There was a non-significant trend towards longer time to remission in the axis II group (10 versus 12 weeks, $P = 0.052$). Subjects with two or more axis II disorders did have a lower response rate, however (62% versus 47%, $P = 0.009$). A smaller study, comparing fluoxetine to nortriptyline, also found that having an axis II disorder did not predict worse outcome (Mulder *et al.*, 2003).

A meta-analysis of the impact of axis II personality disorders on outcome in major depression concluded that antidepressants are as effective in the presence of personality disorders as in their absence (Mulder, 2002). Antidepressant treatment should not be withheld because of the presence of an axis II personality disorder, at least for acute episodes of depression.

Anxiety disorder comorbidity

Comorbid anxiety disorders (but not anxiety symptoms) may predict poorer response to antidepressant treatment for MDD (Walker *et al.*, 2000). No study has prospectively studied the effectiveness of antidepressants with comorbid anxiety disorders in a randomized, double-blind trial. While many antidepressants have shown efficacy for major depression and anxiety disorders, there remains a gap in our knowledge about how to treat patients who present with both disorders. Even as logic would lead one to recommend the use of an antidepressant with efficacy for both disorders individually, there are not enough data to make this recommendation.

Major depressive subtypes

Limited and contradictory information is available to determine if one subtype of depression responds more robustly to one antidepressant versus another. For atypical depression, MAOIs appear in early studies to be more effective than TCAs (Liebowitz *et al.*, 1988). A total of 119 patients were randomized to phenelzine, imipramine, or placebo, with response rates of 71%, 50%, and 28% respectively

(Liebowitz *et al.*, 1988). In later studies SSRIs appear as effective as MAOIs (Pande *et al.*, 1996). In a more recent study, however, fluoxetine was not superior to imipramine in this subtype of depression (McGrath *et al.*, 2000). As MAOIs, TCAs, and SSRIs have not been directly compared (and are not likely to be compared) in an adequately powered trial, and no meta-analysis exists, one cannot with certainty recommend one antidepressant over another for major depression with atypical features.

Few data are available to determine whether one antidepressant or class is preferable to another for more severe and melancholic forms of depression. It is difficult to compare studies due to the lack of a standard definition of severe depression. Using inpatients as a subgroup, one large meta-analysis found TCAs to have a small amount of benefit over SSRIs (Geddes *et al.*, 2002). The authors caution, however, that this difference may be due to chance, and amounts to only 1 HAM-D point. Another meta-analysis found that, while depressed inpatients responded somewhat better to TCAs compared to SSRIs, SSRIs were moderately more tolerable (Anderson, 1998, 2000). This is significant, as the TCA with the highest likelihood of superior efficacy, amitriptyline, is one of the TCAs with the lowest tolerability due to adverse effects. While it is not certain whether one antidepressant is superior for more severe forms of depression, it has become clear that placebo–drug difference increases directly with increased severity (Khan *et al.*, 2002). The more severely ill the patients were who were included in trials, the more likely the drug would be found effective. Higher depression rating scale scores predicted a greater decrease in scores in the treatment group, while higher depression rating scale scores predicted smaller decreases in the placebo group.

Demographics: sex

A small, but statistically significant, increase in response was found to imipramine versus sertraline, an SSRI, for men compared to women in one study of MDD. The results suggest that SSRIs may be preferable to TCAs in premenopausal women (Kornstein *et al.*, 2000). This finding, however, has not been replicated. Wohlfarth *et al.* (2004) found no difference in response to TCAs by sex in a meta-analysis. Quitkin *et al.* (2003) published a meta-analysis of placebo-controlled trials of TCAs, MAOIs, and fluoxetine, and found no differential effect based on age or sex (Quitkin *et al.*, 2002). A small but statistically significant effect favoring MAOIs for women was found, but the authors could not conclude that this effect was clinically significant. Parker *et al.* (2003), in two naturalistic studies of antidepressant treatment of MDD (one retrospective, one prospective) did not find a meaningful difference in response to SSRI or TCA by sex, although there was a trend to better SSRI response in younger subjects and better TCA response in older ones (Parker *et al.*, 2003).

Age

Several studies had found that antidepressants are effective in the elderly (Feighner and Cohn, 1985; Cohn *et al.*, 1990; Bondareff *et al.*, 2000; Schneider *et al.*, 2003). There does not appear to be clear benefit to one versus another in older patients, in spite of the expectation that side-effects of TCAs would limit their usefulness in this group. A meta-analysis of randomized, double-blind studies of antidepressant treatment in the elderly confirms this (Wilson *et al.*, 2003). The authors concluded with caution that, while low-dose treatment with TCAs, ostensibly to reduce the incidence of adverse events in this population, was more effective than placebo in the elderly. They could not, however, recommend this as a treatment strategy as it had not itself been studied prospectively.

How long should pharmacotherapy of MDD continue?

The ideal length of time to continue antidepressant treatment after the resolution of an acute episode has not been definitively determined. In practice this is generally dependent on whether the acute episode is recurrent and – since the older the patient, the more likely that the episode is recurrent – on the age of the patient (American Psychiatric Association, 2000). It is also important to note whether the episode has resolved completely, or whether there are continued or residual symptoms of depression. Residual symptoms after treatment of an episode may predict recurrence (Judd *et al.*, 1998).

Most antidepressants have been studied in continuation after a depressive episode has resolved, and all appear – at least over 4–12 months – better at preventing relapse than placebo (Weihs *et al.*, 2002). Responders to drug are randomized to continue with active drug versus placebo for months to years, and a survival analysis – usually time to relapse or time to given score on a depression rating scale – is performed. Several patterns have emerged which may guide treatment decisions. From these data emerges the recommendation that antidepressants be continued at least 4–6 months after the resolution of an acute episode (American Psychiatric Association, 2000).

It may be the case that antidepressant treatment should be more prolonged. Major depression tends to be a recurrent illness, and the most robust predictor of relapse is having had a previous episode (Keller *et al.*, 1983; Roy-Byrne *et al.*, 1985; Coryell *et al.*, 1991; Maj *et al.*, 1992; Simpson *et al.*, 1997; Mueller *et al.*, 1999). Longitudinal, naturalistic follow-up data of patients who recover from an index episode of major depression found that 85% of subjects had a recurrence over the 15 years of the study, and that even in those who remained well for 5 years there was a 58% risk of relapse (Mueller *et al.*, 1999). The authors suggest that, while there were several predictors of who had a greater likelihood of relapse (female sex, previous episodes of depression, longer index episode length, and never having married), there were no predictors of who would maintain wellness. The limitation of this study is that it is of community-based treatment, and the typical treatment for patients in this study is inadequate. Also, for initial episodes of major depression the majority of subjects had a relapse over the next 5 years, although sex did not predict outcome (Simpson *et al.*, 1997).

A thoughtful and rigorous pooled analysis of 33 trials of antidepressant continuation up to 36 months found that the benefit of antidepressants over placebo was sustained no matter what the length of continuation (Geddes *et al.*, 2003). Most of the studies examined were 12 months in length, so the authors suggest that the data for longer continuation be confirmed. Patients with shorter (1–2 months) and longer (4–6 months) treatment before randomization to continued antidepressant, and from 6 months to 36 months of follow-up after randomized treatment all appeared to have similar reductions in proportional risk. The results for different classes of antidepressants were similar, suggesting that all antidepressants that are effective in treating depression will be effective for maintenance treatment.

The 40-year follow-up by Angst *et al.* (2003) of patients initially hospitalized for unipolar or bipolar depression found steady recurrence rates over the study for this more severely ill population, and suggests that maintenance treatment might be warranted for more severely ill patients. A 10-year follow-up study of 318 subjects after an index episode of depression found that the risk of a recurrence increases with each subsequent episode, and that the risk of recurrence decreased with increasing time as well (Solomon *et al.*, 2000). It also appears that the extent to which an episode is resolved predicts relapse; that is, those patients with complete resolution of their symptoms have a longer time to next episode than those patients who have residual depressive symptoms (Pintor *et al.*, 2003).

While the meta-analyses described by Geddes *et al.* above may provide support for recommending maintenance treatment for all patients, the question of how to proceed for an individual patient remains difficult to answer. Fava has suggested that, for some vulnerable individuals, antidepressant continuation may predispose them to a worse course of illness over their lifetime (Fava, G., 2003). For this reason, and for reasons of cost and side-effect burden, it would be useful to have more certainty about the ideal length of treatment for a given patient.

A substantial percentage of patients in the placebo-controlled arm of maintenance trials never relapse. In examining survival curves in these studies, it appears that most relapses occur in the first few months of follow-up, and beyond that the rate of relapse for both groups is generally similar. This suggests that the vast majority of the benefit of continuation and maintenance of antidepressant treatment is early in treatment, and that beyond that time the relative benefit diminishes greatly. Because it has not been studied, it is not known, for instance, whether patients who have maintained long-term response to maintenance treatment would then be at higher risk of relapse were they switched to active drug or placebo.

Because the risk of recurrence increases with successive episodes, subjects with recurrent MDD should be offered maintenance treatment. For first affective episodes that have completely resolved, it is unclear whether maintenance treatment is warranted. It is not clear that all patients who have a first episode will relapse to a new episode of depression; (Keller *et al.*, 1983) describe the risk of relapse as greatest for those patients who have had three previous episodes. At a minimum, continuation treatment is recommended, with antidepressants continued for at least 4–6 months after the resolution of the index episode. As many episodes do not remit for several months, this would more often than not be more than 6 total months of treatment.

What is the best pharmacotherapy approach to resistant MDD?

Many patients do not respond or only partially respond to initial antidepressant treatment. This is not surprising, as the effectiveness of antidepressants in controlled trials is limited to 40–60%. Many strategies have been used to remedy this problem, but few have undergone rigorous assessment in blinded trials. For the purposes of this chapter, we will only examine strategies – be they drug-switching or augmentation – that have been adequately tested in blinded parallel-group studies.

Before switching antidepressants or augmenting them with another drug, initial treatment must be optimized; underutilization and underdosing of antidepressants for major depression has been documented repeatedly. Pseudoresistance, as this has been called, is the result of inadequate doses or inadequate treatment duration and must be differentiated from true treatment resistance (Nierenberg and Amsterdam, 1990). Patients must be prescribed adequate doses of drug, and underprescribing is as ineffective over the long term as not being prescribed at all (Leon *et al.*, 2003). There is also a direct relationship between treatment non-adherence and poor outcome; both patients and prescribers generally overestimate the extent to which patients actually take their medications (Demyttenaere *et al.*, 2001).

It is also important to determine as much as is possible whether the depressive episode is unipolar as opposed to bipolar. Bowden (2001) has suggested that a bipolar family history disorder, previous episodes of antidepressant-induced or spontaneous mood elevation, a high frequency of depressive episodes, and a greater percentage of time ill may point to a bipolar diagnosis (Bowden, 2001).

Early non-response to antidepressant treatment may predict continued non-response, although it is impossible to determine with certainty who will be responders or non-responders. It has been suggested that those patients with poor response (i.e., nearly no response) to antidepressant treatment by week 4 and certainly by week 6 of treatment are not likely to respond to that antidepressant (Nierenberg *et al.*, 1995). In an open-label study of fluoxetine, only 36% of subjects who had less than a 20% reduction in depression rating scale scores at 2 weeks responded by the 8th week of the trial (Nierenberg *et al.*, 1995). On the other hand, a recent study suggests that a fluoxetine trial should not be considered failed until 8 weeks of non-response (Quitkin *et al.*, 2003). In this analysis, patients without improvement by week 6 in a 12-week open trial of 20 mg fluoxetine had a remission rate at week 12 of 31% (using last observation carried-forward analysis) or 41% (using completer analysis); for those unimproved by week 8, only 23% had remissions by week 12. Even fewer of those unimproved by week 10 ultimately responded.

Antidepressant switching

A first strategy for non-response to initial antidepressant treatment can be switch to another antidepressant, either to an antidepressant of the same class or to one of a different class. Unfortunately, only one randomized trial is published to date. A study of subjects who had failed two previous antidepressants showed somewhat increased benefit from switching to venlafaxine than to paroxetine. The response rate was 51.9% for venlafaxine and 32.7% for paroxetine ($P = 0.044$), and remission was achieved in 42.3% of the venlafaxine subjects versus 20.0% of the paroxetine subjects ($P = 0.01$) (Poirer and Boyer, 1999). Open trials do suggest benefit from switch from one SSRI to another, and a trial of treatment-refractory patients on sertraline or imipramine switched to the opposing drug showed equivalent benefit for each (Thase *et al.*, 2002).

Augmentation

Lithium

The best-studied drug augmentation for the treatment of treatment-resistant depression is lithium carbonate. There have been 13 controlled trials of lithium augmentation of antidepressants for treatment-resistant depression. Early studies of lithium augmentation demonstrated benefit compared to placebo when added to TCAs, but the most recent study showed no benefit of lithium over placebo for 35 treatment-resistant subjects who had tolerated but failed to respond to an open 6-week trial of nortriptyline (Nierenberg *et al.*, 2003). Response was defined as $\geq 50\%$ decrease in HAM-D17 scores. After 6 weeks of double-blind augmentation, 12.5% of subjects responded to lithium and 20.0% to placebo. This suggests that, while lithium augmentation may be helpful for patients who fail to respond to a single drug, it appears not to be effective for those subjects non-responsive to two or more antidepressants.

Thyroid hormone

The other most studied drug for antidepressant non-response is thyroid hormone, specifically triiodothyronine (T_3). A meta-analysis by Altshuler *et al.* (2001) found that the pooled, weighted effect size of the addition of T_3 to TCAs in non-refractory patients was 0.58. Five of the six randomized trials of T_3 found benefit in augmentation. All the trials, however, took place between 1969 and 1974 in patients prescribed relatively low doses of TCAs. Whether the effect would have been apparent in subjects with higher TCA dosing is not clear. The results are not necessarily generalizable to SSRIs and other non-TCAs.

Additional antidepressants

Antidepressants themselves have been studied for augmentation, although no meta-analyses exist to guide recommendations. The antidepressant mianserin was studied in non-responders to sertraline. Two hundred and ninety-five non-responders to 4 weeks of 50 mg sertraline who then had their doses increased to 100 mg for 2 additional weeks were randomized to three arms: (1) 100 mg of open-label sertraline plus placebo; (2) 100 mg of open-label sertraline plus the antidepressant mianserin; or (3) 200 mg of open-label sertraline. The group increased to 200 mg, interestingly, fared the worst, with significantly fewer responders than the other two groups. Adding mianserin did not improve outcomes compared to placebo in a study that was adequately powered to show a difference (Licht and Qvitzau, 2002).

A double-blind, placebo-controlled trial of mirtazapine augmentation of patients who remained depressed on antidepressant monotherapy was performed. Twenty-six patients whose HAM-D17 scores remained $\geq$ 12 after 4 weeks of maximally tolerated antidepressant treatment were randomized to receive mirtazapine (15 mg, to be raised at the clinician's discretion after 1 week to a maximum of 30 mg) or placebo for 4 weeks. Response was defined as CGI change score of "much improved" or "very much improved" and a 50% or greater reduction in HAM-D score, with remission defined as HAM-D score < 8. Response to mirtazapine was marked, with a response rate of 64% (7/11) for those on drug compared to 20% for placebo (3/15)($P = 0.043$). The remission rate was 45.4% for drug and 13.3% for placebo. Nine of the 15 in the placebo group were offered open-label mirtazapine in the study, and 55.5% (5/9) had a positive response; all of these went on to remission (Carpenter *et al.*, 2002).

Aside from its small size, a limitation of this study is the wide range of doses of a broad array of antidepressants (bupropion, citalopram, fluoxetine, paroxetine, fluvoxamine, sertraline, and venlafaxine) that were augmented with mirtazapine. It is difficult, then, to state whether an antidepressant or class of antidepressant is likely to benefit from mirtazapine augmentation.

Interestingly, Fava's double-blind study of 101 partial- or non-responders to 8 weeks of 20 mg of fluoxetine compared fluoxetine dosage increased to 40 mg, desipramine augmentation, and lithium augmentation, and found no significant difference in any strategy (Fava *et al.*, 2002). There was a non-significant increase in the percentage of responders to higher-dose fluoxetine, although this may be enough of a difference to make the recommendation that SSRI doses be increased as an initial strategy for limited response to initial therapy. The study may be most limited by not having a comparison group of subjects who remained on 20 mg of fluoxetine, although the authors suggest that adding a placebo comparison group might not be acceptable to subjects who had already been on the drug for 8 weeks.

Lack of adequate data hampers the ability to make recommendations with any degree of certainty regarding the strategies to follow for initial antidepressant resistance. Numerous strategies to augment antidepressant response have been evaluated in open or small randomized trials with some effect, including bupropion, buspirone, atypical antipsychotics, nefazodone, and modafinil, but the data are too scant to make any reasonable recommendations regarding their use. One double-blind trial of olanapine, fluoxetine, or the combination in treatment-resistant depression found significant benefit for the combination of the two. The study included only 28 subjects, however, making it too small to use for making recommendations (Shelton *et al.*, 2001). It is clear that larger randomized trials of next-step strategies for the significant proportion of patients who do not respond to initial antidepressant therapy are necessary.

Conclusion

Safety and patient choice are the driving factors dictating first-line therapy for MDD, as no antidepressant agent of any class has demonstrated clear superiority in the treatment of this illness. Although TCAs and MAOIs are effective for many patients with major depression, these medications have properties that can limit their utility. TCAs have significant rates of side-effects (for example, sedation, orthostasis, and anticholinergic effects) and a narrow therapeutic index with a high risk of death in overdose. MAOIs, despite their efficacy, require dietary restrictions and carry a risk of hyperadrenergic crisis; these factors can make them less attractive to patients and physicians alike. SSRIs and newer drugs, such as the dual-action agents bupropion, mirtazapine, and venlafaxine, have proven to be safe and effective alternatives to these older antidepressants; these agents are all suitable for first-line use in patients with MDD. As each of these newer drugs has a unique side-effect profile, the risk of one side-effect versus another should guide drug selection.

Some interest has been given to determining whether drugs have differential effects in different groups of patients categorized, for instance, by sex, age, depressive subtype, or some other measure. Data definitively showing benefits for different drugs when examined in this way are too limited to allow for clear recommendations. While more severe depressions (e.g., in inpatient settings) may have responded better to TCAs, mirtazapine, or venlafaxine in several studies, consideration must be given to the long-term tolerability of the drug, and recommending one drug over another.

It is prudent to recommend continuation treatment for single episodes of MDD. Repeated trials comparing continuation of active drug to placebo for episodes of MDD responsive to treatment suggest that patients should remain on antidepressant for at least 3–6 months following remission of an episode, as antidepressant drugs have repeatedly shown superiority to placebo in preventing the reemergence of depressive symptoms after remission from an acute episode. For episodes of recurrent or chronic depression, maintenance treatment is the most appropriate data-based recommendation.

For depressions that do not respond to initial drug therapy, no single strategy – be it dosage increase, switch to a different drug of the same class, switch to a different class of drug, or augmentation with an additional antidepressant, lithium, thyroid hormone, atypical antipsychotic drug, or other agent – has shown greater efficacy than another. It is important not to declare a trial failed prematurely, as significant percentages of patients with even no response within 6–8 weeks of initiation of treatment ultimately do respond, so maintaining treatment with an adequate dose of an antidepressant for at least that long is the primary recommendation.

As most refractory depression trials have been small, the effect size of any option is small. Lithium and T_3 have been studied the most extensively and can be recommended the most strongly on the basis of placebo-controlled data of TCA augmentation, although their risks and side-effect profiles may make them less attractive to patients. As it stands at the time of this writing, it is best to weigh the data regarding a given treatment's likely benefit against its inevitable increase in adverse effects. Patient preference and safety should determine treatment decisions for refractory or chronic MDD. Any augmentation strategy for refractory depression that results in remission should be continued for at least 9 months, and probably longer.

The limited data available to recommend continuation and maintenance treatment for responders and refractory treatment strategies for non-responders or partial responders may be greatly broadened by the completion of the STAR*D study. STAR*D aims to enroll 4000 subjects with major depression or dysthymia for treatment with the SSRI citalopram. Given historical response rates, it is expected that about 2000 treatment-refractory subjects will then be randomly assigned to one of six further treatment options:

1. augmenting the first antidepressant with other medications or psychotherapy
2. changing to a different antidepressant or psychotherapy
3. adding psychotherapy or discontinuing the first antidepressant medication while switching to psychotherapy
4. switching to another antidepressant
5. augmenting the first antidepressant with other medications
6. augmenting the first antidepressant with other medications or switching to another antidepressant

Other attempts to study the effectiveness of antidepressants in clinical settings such as TMAP and other algorithm-based studies may provide some needed data to direct clinical decision-making. As a randomized trial, though, STAR*D will have the statistical power to differentiate between treatment options for non-responders. The NIMH is hopeful that a study of this design and magnitude will provide more evidence on which to base treatment choices.

All current antidepressants are hampered in their utility by their limited effectiveness, treatment-emergent adverse effects, and the delay to onset of antidepressant response. Future drug development, if it is to improve the care of patients with MDD, must address these limitations. To have advantages over existing drugs, novel antidepressants must have a more rapid onset of action, higher rates of response and remission, or marked improvements in tolerability and ease of use.

REFERENCES

Altshuler, L. L., Bauer, M., Fry, M. A., *et al.* (2001). Does thyroid supplementation accelerate tricyclic antidepressant response? A review and meta-analysis of the literature. *American Journal of Psychiatry*, **158**, 1617–22.

American Psychiatric Association (2000). Practice guideline for the treatment of patients with major depressive disorder (revision). *American Journal of Psychiatry*, **157** (suppl. 4), 1–45.

Anderson, I. M. (1998). SSRIs versus tricyclic antidepressants in depressed inpatients: a meta-analysis of efficacy and tolerability. *Depression and Anxiety*, **7** (suppl. 1), 11–17.

(2000). Selective serotonin reuptake inhibitors versus tricyclic antidepressants: a meta-analysis of efficacy and tolerability. *Journal of Affective Disorders*, **58**, 19–36.

Angst, J., Gamma, A., Sellaro, R., Lavori, P. W., and Zhang, H. (2003). Recurrence of bipolar disorders and major depression. A life-long perspective. *European Archives of Psychiatry and Clinical Neuroscience*, **253**, 236–40.

Baker, C. B., Tweedie, R., Duval, S., and Woods, S. W. (2003). Evidence that the SSRI dose response in treating major depression should be reassessed: a meta-analysis. *Depression and Anxiety*, **17**, 1–9.

Barbui, C., Hotopf, M., Freemantle, N., *et al.* (2003). Treatment discontinuation with selective serotonin reuptake inhibitors (SSRIs) versus tricyclic antidepressants (TCAs) (Cochrane Review). In: *The Cochrane Library*, issue 4. Chichester, UK: John Wiley.

Bondareff, W., Alpert, M., Friedhoff, A. J., *et al.* (2000). Comparisons of sertraline and nortriptyline in the treatment of major depressive disorder in late life. *American Journal Psychiatry*, **157**, 729–36.

Bowden, C. L. (2001). Strategies to reduce misdiagnosis of bipolar depression. *Psychiatric Services*, **52**, 51–5.

Carpenter, L. L., Yasmin, S., and Price, L. H. (2002). A double-blind, placebo-controlled study of antidepressant augmentation with mirtazapine. *Biology and Psychiatry*, **51**, 183–8.

Cohn, C. K., Shrivastava, R., Mendels, J., *et al.* (1990). Double-blind, multicenter comparison of sertraline and amitriptyline in elderly depressed patients. *Journal of Clinical Psychiatry*, **51**(suppl. B), 28–33.

Coryell, W., Endicott, J., Keller, M. B. (1991). Predictors of relapse into major depressive disorder in a nonclinical population. *American Journal of Psychiatry*, **148**, 1353–8.

Crismon, M. L., Trivedi, M., Pigott, T. A., *et al.* (1999). The Texas Medication Algorithm Project: report of the Texas Consensus Conference Panel on medication treatment of major depressive disorder. *Journal of Clinical Psychiatry*, **60**, 142–56.

Demyttenaere, K., Mesters, P., Boulanger, B., *et al.* (2001). Adherence to treatment regimen in depressed patients treated with amitriptyline or fluoxetine. *Journal of Affective Disorders*, **65**, 243–52.

Fava, G. A. (2003). Can long-term treatment with antidepressant drugs worsen the course of depression? *Journal of Clinical Psychiatry*, **64**, 123–33.

Fava, M., Alpert, J., Nierenberg, A., *et al.* (2002). Double-blind study of high-dose fluoxetine versus lithium or desipramine augmentation of fluoxetine in partial responders and nonresponders to fluoxetine. *Journal of Clinical Psychopharmacology*, **22**, 379–87.

Fava, M., Rush, A. J., Trivedi, M. H., *et al.* (2003). Background and rationale for the sequenced treatment alternatives to relieve depression (STAR*D) study. *Psychiatric Clinics of North America*, **26**, 457–94.

Feighner, J. P. and Cohn, J. B. (1985). Double-blind comparative trials of fluoxetine and doxepin in geriatric patients with major depressive disorder. *Journal of Clinical Psychiatry*, **46**, 20–5.

Freemantle, N., Anderson, I. M., and Young, P. (2000). Predictive value of pharmacological activity for the relative efficacy of antidepressant drugs. *British Journal of Psychiatry*, **177**, 292–302.

Geddes, J. R., Carney, S. M., Davies, C., *et al.* (2003). Relapse prevention with antidepressant drug treatment in depressive disorders: a systematic review. *Lancet*, **361**, 653–61.

Geddes, J. R., Freemantle, N., Mason, J., Eccles, M. P., and Boynton, J. (2002). Selective serotonin reuptake inhibitors (SSRIs) for depression (Cochrane Review). In: *The Cochrane Library*, issue 3. Oxford: Update Software.

Gill, D. and Hatcher, S. (1999). A systematic review of the treatment of depression with antidepressant drugs in patients who also have a physical illness. *Journal of Psychosomatic Research*, **47**, 131–43.

(2003). Antidepressants for depression in medical illness. *Cochrane Database Systematic Review*, 4, CD001312.

Judd, L. L., Akiskal, H. S., Maser, J. D., *et al.* (1998). A prospective 12-year study of subsyndromal and syndromal depressive symptoms in unipolar major depressive disorders. *Journal of Affective Disorders*, **50**, 97–108.

Keller, M. B., Lavori, P. W., Lewis, C. E., and Klerman, G. L. (1983). Predictors of relapse in major depressive disorder. *Journal of the American Medical Association*, **250**, 3299–304.

Kessler, R. C., McGonagle, K. A., Zhao, S., *et al.* (1994). Lifetime and 12 month prevalence of DSM III-R psychiatric disorders in the United States. *Archives of General Psychiatry*, **51**, 8–19.

Khan, A., Leventhal, R. M., Khan, S. R., and Brown, W. A. (2002). Severity of depression and response to antidepressants and placebo: an analysis of the Food and Drug Administration database. *Journal of Clinical Psychopharmacology*, **22**, 40–5.

Khan, A., Khan, S. R., Walens, G., Kolts, R., and Giller, E. L. (2003). Frequency of positive studies among fixed and flexible dose antidepressant clinical trials: an analysis of the food and drug administration summary basis of approval reports. *Neuropsychopharmacology*, **28**, 552–7.

Koenig, H. G., Goli, V., Shelp, F., *et al.* (1989). Antidepressant use in elderly medical inpatients: Lessons from an attempted clinical trial. *Journal of General Internal Medicine*, **4**, 498–505.

Kornstein, S. G., Schatzberg, A. F., Thase, M. E., *et al.* (2000). Gender differences in treatment response to sertraline versus imipramine in chronic depression. *American Journal of Psychiatry*, **157**, 1445–52.

Leon, A. C., Solomon, D. A., Mueller, T. I., *et al.* (2003). A 20-year longitudinal observational study of somatic antidepressant treatment effectiveness. *American Journal of Psychiatry*, **160**, 727–33.

Licht, R. W. and Qvitzau, S. (2002). Treatment strategies in patients with major depression not responding to first-line sertraline treatment. A randomised study of extended duration of treatment, dose increase or mianserin augmentation. *Psychopharmacology (Berlin)* **161**, 143–151.

Liebowitz, M. R., Quitkin, F. M., Stewart, J. W., *et al.* (1988). Antidepressant specificity in atypical depression. *Archives of General Psychiatry*, **45**, 129–37.

Maj, M., Veltro, F., Pirozzi, R., Lobrace, S., and Magliano, L. (1992). Pattern of recurrence of illness after recovery from an episode of major depression: a prospective study. *American Journal of Psychiatry*, **149**, 795–800.

McGrath, P. J., Stewart, J. W., Janal, M. N., *et al.* (2000). A placebo-controlled study of fluoxetine versus imipramine in the acute treatment of atypical depression. *American Journal of Psychiatry*, **157**, 344–50.

Mueller, T. I., Leon, A. C., Keller, M. B., *et al.* (1999). Recurrence after recovery from major depressive disorder during 15 years of observational follow-up. *American Journal of Psychiatry*, **156**, 1000–6.

Mulder, R. T. (2002). Personality pathology and treatment outcome in major depression: a review. *American Journal of Psychiatry*, **159**, 359–71.

Mulder, R. T., Joyce, P. R., and Luty, S. E. (2003). The relationship of personality disorders to treatment outcome in depressed outpatients. *Journal of Clinical Psychiatry*, **64**, 259–64.

Nierenberg, A. A. and Amsterdam, J. D. (1990). Treatment-resistant depression: definition and treatment approaches. *Journal of Clinical Psychiatry*, **51** (suppl.), 39–47.

Nierenberg, A. A., McLean, N. E., Alpert, J. E., *et al.* (1995). Early nonresponse to fluoxetine as a predictor of poor 8-week outcome. *American Journal of Psychiatry*, **152**, 1500–3.

Nierenberg, A. A., Papakostas, G. I., Petersen, T., *et al.* (2003). Lithium augmentation of nortriptyline for subjects resistant to multiple antidepressants. *Journal of Clinical Psychopharmacology*, **23**, 92–5.

Pande, A. C., Birkett, M., Fechner-Bates, S., Haskett, R. F., and Greden, J. F. (1996). Fluoxetine versus phenelzine in atypical depression. *Biology and Psychiatry*, **40**, 1017–20.

Papakostas, G. I., Petersen, T., Iosifescu, D. V., *et al.* (2003). Axis III disorders in treatment-resistant major depressive disorder. *Psychiatry Research*, **118**, 183–8.

Parker, G., Parker, K., Austin, M. P., Mitchell, P., and Brotchie, H. (2003). Gender differences in response to differing antidepressant drug classes: two negative studies. *Psychological Medicine*, **33**, 1473–7.

Pintor, L., Gasto, C., Navarro, V., Torres, X., and Fananas, L. (2003). Relapse of major depression after complete and partial remission during a 2-year follow-up. *Journal of Affective Disorders*, **73**, 237–44.

Poirer, M. F. and Boyer, P. (1999). Venlafaxine and paroxetine in treatment-resistant depression. Double-blind, randomised comparison. *British Journal of Psychiatry*, **175**, 12–16.

Popkin, M. K., Callies, A. L., and Mackenzie, T. B. (1985). The outcome of antidepressant use in the medically ill. *Archives of General Psychiatry*, **42**, 1160–3.

Quitkin, F. M., Stewart, J. W., McGrath, P. J., *et al.* (2002). Are there diferences between women's and men's antidepressant responses? *American Journal of Psychiatry*, **159**, 1848–54.

Quitkin, F. M., Petkova, E., McGrath, P. J., *et al.* (2003). When should a trial of fluoxetine for major depression be declared failed? *American Journal of Psychiatry*, **160**, 734–40.

Roy-Byrne, P., Post, R. M., Uhde, T. W., Porcu, T., and Davis, D. (1985). The longitudinal course of recurrent affective illness: life chart data from research patients at the NIMH. *Acta Psychiatrica Scandinavica* **7** (suppl.), 3–34.

Russell, J. M., Kornstein, S. G., Shea, M. T., *et al.* (2003). Chronic depression and comorbid personality disorders: response to sertraline versus imipramine. *Journal of Clinical Psychiatry*, **64**, 554–61.

Schneider, L. S., Nelson, J. C., Clary, C. M., *et al.* (2003). An 8-week multicenter, parallel-group, double-blind, placebo-controlled study of sertraline in elderly outpatients with major depression. *American Journal of Psychiatry*, **160**, 1277–85.

Shelton, R. C., Tollefson, G. D., Tohen, M., *et al.* (2001). A novel augmentation strategy for treating resistant major depression. *American Journal of Psychiatry*, **158**, 131–4.

Simpson, H. B., Nee, J. C., and Endicott, J. (1997). First-episode major depression: few sex differences in course. *Archives of General Psychiatry*, **54**, 633–9.

Solomon, D. A., Keller, M. B., Leon, A. C., *et al.* (2000). Multiple recurrences of major depressive disorder. *American Journal of Psychiatry*, **157**, 229–33.

Thase, M. E., Entsuah, A. R., and Rudolph, R. L. (2001). Remission rates during treatment with venlafaxine or selective serotonin reuptake inhibitors. *British Journal of Psychiatry*, **178**, 234–41.

Thase, M. E., Rush, A. J., Howland, R. H., *et al.* (2002). Double-blind switch study of imipramine or sertraline treatment of antidepressant-resistant chronic depression. *Archives of General Psychiatry*, **59**, 233–9.

Walker, E. A., Katon, W. J., Russo, J., *et al.* (2000). Predictors of outcome in a primary care depression trial. *Journal of General Internal Medicine*, **15**, 859–67.

Weihs, K. L., Houser, T., Batey, S. R., *et al.* (2002). Continuation phase treatment with bupropion SR effectively decreases the risk for relapse of depression. *Biology and Psychiatry*, **51**, 753–61.

Williams, J. W. Jr, Mulrow, C. D., Chiquette, E., *et al.* (2000). A systematic review of newer pharmacotherapies for depression in adults: evidence report summary. *Annals of Internal Medicine*, **132**, 743–56.

Wilson, K., Mottram, P., Sivanranthan, A., and Nightingale, A. (2003). Antidepressants versus placebo for the depressed elderly. In: *The Cochrane Library*, issue 3. Oxford: Update Software.

Wohlfarth, T., Storosum, J. G., Elferink, A. J. A., *et al.* (2004). Response to tricyclic antidepressants: independent of gender? *American Journal of Psychiatry*, **161**, 370–2.

Workman, E. A., and Short, D. D. (1993). Atypical antidepressants versus imipramine in the treatment of major depression: a meta-analysis. *Journal of Clinical Psychiatry*, **54**, 5–12.

2

Evidence-based pharmacotherapy of bipolar disorder

S. Nassir Ghaemi and Douglas J. Hsu

Cambridge Hospital and Harvard University, Boston, MA, USA

Conventional wisdom regarding the prevalence of bipolar disorder in the general population is most commonly derived from the Epidemiological Catchment Area (ECA) study, which reported that mania and hypomania occur in 1.2% of the population over a lifetime (Regier *et al.*, 1988). Follow-up studies, however, have called into question the diagnostic validity of the ECA study (Anthony *et al.*, 1985; Helzer *et al.*, 1985). The reported 4:1 ratio of unipolar to bipolar disorder in the ECA study has been called into doubt by suggesting a 2:1 ratio (Goodwin and Jamison, 1990) or even a 1:1 ratio of unipolar to bipolar disorder (Weissman *et al.*, 1988). Regardless of the overall prevalence of bipolar disorder, the associated risk factors for individuals with bipolar disorder are high. Bipolar disorder is associated with a high lifetime suicide rate (19%), comorbid conditions such as substance abuse (60%), and high rates of social stressors such as divorce leading to chaotic life histories.

This chapter will review the evidentiary basis of treatments for acute mania, acute bipolar depression, and prophylaxis of mood episodes in bipolar disorder, including an evidence-based discussion of polypharmacy. Tables summarize the levels of evidence data, organized by treatment indication.

Relevant studies were identified by MEDLINE (1966–current) searches using the keywords: bipolar disorder, treatment, pharmacology, mood stabilizers, neuroleptics, antidepressants, mania, bipolar depression, and prevention. Keywords for each agent combined with bipolar disorder were also used. Articles were screened in abstract form and reviewed in detail when they met study inclusion criteria. Further articles were obtained through bibliographic cross-referencing, consultation of major texts in the field (such as Goodwin and Jamison's *Manic-Depressive Illness*, 1990), and discussion with experts in the field. Abstracts from conference proceedings for the past 5 years were reviewed from meetings of the American Psychiatric Association, the American College of Neuropsychopharmacology, the International Conferences on Bipolar Disorder (Pittsburgh), the New Clinical Drug Evaluation Unit (NCDEU), the European College of Neuropsychopharmacology, the European Stanley Foundation Conference on Bipolar Disorder, and the Collegium International Neuro-psychopharmacologicum. Inclusion criteria for the study were purposefully broad: (1) identification of the diagnosis of bipolar disorder or manic-depressive illness; (2) identification of sample size; and (3) identification of treatments used.

What is the first-line pharmacotherapy of acute mania?

Lithium

Initial studies of acute mania date to the first randomized controlled trials (RCTs) in psychiatry, with a placebo-controlled trial of lithium conducted by Schou and colleagues in 1954, followed by three other placebo-controlled trials up to 1971 (Maggs, 1963; Goodwin *et al.*, 1969; Stokes *et al.*, 1971). These studies were all of the small, crossover variety, however, and thus did not convince some who were skeptical about this new agent which was claimed by some to be the first effective treatment for manic-depressive illness. A number of other non-placebo-controlled comparisons with traditional neuroleptic agents were also conducted (Platman, 1970; Spring *et al.*, 1970; Johnson *et al.*, 1971; Prien *et al.*, 1972; Shopsin *et al.*, 1975; Takahashi *et al.*, 1975). Generally, lithium was equally effective as traditional neuroleptic agents, especially chlorpromazine, but less rapid in its efficacy. Since mania resolves spontaneously in 2–3 months, and in the meantime can lead to many problems, this slow onset of effect led to the common use of neuroleptics for mania.

RCTs of lithium in mania continued to be conducted in the 1980s and beyond, but mostly as a reference group in protocols designed to test other new agents, such as carbamazepine (Lerer *et al.*, 1987; Small *et al.*, 1991), valproate (Freeman *et al.*, 1992; Bowden *et al.*, 1994), risperidone (Segal *et al.*, 1998), and olanzapine (Berk *et al.*, 1999). These newer studies are expanding and confirming the evidence regarding lithium's efficacy in mania. For instance, in the valproate study (Bowden *et al.*, 1994), a parallel-design RCT clearly demonstrated that lithium was as effective as valproate for pure mania, but about half as effective for mixed episodes. Further, in a secondary analysis, it appeared that in those persons with previous lithium response by history, lithium was quite effective, but valproate was less so. This finding suggests possible subtyping, with some persons being better lithium-responders and others being better valproate-responders. It can be difficult to know to which group one individual belongs short of simply trying both agents. Mixed episodes, however, are rather clear indications for preference of valproate over lithium.

Anticonvulsants

As just mentioned, valproate has been studied carefully in acute mania (Table 2.1). There is one small (Pope *et al.*, 1991) and one large (Bowden *et al.*, 1994)

Table 2.1 Studies of acute mania

Agent	Number of studies	Total patients	Findings
Lithium	5	358	More effective than placebo
	16	775	Equivalent to neuroleptics or valproate
Valproate	2	215	More effective than placebo
	6	620	Equivalent to lithium or neuroleptics
Carbamazepine	4	72	More effective than placebo
	5	230	Equivalent to neuroleptics
Oxcarbazepine	1	6	More effective than placebo
	2	72	Equivalent to haloperidol/lithium
Phenytoin	1	39	Mild benefit over placebo
Lamotrigine	2	444	Equivalent to placebo
	2	46	Equivalent to lithium
Gabapentin	2	142	Equivalent to placebo
Topiramate	1	97	Equivalent to placebo
Zonisamide	1	15	Mild benefit
Haloperidol	1	27	More effective than placebo
	9	901	Equivalent to lithium, atypical neuroleptics
Clozapine	1	27	Equivalent to chlorpromazine
Risperidone	3	307	Equivalent to lithium
Olanzapine	2	254	More effective than placebo
	5	1195	Equivalent to haloperidol/lithium/ valproate
Quetiapine	2	221	More effective than placebo as adjunct to lithium/valproate
Ziprasidone	1	195	More effective than placebo
Aripiprazole	1	262	More effective than placebo
Verapamil	1	32	Equivalent to placebo
Clonazepam	4	92	Equivalent to lorazepam or placebo when combined with neuroleptics; may reflect agitation benefit rather than core manic symptoms
Lorazepam	1	24	Equivalent to clonazepam
Chlorpromazine	8	521	More effective than or equivalent to lithium
ECT	2	64	Equivalent to lithium for acute mania; ECT + chlorpromazine more effective than ECT alone

ECT, electroconvulsive therapy.

placebo-controlled study demonstrating that valproate is as effective as lithium, and more effective than placebo. Valproate added to traditional neuroleptics has also been shown in one RCT to be more effective than traditional neuroleptics alone (Muller-Oerlinghausen *et al.*, 2000). Two RCTs appear to indicate that olanzapine may be somewhat more effective than valproate for acute mania (Zajecka *et al.*, 2002; Tohen *et al.*, 2002a), though the somewhat lower efficacy shown in one of the olanzapine comparison studies (Tohen *et al.*, 2002a) may partially reflect low and slow dosing of valproate in that study (mean level 79 ng/dl). In the largest valproate study, the mean level found effective in acute mania was 93.2 ng/dl (Bowden *et al.*, 1994). Thus, in acute mania, the therapeutic range has been broadened from 50 to 120 ng/dl, but optimal efficacy is achieved in the higher end of that range, if tolerated.

For acute mania, carbamazepine has been shown effective in one crossover RCT versus placebo (Post *et al.*, 1987), in three RCTs versus lithium (Lerer *et al.*, 1987; Lusznat *et al.*, 1988; Small *et al.*, 1991), and two RCTs versus chlorpromazine (Okuma *et al.*, 1979; Grossi *et al.*, 1984). Carbamazepine has also been reported to be effective as adjunctive therapy with haloperidol (Klein *et al.*, 1984; Muller and Stoll, 1984; Moller *et al.*, 1989). While this body of evidence suggests efficacy with carbamazepine, because most studies did not have a placebo control, efficacy has not been established as cleanly as if parallel-design, placebo-controlled studies had been conducted.

Oxcarbazepine, a chemical analog of carbamazepine, has been shown to be more effective than placebo in one small RCT crossover study of 6 patients (Emrich *et al.*, 1983). Small RCTs have also found oxcarbazepine to be as effective as lithium (Emrich, 1990) and haloperidol (Muller and Stoll, 1984; Emrich, 1990). A large observational comparison of oxcarbazepine with valproate also suggests equal efficacy to that agent (Reinstein *et al.*, 2002). The same limitations mentioned above apply for these oxcarbazepine studies. Among older anticonvulsants, it is also noteworthy that one small placebo-controlled RCT study of phenytoin found benefit when added to haloperidol (Mishory *et al.*, 2000).

Among novel anticonvulsants, none has been shown to be effective in acute mania in placebo-controlled RCTs. Two large studies of lamotrigine for acute mania were ineffective (GlaxoSmithKline, data on file). A large RCT parallel-design add-on study of 114 outpatients found that gabapentin was not more effective than placebo when added to valproate or lithium for acute mania (Pande *et al.*, 2000), and a RCT study of topiramate monotherapy failed to find efficacy greater than placebo (Calabrese, 2000).

Neuroleptic agents

Neuroleptic agents have been studied extensively in acute mania. Traditional neuroleptics have been shown effective, but mainly as comparison arms to lithium in non-placebo-controlled studies from the 1970s. Only one early study was placebo-controlled (Klein, 1967). Most placebo-controlled studies with traditional neuroleptic agents were conducted in the 1990s, where these agents were used as reference groups for protocols designed to examine atypical neuroleptic agents (Tohen *et al.*, 2003; Sachs *et al.*, 2002b). As mentioned previously, the early studies suggested equal but more rapid efficacy compared to lithium. The recent placebo-controlled studies, all of which used haloperidol, demonstrated better efficacy than placebo, when used as add-on treatment to lithium or valproate for acute mania. The recent studies also demonstrate that haloperidol possesses equal antimanic efficacy compared with risperidone or olanzapine, either as add-on to valproate or lithium or in monotherapy treatment of mania. However, these studies also suggest that, while haloperidol may lead to increased depressive symptoms, or a postmanic depression, olanzapine and risperidone do not have as much of this effect. Furthermore, the atypical neuroleptics produced much fewer extrapyramidal symptoms (EPS). In summary, traditional neuroleptic agents are effective for acute mania, but tend to exacerbate or induce postmanic depression and lead to more EPS than atypical neuroleptics.

Atypical neuroleptics are now standard treatments for acute mania. Clozapine was the first to be studied, but there is only one small ($n = 27$), open randomized study comparison with chlorpromazine in acute mania (Barbini *et al.*, 1997). An RCT study of risperidone in acute mania suggested that it has equivalent efficacy compared to lithium and haloperidol (Segal *et al.*, 1998). Risperidone has also been shown to be effective in two RCTs as adjunctive treatment with valproate or lithium (Yatham *et al.*, 2003; Sachs *et al.*, 2002b). Interestingly, adjunctive use of risperidone with carbamazepine did not demonstrate efficacy compared to placebo, probably due to hepatic cytochrome P450 enzyme induction leading to serum levels of risperidone and its active metabolite 9-OH-risperidone. One small non-placebo-controlled monotherapy study suggested that risperidone had equal efficacy to lithium for acute mania (Segal *et al.*, 1998). Olanzapine, used as monotherapy as well as adjunctive therapy, has been extensively studied for acute mania in both placebo-controlled protocols and in comparison to other active agents like lithium, valproate, or haloperidol (Berk *et al.*, 1999; Tohen *et al.*, 1999, 2000, 2002a, 2002b, 2003; Zajecka *et al.*, 2002). In every published case, olanzapine demonstrates efficacy in acute mania that is better than placebo and at least equivalent to standard comparison agents. Its efficacy was slightly better than valproate in one study (Tohen *et al.*, 2002a), which, as mentioned, may have been influenced by other methodological issues such as dosing regimen.

While the number of patients studied in these RCTs demonstrating olanzapine efficacy is extensive, olanzapine consistently demonstrated more weight gain than placebo or standard comparison agents. One case of fatal diabetic ketoacidosis occurred with olanzapine in one of these studies (Zajecka *et al.*, 2002). Other issues recently raised, such as worsened lipid profiles and increased long-term risk of diabetes, have not generally been derived from RCTs, but rather from large and small open randomized comparisons, based on observational clinical databases (McIntyre *et al.*, 2001). Those reports tend to be rather consistent in suggesting that such risks are more commonly seen with clozapine and olanzapine than with other agents, but they are not definitive. The only RCT to look at this issue, which was conducted in schizophrenia, found increased serum glucose levels with clozapine and olanzapine compared to risperidone (Lindenmayer *et al.*, 2003). This study, however, was not long enough to ascertain whether this effect led to long-term development of diabetes mellitus.

Quetiapine, added to valproate, has been shown to be more effective than placebo in treating adolescent mania in one small RCT (Delbello *et al.*, 2002). Recent results from the first large, multicenter, placebo-controlled RCT also support the effectiveness of quetiapine as an adjunct to lithium or valproate for the treatment of mania (Sachs *et al.*, 2002a). Ziprasidone monotherapy has been shown to be more effective than placebo in one RCT (Keck *et al.*, 2003). Aripiprazole has been demonstrated to be more effective than placebo in monotherapy of mania in one study (Keck *et al.*, 2002).

One of the concerning issues with atypical neuroleptics is that negative studies of mania are not always publicly presented or available for evaluation since almost all of these studies are proprietary clinical trials conducted by the pharmaceutical industry. Hence, in assessing evidence for or against efficacy, we clearly have a problem of bias toward positive studies. One is tempted to call this the "private-industry" bias against negative studies, rather than the more commonly cited "file drawer" bias (where academic investigators lose interest in their negative data), and it is important to keep this fact in mind. We really do not know exactly how many negative studies might exist with these agents. However, it is also relevant that negative studies do not always entail inefficacy; studies can fail for various reasons, including unusual samples, insufficient statistical power, or other factors. Nonetheless, complete access to negative studies is needed to assess the evidence fully on any agent.

Other agents

Other agents studied in acute mania include calcium channel blockers and benzodiazepines. Verapamil was not effective in treating acute mania in one placebo-controlled RCT ($n = 32$) (Janicak *et al.*, 1998). While clonazepam has been reported effective, mainly in high doses, in acute mania in four RCTs (Chouinard *et al.*, 1983, 1993; Bradwejn *et al.*, 1990; Edwards *et al.*, 1991), it is difficult to tell whether this effect is simply an antiagitation effect or a more direct effect on core mood symptoms of mania.

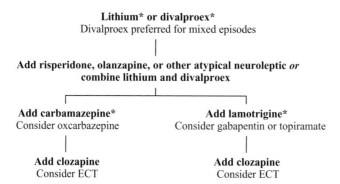

Figure 2.1   An algorithm for the polypharmacy of bipolar disorder, type I. ECT, electroconvulsive therapy.
* Meet conservative criteria for mood stabilizer.

ECT

In two RCTs, electroconvulsive therapy (ECT) has been reported as effective as lithium for acute mania ($n = 34$) (Small *et al.*, 1988), and ECT combined with chlorpromazine was more effective than sham ECT added to chlorpromazine ($n = 30$) (Sikdar *et al.*, 1994).

Summary of acute mania studies

As shown in Table 2.1, the largest number of studies have been conducted with lithium ($n = 21$), and the largest number of patients studied with olanzapine ($n = 1449$). Given the added factor of the years of experience with using lithium, its large biological base of plausibility for use in bipolar disorder, and the potential private-industry bias problem in relation to negative studies, we would conclude that, solely on efficacy-based evidence, lithium remains the first-line treatment for acute mania. Following lithium are olanzapine, haloperidol, valproate, carbamazepine, and risperidone in order of amount of RCT evidence.

In the case of acute mania, polypharmacy with mood stabilizer plus neuroleptic appears to be more effective than either mood stabilizer or neuroleptic monotherapy. Recent treatment guidelines for acute mania have focused on the use of atypical neuroleptics and novel anticonvulsants as adjuncts to mood stabilizers. Figure 2.1 is an example of an algorithm in treating bipolar mania, including the advice to use valproate for mixed episodes.

What is the first-line pharmacotherapy of acute bipolar depression?

Lithium

A classic review of pre-1980 studies identified nine placebo-controlled RCTs of lithium in acute bipolar depression (Zornberg and Pope, 1993). Eight of nine studies reported lithium as more effective than placebo, with the last study reporting similar efficacy between lithium and placebo. While all studies were of crossover design, it was only possible to obtain "unequivocal" response data from five studies (Fieve *et al.*, 1968; Goodwin *et al.*, 1972; Noyes *et al.*, 1974; Baron *et al.*, 1975; Mendels, 1976). Unequivocal response, defined as patients with good or moderate response to lithium with ensuing relapse when switched back to placebo, was reported in only 36% of patients. This is in comparison to the 69% of patients with any positive response to lithium, regardless of degree of improvement or placebo relapse.

Recent parallel-design studies are somewhat more interpretable. In a recent RCT, 117 acutely depressed patients, lithium-refractory, bipolar I patients were randomized to the addition of placebo, paroxetine, or imipramine. The addition of those antidepressants was not more effective than lithium plus placebo in patients with a therapeutic lithium serum level (≥ 0.8 ng/dl). In patients with subtherapeutic lithium levels, however, paroxetine and imipramine did provide significant antidepressant benefit (Nemeroff *et al.*, 2001).

In another RCT, 27 patients who were refractory to either lithium or valproate were randomized to the addition of either paroxetine, or combination with the other mood stabilizer (lithium and valproate). While the paroxetine plus mood stabilizer group led to lower dropouts and fewer side-effects, there was an equivalent magnitude of antidepressant effect in the two groups (Young *et al.*, 2000).

The available RCT data suggest that therapeutic use of lithium, alone or in combination with valproate, likely provides equal acute antidepressant efficacy to the addition of a tricyclic antidepressant (TCA) or serotonin reuptake inhibitor (SRI).

Valproate and carbamazepine

In a placebo-controlled RCT of valproate in acute bipolar depression ($n = 45$) (Sachs *et al.*, 2001), 43% response was noted with valproate versus 27% with placebo (using the Hamilton Depression Rating Scale (HDRS)). While non-significant by *P*-value, use of confidence intervals (CI) suggests that some possibility of a benefit exists, with relative risk of benefit with valproate being 1.50 (95% CI 0.64, 3.50). In other words, 50% greater benefit was observed with valproate, and while this may have been due to chance, the possibility also exists that up to three times more benefit exists with valproate than with placebo. It is important when interpreting such small negative studies to note the high risk of type II error, with false-negative findings due to small sample size. In such cases, failure to find a difference between drug and placebo is not at all the same thing as demonstrating lack of benefit with drug versus placebo (also called non-equivalence). The confidence intervals suggest that if this experiment were repeated numerous times, benefit is likely to be shown with valproate more often than not. Until further studies are done, one cannot rule in, but also one cannot rule out, acute antidepressant efficacy with valproate.

One other RCT is available, though not yet published, in which valproate was compared to placebo in 25 patients, with statistical benefit using random regression methods. Based on limited data availability, a preliminary interpretation conducted by us suggests that absolute HDRS scores improved from 21.6 initially to approximately 3.6 after 9 weeks with valproate, versus 19.4 to 11.9 with placebo (Petty *et al.*, 2002, personal communication).

As mentioned previously, another RCT which combined lithium and valproate found that the combination demonstrated excellent acute antidepressant benefit (Young *et al.*, 2000). Furthermore, data from large observational studies, including one with a 9-month prospective follow-up using HDRS scales (Ghaemi and Goodwin, 2001b), support acute and long-term antidepressant benefits with valproate. Lastly, there is a small literature on unipolar depression that suggests acute antidepressant benefit with valproate (Vinar *et al.*, 1989; Davis *et al.*, 1996).

Three placebo-controlled RCTs of carbamazepine treatment for bipolar depression have been conducted. Two studies reported carbamazepine as more effective than placebo (Ballenger and Post, 1978; Post *et al.*, 1983), with the third study reporting carbamazepine plus lithium as more effective than carbamazepine plus placebo (Kramlinger and Post, 1989). Data from a small observational study also suggest acute antidepressant benefit with this agent (Dilsaver *et al.*, 1996), which, notably, shares the basic tricyclic chemical structure with tricyclic antidepressants.

Lamotrigine

One RCT demonstrated efficacy with lamotrigine at both 50 and 200 mg/day compared to placebo for acute bipolar depression ($n = 195$), though somewhat more efficacy at the higher dose was noted (Calabrese *et al.*, 1999). A follow-up RCT in 206 patients failed to find a difference with placebo (both groups being about 50% in response) (Bowden, 2001). A small crossover RCT ($n = 31$) also found lamotrigine more effective than placebo, while gabapentin was not different from placebo, for refractory acute bipolar depression (Frye *et al.*, 2000). It is relevant that a placebo-controlled RCT of the antidepressive properties of lamotrigine in unipolar-depressed patients ($n = 40$) found that lamotrigine may accelerate the onset of action when used adjunctively with antidepressants (Normann *et al.*, 2002).

Other novel anticonvulsants

An open randomized study suggests that topiramate, when used adjunctively with lithium, may have as much acute antidepressant efficacy as bupropion for refractory bipolar depression ($n = 36$) (McIntyre *et al.*, 2002). Other data from large observational studies also support a possible benefit for this agent (Marcotte, 1998; Ghaemi *et al.*, 2001b), as well as for gabapentin (Ghaemi *et al.*, 1998; De Leon, 2001; Ghaemi and Goodwin, 2001a). As mentioned above, however, gabapentin was not effective in one crossover RCT of refractory bipolar depression (Frye *et al.*, 2000).

Oxcarbazepine has been reported useful in two small observational studies for bipolar depressive symptoms (Berv *et al.*, 2002; Ghaemi *et al.*, 2002b). Data for other agents like levetiracetam and zonisamide are still at the case-series level.

Olanzapine

One large ($n = 647$) placebo-controlled, monotherapy RCT reported that olanzapine is superior to placebo in treating bipolar depression (Tohen *et al.*, 2002d). In addition to the 647 patients randomized to either olanzapine or placebo, an additional 86 received an olanzapine–fluoxetine combination (OFC) as an active control. Although olanzapine was shown to be superior to placebo, greater magnitude of improvement was seen with OFC treatment. Most of the magnitude of improvement in olanzapine monotherapy was seen in neurovegetative symptoms of sleep and appetite, while OFC treatment demonstrated about 50% or greater benefit than placebo in all items of the Montgomery Asberg Depression Rating Scale (MADRS). Statistical benefit was shown with olanzapine monotherapy for depressed mood and suicidality, but the magnitude of this benefit over placebo was minimal (0.2–0.4 points on each item) and thus not likely of clinical significance. No benefit was seen with olanzapine in anhedonia items.

The size of this study is its most impressive feature, as it is, by far, the largest study ever conducted in bipolar depression research. The impressive size, however, also raises the potential of establishing statistical significance where a clinical benefit might be small. Overall, a conservative interpretation is that the OFC arm of this study clearly shows antidepressant efficacy with a low mania switch rate, and that olanzapine monotherapy provided primarily neurovegetative, rather than core mood, depressive benefits.

Other atypical neuroleptic agents

An RCT examining the effect of risperidone and paroxetine concurrent therapy, risperidone monotherapy, and paroxetine monotherapy found a moderate benefit in the risperidone group, though these differences were not statistically significant in this small sample ($n = 22$) (Shelton, 2001). Ziprasidone, with a marked norepinephrine (noradrenaline) and serotonin blockade, could be an especially beneficial atypical neuroleptic in the treatment of bipolar depression. Clinical data, however, are not yet available to test this biochemical possibility.

ECT

Three small observational studies have reported ECT as effective treatment for acute bipolar depression (Abrams and Taylor, 1974; Gagne *et al.*, 2000; Ciapparelli *et al.*, 2001).

Antidepressants

One placebo-controlled RCT ($n = 56$) has shown that the monoamine oxidase inhibitor (MAOI) tranylcypromine has better acute antidepressant efficacy than the TCA imipramine, without an increased risk of manic switching (Himmelhoch *et al.*, 1991; Thase *et al.*, 1992). Four other small crossover placebo-controlled RCTs comparing the effectiveness of tricyclics to lithium have found mixed results, without clear evidence of greater efficacy of TCAs over lithium (Fieve *et al.*, 1968; Mendels *et al.*, 1972; Watanabe *et al.*, 1975; Worrall *et al.*, 1979). The reversible MAOI moclobemide has been shown to have a lower acute mania switch rate than imipramine. Moclobemide, however, did not have a better efficacy compared to imipramine in a placebo-controlled RCT of 381 bipolar depressed patients who did *not* receive lithium (Baumhackl *et al.*, 1989). Another placebo-controlled RCT confirms these results, suggesting that moclobemide is equal in effectiveness to imipramine and less likely to precipitate mania (Silverstone, 2001).

Among SRIs, only paroxetine has been definitively shown to have a lower acute mania switch rate than imipramine in a study of 117 bipolar type I depressed patients in a placebo-controlled RCT (Nemeroff *et al.*, 2001). Paroxetine was not more effective than placebo when added to therapeutic serum levels of lithium (≥ 0.8) but better efficacy as compared to lithium plus placebo was seen with subtherapeutic serum levels of lithium (≤ 0.8). A non-placebo-controlled RCT has suggested that paroxetine used adjunctively with a mood stabilizer is of equal effectiveness to mood stabilizers alone (Young *et al.*, 2000). A comparison of the efficacy of venlafaxine and paroxetine as adjunctive treatment along with mood stabilizers was also examined in an open randomized study ($n = 60$). The data from this study suggest that venlafaxine and paroxetine have equal efficacy, but venlafaxine had a higher manic switch rate (12% versus 2%, though not statistically significant) (Vieta *et al.*, 2002).

Fluoxetine has been shown to have similar acute mania switch rates to imipramine in another placebo-controlled RCT study of 89 patients with bipolar depression (Cohn *et al.*, 1989). Although this study reported efficacy of fluoxetine superior to imipramine, many fluoxetine-treated patients also received lithium, whereas many of the imipramine group did not receive lithium, thus biasing any direct comparison of efficacy. As stated earlier, another study reports that OFC treatment was superior to both olanzapine monotherapy and placebo, with mania switch rates equivalent to placebo (Tohen *et al.*, 2002d).

There have been two non-placebo-controlled RCTs on the efficacy of bupropion treatment of acute bipolar depression. In one, bupropion had a much lower acute mania switch rate than desipramine (11% versus 50%), but that study was limited to only 19 treatment trials in 15 patients (Sachs *et al.*, 1994b). Another study compared bupropion with the β_2-antagonist idazoxan, and reported equal efficacy and manic switch rates (Grossman *et al.*, 1999).

Two other reports are commonly cited as providing RCT evidence of safety or efficacy with SRIs in bipolar disorder. In one report (Peet, 1994), SRIs were reported to have acute manic switch rates that were lower than TCAs and equal to placebo. In another report (Amsterdam and Garcia-Espana, 2000), fluoxetine was reported to have a low manic switch rate (about 5%) compared to placebo (about 0.5%, though this 10-fold increased risk is significant). Both of these reports, however, were post-hoc exploratory analyses of unipolar depression clinical trials. The authors reanalyzed the data by retrieving information based on patients identified as having been included in those trials with the diagnosis of bipolar type II depression. These reports have the drawback of at best being applicable to patients with bipolar disorder type II, not type I, and further of not having been designed to assess safety of antidepressants in bipolar disorder. Manic rating scales were not conducted and reports of manic switch rates are based only on spontaneously reported side-effects, and this is likely to lead to underreporting of those symptoms (sexual dysfunction is a classic example). Also, none of these patients was taking a concomitant mood stabilizer such as lithium. Thus, despite being based on RCT data, these studies are exploratory at best and limited in generalizability to type II bipolar illness.

Sertraline and venlafaxine are being studied in a non-placebo-controlled RCT comparison with bupropion for bipolar depression, with preliminary data before unblinding suggesting similar 2-month acute mania/hypomania switch rates in all three groups (around 14%) (Post *et al.*, 2001).

The above studies found that antidepressants can be helpful in the treatment of acute depressive symptoms in bipolar disorder, but only marginally better than lithium when used in full therapeutic doses. On the other hand, antidepressants use along with lithium may allow a lower overall lithium dose, which can be better tolerated than full-dose lithium monotherapy. These studies also demonstrate that standard antidepressants cause acute mania to a greater extent than placebo, and this risk seems highest with the TCAs. In type I bipolar depression, the only two antidepressants that have been shown to have a low risk of causing mania are paroxetine and bupropion. SRIs as a whole may be safer in type II bipolar depression based on exploratory analysis of unipolar depression clinical trials, though this hypothesis has not been adequately tested in prospectively designed RCTs of bipolar type II depression.

Table 2.2 Studies of acute depression

Agent	Number of studies	Total patients	Findings
Lithium	10	179	More effective than placebo
	2	144	Equivalent to imipramine and paroxetine
Valproate	2	70	Possible benefit
	1	27	Valproate plus lithium equivalent to addition of paroxetine to either single mood stabilizer
Carbamazepine	3	30	Mildly effective
Lamotrigine	3	432	More effective than placebo
Gabapentin	1	31	Equivalent to placebo
Topiramate	1	36	Equivalent to bupropion when added to lithium
Oxcarbazepine	1	13	Suggested uncontrolled adjunctive benefit
Olanzapine	1	833	Mildly effective versus placebo, more for neurovegetative than core mood symptoms
Risperidone	1	22	Possibly speeds onset of response when added to paroxetine
ECT	3	50	Possible uncontrolled benefit
Paroxetine	2	144	Equivalent to therapeutic lithium levels, proven low acute mania switch rate
Fluoxetine	3	255	Poor methodologies limit efficacy assessment. Probably equivalent to TCAs in both efficacy and acute mania switch rate
Bupropion	3	99	Equivalent to desipramine, proven low acute mania switch rate
Sertraline	1	64	Blind not yet broken in one study
Venlafaxine	1	64	Blind not yet broken in one study
Moclobemide	2	537	Low acute mania switch rate; data only in bipolar type II disorder in patients not taking mood stabilizers
Imipramine	5	638	Equivalent to lithium in efficacy; high acute mania switch rate
	3	191	Equivalent to lithium in efficacy
Desipramine	1	12	Equivalent to lithium in efficacy
	1	15	Equivalent to bupropion when added to lithium; high acute mania switch rate
Tranylcypromine	1	56	More effective than imipramine when added to lithium; equivalent acute mania switch rate to imipramine
Pramipexole	1	24	More effective than placebo when added to lithium; probable low acute mania switch rate

ECT, electroconvulsive therapy; TCAs, tricyclic antidepressants.

Dopamine agonists, with their potential antidepressant properties, are now beginning to be studied for the treatment of bipolar depression. One placebo-controlled RCT of 24 bipolar depressed patients showed antidepressant efficacy for the dopamine agonist pramipexole when added to lithium plus placebo, and acute mania switch was relatively low (8%) (Goldberg *et al.*, 2004).

Summary of acute bipolar depression studies

As shown in Table 2.2, the largest number of studies demonstrating efficacy have been conducted with lithium ($n = 12$), while the largest number of patients studied was with olanzapine ($n = 833$). Again, given the breadth and range of the available data with lithium, it seems most reasonable to conclude that it is the first-line agent for the treatment of bipolar depression. Anticonvulsants and possibly atypical neuroleptics are also useful. Standard antidepressants are important options, though usually second- or third-line rather than first-line choices due to the fact that the evidence basis for their efficacy and safety is much less impressive than is often assumed. Among standard antidepressants, there does not appear to be evidence of better efficacy than lithium, and only paroxetine and bupropion (and perhaps pramipexole) show some evidence of short-term safety (i.e., proven low acute mania switch rates in bipolar disorder type I) (Figure 2.1).

What is the best pharmacotherapy approach to prophylaxis in bipolar disorder?

Lithium

There have been at least 13 placebo-controlled RCTs (total $n = 509$) that have demonstrated benefit with lithium in the prevention of manic and depressive episodes in bipolar disorder (Laurell and Ottosson, 1968; Baastrup *et al.*, 1970; Melia, 1970; Cundall *et al.*, 1972; Coppen *et al.*, 1973, 1976; Prien *et al.*, 1973a, 1973b; Stallone *et al.*, 1973; Dunner *et al.*, 1976; Fieve *et al.*, 1976; Quitkin *et al.*, 1981; Kane *et al.*, 1982) (Table 2.3). A Cochrane Collaboration meta-analysis (Figure 2.2) has demonstrated benefit in these studies with marked reduction of risk of relapse (odds ratio 0.21). These studies generally consisted of initial treatment with lithium (plus or minus an antidepressant or neuroleptic) for acute mood symptoms, followed by double-blind randomization to continuation of lithium or switch to placebo. It is now generally felt that this kind of sudden discontinuation design may have overestimated the benefit of lithium due to increased risk of withdrawal mania in patients in whom lithium is stopped abruptly (Suppes *et al.*, 1991). Three RCTs have controlled for this risk either by gradual discontinuation of lithium or by avoiding the use of lithium in the initial acute treatment phase before double-blind randomization for prophylaxis. In these three studies (total $n = 110$),

Table 2.3 Prophylaxis

Agent	Number of studies	Total patients	Findings
Lithium	14	541	More effective than placebo; sudden discontinuation studies
	3	1010	More effective than placebo; gradual discontinuation studies
	5	261	More effective than imipramine
Valproate	1	372	Equivalent to placebo and lithium in a probable failed study
	1	251	Equivalent to olanzapine
Carbamazepine	2	32	Mild benefit over placebo
	2	64	Mildly less effective than lithium in one study; mildly more effective than lithium in another study
Lamotrigine	2	645	More effective than placebo. Equivalent to lithium with somewhat greater benefit in depressive prophylaxis
	1	182	Equivalent to placebo in rapid-cycling, though possible benefit in bipolar type II subgroup
Gabapentin	1	18	Possible monotherapy uncontrolled benefit
Topiramate	1	76	Possible adjunctive uncontrolled benefit
Oxcarbazepine	1	15	Equivalent to lithium
Flupenthixol	2	53	No added benefit versus placebo when added to lithium
Olanzapine	3	778	Equivalent to lithium or valproate. More effective than placebo when added to lithium or valproate
Risperidone	1	358	Suggested uncontrolled benefit
Clozapine	1	38	Mildly more effective when added to mood stabilizers than mood stabilizer combinations without clozapine
Imipramine	2	66	Equivalent to or worse than placebo
	2	192	No added benefit versus placebo when combined with lithium. More manic episodes over time in one study
Fluoxetine	1	10	Possible benefit in retrospective post-hoc analysis of bipolar II subsample from a unipolar depression cohort
ECT	1	58	More benefit if continued long-term in those with acute benefit, added to pharmacotherapy, than in those in whom ECT was discontinued after acute benefit
Omega-3 fatty acids	1	30	Mildly more effective than placebo when added to standard mood stabilizers in a rapid-cycling sample
Clonazepam	1	28	Equivalent to placebo when added to lithium

ECT, electroconvulsive therapy.

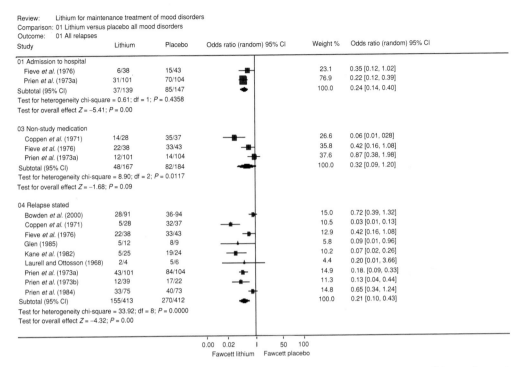

Review: Lithium for maintenance treatment of mood disorders
Comparison: 01 Lithium versus placebo all mood disorders
Outcome: 01 All relapses

Study	Lithium	Placebo	Odds ratio (random) 95% CI	Weight %	Odds ratio (random) 95% CI
01 Admission to hospital					
Fieve et al. (1976)	6/38	15/43		23.1	0.35 [0.12, 1.02]
Prien et al. (1973a)	31/101	70/104		76.9	0.22 [0.12, 0.39]
Subtotal (95% CI)	37/139	85/147		100.0	0.24 [0.14, 0.40]
Test for heterogeneity chi-square = 0.61; df = 1; P = 0.4358					
Test for overall effect Z = –5.41; P = 0.00					
03 Non-study medication					
Coppen et al. (1971)	14/28	35/37		26.6	0.06 [0.01, 028]
Fieve et al. (1976)	22/38	33/43		35.8	0.42 [0.16, 1.08]
Prien et al. (1973a)	12/101	14/104		37.6	0.87 [0.38, 1.98]
Subtotal (95% CI)	48/167	82/184		100.0	0.32 [0.09, 1.20]
Test for heterogeneity chi-square = 8.90; df = 2; P = 0.0117					
Test for overall effect Z = –1.68; P = 0.09					
04 Relapse stated					
Bowden et al. (2000)	28/91	36-94		15.0	0.72 [0.39, 1.32]
Coppen et al. (1971)	5/28	32/37		10.5	0.03 [0.01, 0.13]
Fieve et al. (1976)	22/38	33/43		12.9	0.42 [0.16, 1.08]
Glen (1985)	5/12	8/9		5.8	0.09 [0.01, 0.96]
Kane et al. (1982)	5/25	19/24		10.2	0.07 [0.02, 0.26]
Laurell and Ottosson (1968)	2/4	5/6		4.4	0.20 [0.01, 3.66]
Prien et al. (1973a)	43/101	84/104		14.9	0.18. [0.09, 0.33]
Prien et al. (1973b)	12/39	17/22		11.3	0.13 [0.04, 0.44]
Prien et al. (1984)	33/75	40/73		14.8	0.65 [0.34, 1.24]
Subtotal (95% CI)	155/413	270/412		100.0	0.21 [0.10, 0.43]
Test for heterogeneity chi-square = 33.92; df = 8; P = 0.0000					
Test for overall effect Z = –4.32; P = 0.00					

0.00   0.02   50   100
Fawcett lithium   Fawcett placebo

Figure 2.2   Meta-analysis of lithium versus placebo prophylaxis treatment. CI, confidence interval. Reprinted with permission from Burgess *et al.* (2002). Copyright Cochrane Library, reproduced with permission.

lithium has again been shown to be beneficial, slightly more for prevention of mania than for prevention of depression (Bowden *et al.*, 2000, 2002; Calabrese *et al.*, 2002).

Despite these RCT data, a number of large observational studies from the 1980s and 1990s reported much lower remission rates with lithium than expected from the RCTs (Harrow *et al.*, 1990; Sachs *et al.*, 1994a; Goldberg *et al.*, 1995; Goldberg and Harrow, 1999). These other studies led to a widespread perception, particularly in the USA, that lithium may have lost its efficacy as more diverse forms of mood illness were being diagnosed within the bipolar paradigm. A number of factors may have accounted for these studies, such as the study of refractory patients in tertiary care academic centers, the widespread use of antidepressants in the 1990s that may have led to long-term mood destabilization, and the use of lithium in patients with other reasons for poor prognosis (such as substance abuse and psychosis). Other recent large observational studies, conducted in the community setting and minimizing antidepressant use, suggest that these reports of lithium's inefficacy were probably premature (Tondo *et al.*, 1998b; Baldessarini and Tondo, 2000).

Another important aspect of the prophylactic utility of lithium is its effect on suicide and mortality. Lithium is the only psychotropic agent that has been definitively shown to reduce mortality and suicide rates in any psychiatric illness (Tondo *et al.*, 1998a; Baldessarini and Jamison, 1999). It not only reduces suicide rates in bipolar disorder, but it also reduces mortality due to cardiovascular disease, which is the top cause of death in patients with bipolar disorder (Tondo and Baldessarini, 2000; Tondo *et al.*, 2001). The most rigorous data on this difficult-to-study topic is from an open randomized study which supported the superiority of lithium in its anti-suicide effect compared to carbamazepine in 2.5-year outcome (Thies-Flechtner *et al.*, 1996). In this study, antisuicide benefit with lithium was not specifically related to efficacy in prevention of mood episodes, and thus whether or not lithium reduced mood episode relapse rates, it appeared to reduce suicide rates.

Valproate and carbamazepine

One RCT of valproate compared to lithium and placebo has been conducted ($n = 372$) (Bowden *et al.*, 2000). In this study, there was no overall benefit with valproate versus placebo, although since only about one-third of patients relapsed in 1 year in each arm of this study, these low relapse rates made it difficult to demonstrate benefit. Two open randomized comparisons with lithium (total $n = 114$) (Lambert and Venaud, 1992; Hirschfeld *et al.*, 1999) suggest equal or better efficacy with valproate, as do large observational comparative studies (Calabrese and Delucchi, 1990; Ghaemi and Goodwin, 2001b).

Two placebo-controlled RCTs have been conducted on the prophylactic effects of carbamazepine (Ballenger and Post, 1978; Okuma *et al.*, 1981), with carbamazepine being superior to placebo. In addition, two non-placebo-controlled RCTs have reported similar efficacies between carbamazepine and lithium (Watkins *et al.*, 1987; Lusznat *et al.*, 1988).

Lamotrigine

Two large recent prophylaxis studies ($n = 1315$) have now demonstrated that lamotrigine is more effective than placebo in prevention of depressive episodes in bipolar disorder. In the two studies, lamotrigine seemed mildly more effective than lithium for depressive prophylaxis, though the difference with lithium was not statistically significant (Calabrese *et al.*, 2002; Bowden *et al.*, 2002).

Other novel anticonvulsants

Data from small observational studies suggest potential long-term benefit with gabapentin (Schaffer and Schaffer, 1999) and with topiramate (Ghaemi *et al.*, 2001b), mainly as adjunctive agents, in bipolar disorder. These studies, however, are limited in number and difficult to interpret in the absence of more rigorous data supporting acute benefit with these agents. A small, open randomized study ($n = 15$) of oxcarbazepine reported some benefit compared to lithium in prophylaxis of bipolar disorder (Cabrera *et al.*, 1986).

Typical neuroleptic agents

There are two RCTs (one crossover) of typical neuroleptic agents in prevention of mania in bipolar disorder (total $n = 53$) (Ahlfors *et al.*, 1981; Esparon *et al.*, 1986). In both small studies, neuroleptics added to lithium were not more effective than lithium plus placebo in preventing manic episodes, and, in contrast, neuroleptic use was associated with increased occurrence of depressive morbidity. These studies suggest that typical neuroleptics do not possess mood-stabilizing properties, but rather seem to be purely antimanic agents, bringing mood down when it is elevated, but continuing to bring mood down below euthymia.

Olanzapine

There are four RCTs of olanzapine in the prevention of mood episodes in bipolar disorder – one study in which olanzapine is used as an adjunct to mood stabilizer, two in monotherapy comparison with mood stabilizers (divalproex and lithium), and one in monotherapy comparison with placebo. At the time of writing, the placebo-controlled study had not yet been publicly presented.

The first study (Tohen *et al.*, 2004) examined whether continuation of olanzapine in patients who had initially responded to olanzapine plus mood stabilizer for acute mania was effective in preventing remission. In this study, patients who had responded to olanzapine plus lithium or valproate for acute mania after a 6-week treatment period were then re-randomized to either olanzapine plus mood stabilizer or placebo plus mood stabilizer for up to 18 months. Survival analysis demonstrated much longer time to recurrence of either mania or depression in the group maintained on olanzapine plus valproate or lithium compared to the mood stabilizer plus placebo group. Unfortunately, 19.6% of patients in the olanzapine-plus-mood-stabilizer group gained a clinically important amount of body weight (>7% increase in baseline body mass index, BMI) compared to only 6.3% in the valproate/lithium monotherapy group. This is the first RCT to demonstrate long-term adjunctive mood-stabilizing benefit from continuation of a neuroleptic after recovery from acute mania.

In another RCT report (Tohen *et al.*, 2002a), acutely manic patients were randomized to olanzapine or valproate, with somewhat better responses acutely (at 2 months) with olanzapine. All patients were then continued on their original double-blind randomization for up to 1 year, with some apparent marginal clinical benefit with olanzapine versus valproate, although there were no statistically significant differences regarding efficacy. Both groups, however, had very high dropout rates (near 85%), with more sedation and weight gain with olanzapine compared to more gastrointestinal upset with valproate.

In a third RCT report (Tohen *et al.*, 2002c), acutely manic patients were randomized to olanzapine or lithium for 2 months, and then continued on their original double-blind randomization for each drug for up to a year. This study, designed and powered to be an equivalence study, demonstrated overall similar benefit clinically and statistically in both groups. Dropout rates were low (about 40%) compared to the valproate comparison study, and olanzapine was again associated with more weight gain than lithium.

The above two studies are not definitive due to the absence of a placebo group and thus the studies could be demonstrating that olanzapine is equally effective, or equally ineffective, as valproate or lithium in these samples. While a placebo arm would have markedly strengthened both studies, the high dropout rate in the valproate study raises concerns regarding mutual inefficacy, while the low dropout rate in the lithium study is reassuring. A fourth study was conducted directly comparing olanzapine to placebo, which is quite useful, although in that sample it too would have been ideal to have an active control arm (lithium or valproate). The results of this last study are pending, but if they support the efficacy of olanzapine compared to placebo for prevention of manic or depressive episodes, the trend of the data would appear to be supportive of long-term prophylactic benefit with olanzapine.

It is noteworthy that tardive dyskinesia (TD) was not observed in any of these long-term prophylaxis studies of olanzapine, supporting the long-term schizophrenia clinical trial literature that indicates that TD risk with atypical neuroleptics is significantly lower than the rates observed with typical neuroleptics.

Other large observational studies support the generalizability of the above RCT findings, particularly regarding adjunctive long-term benefit with olanzapine added to standard mood stabilizers like lithium or valproate (Sanger *et al.*, 2001; Vieta *et al.*, 2001b).

Other atypical neuroleptic agents

A large ($n = 358$) observational study with risperidone (Vieta *et al.*, 2001a) found excellent long-term adjunctive mood-stabilizing benefit when combined with standard mood stabilizers for bipolar disorder, with only 25% recurrence at up to 1 year follow-up (mean 6 months).

A small open randomized study ($n = 38$) with clozapine added to standard mood stabilizers versus usual treatment (standard mood stabilizers in the absence of clozapine) found evidence of a mild amount of marginal mood-stabilizing benefit in the clozapine group (Suppes *et al.*, 1999).

Other agents

In one small RCT, clonazepam, added to lithium compared to placebo in 28 stable euthymic bipolar patients, was not found to have a prophylactic effect (Cosgrove *et al.*, 1999). Time to relapse did not differ between the clonazepam and placebo groups, though somewhat less rescue medication was needed in the clonazepam group. Since this study was small, the possibility of type II false-negative error cannot be discounted.

Standard antidepressants

Five placebo-controlled RCTs of TCAs (total $n = 263$) failed to find any benefit with use of tricyclics in conjunction with lithium for the prevention of depressive episodes in bipolar disorder, type I or II (Ghaemi *et al.*, 2001a). Two RCTs of the newer antidepressants buproprion (Sachs *et al.*, 1994b) and fluoxetine (Amsterdam *et al.*, 1998) have been conducted. The limited total number of subjects available for assessment at 1 year follow-up, 6 in the bupropion study and 10 in the fluoxetine study, precludes a meaningful statistical analysis.

One (Quitkin *et al.*, 1981) of these studies on TCAs found evidence of long-term worsening with antidepressants, with more manic episodes over time compared to lithium alone (and no benefit in terms of reduction of depressive episodes).

These data would seem to support the recommendation, recently gaining in popularity among researchers (Sachs, 1996), that antidepressants be discontinued after use for the acute major depressive episode in bipolar disorder, given the lack of evidence of long-term preventive benefit.

A large, non-randomized, controlled observational comparison study has reported increased 1-year depressive relapse rates in patients in whom antidepressants are discontinued after recovery from the acute major depressive episode, compared to those in whom mood stabilizer plus antidepressant combination treatment is continued long-term (Altshuler *et al.*, 2001). In contrast, it is important to note that larger, more rigorous RCT data are available from another study (Prien *et al.*, 1984), clearly demonstrating that, after recovery from an acute major depressive episode with lithium plus imipramine, discontinuation of imipramine did not lead to increased 1-year relapse rates compared to continuation of imipramine plus lithium.

Overall, these studies fail to provide any rigorous evidence of long-term benefit with antidepressants in the prevention of depression in patients with bipolar disorder.

ECT

The largest and longest controlled follow-up study of maintenance ECT in bipolar disorder is a small, non-randomized, observational study of major depression ($n = 58$), which included bipolar ($n = 12$) and unipolar ($n = 46$) types (Gagne *et al.*, 2000). Patients who responded to ECT for acute depression tended to maintain response much more strongly at 2-year follow-up if ECT was continued into the maintenance phase than those in whom ECT was discontinued (93% versus 52% 2-year remission rate; 73% versus 18% 5-year remission rate). This finding may be interpreted in the setting of the common use of ECT as near last-resort treatment in patients who are highly refractory to pharmacotherapy. In such patients, this study suggests, resumption of pharmacotherapy after ECT may not be beneficial compared to commitment to long-term ECT treatment. Unfortunately, no randomized data with maintenance ECT for bipolar disorder exist.

Novel agents: omega-3 fatty acids, vitamin/mineral supplements

When omega-3 fatty acids versus placebo were added to standard mood stabilizers in a small RCT, investigators found shorter time to need for intervention with other medication in the placebo-treated group (Stoll *et al.*, 1999). Patients, however, were only moderately symptomatic with a mixture of manic and depressive symptoms, and no statistical differences in mood ratings scales or episode frequency was demonstrated. No follow-up RCT data have been made public, and thus, at this point, the putative mood-stabilizing benefit of omega-3 fatty acids remains a matter of controversy. Significant data from open randomized or large observational studies are also unavailable.

Recently, a prospective small observational study suggested some benefit with a multivitamin, multimineral supplement for acute mania (Kaplan *et al.*, 2001), and an accompanying commentary describes cases of long-term benefit (Popper, 2001). An RCT of this agent is currently underway.

Rapid-cycling bipolar disorder as a proxy for prophylaxis

Unfortunately, no agent has been shown to be effective in a primary outcome analysis of an RCT study in rapid-cycling bipolar disorder. The only RCT study conducted to date has been with lamotrigine (Calabrese *et al.*, 2000). In that study, efficacy with lamotrigine versus placebo was not demonstrable in the total sample primary outcome measure of time to relapse into an episode. However, in a post-hoc secondary analysis, there was a suggestion that the observed lack of efficacy was due to the subgroup with bipolar I disorder, with statistically significant benefit noted in the bipolar II subgroup. This observation is the only positive RCT treatment shown to provide benefit in this difficult-to-treat population.

Indeed, the only intervention that has been demonstrated in an RCT to improve rapid-cycling in bipolar I disorder is the discontinuation of antidepressants. Two different small studies (total $n = 15$), using an on-off-on paradigm, found that TCAs tended to be associated with rapid-cycling, and discontinuation of TCAs led to reduction in cycling rate and/or resolution of rapid-cycling (Wehr and Goodwin, 1979; Wehr et al., 1988). Some (Koukopoulos et al., 2000), but not all (Turvey et al., 1999), small observational reports also suggest that discontinuation of antidepressants is a potentially important intervention in recovery from a rapid-cycling course.

Despite a widespread conception that anticonvulsants have been shown to be more effective than lithium in treating rapid-cycling, this view is based on small observational study data only (Calabrese et al., 1993). In fact, data from another small observational study (Baldessarini et al., 2000) indicate that lithium, in the context of minimization of antidepressant use, may be effective in the treatment of rapid-cycling.

In summary, no definitive randomized data support any agent for treatment of rapid-cycling bipolar disorder, with the exception of discontinuation of antidepressants.

Summary of prophylaxis studies

As shown in Table 2.3, as with acute mania and acute depression, the largest number of studies demonstrating efficacy have been conducted with lithium. In this case, there is clear and widely accepted superiority to the lithium data regarding efficacy as a first-line agent. Anticonvulsants and possibly atypical neuroleptics are also useful. Standard antidepressants and typical neuroleptics appear to be ineffective at best and potentially harmful at worst.

Polypharmacy in psychiatry is a large topic that we have examined in detail elsewhere (Ghaemi, 2002). It is fairly common in bipolar disorder, with long-term mood stabilizer monotherapy usually in no greater than one-third of patients (Denicoff et al., 1997). The larger question is whether polypharmacy, and with what agents, is supported by evidence in long-term prophylaxis of bipolar disorder. There is only one RCT of polypharmacy with lithium plus valproate in the maintenance treatment of bipolar I disorder, in which 12 patients followed for 1 year were randomly assigned either placebo or valproate added to lithium. The combination treatment was associated with less relapse but more side-effects (Solomon et al., 1997). In an open randomized 1-year outcome study, 52 patients were followed on lithium alone, carbamazepine alone, or the combination for up to 3 years. While treatment response (based on moderate to marked improvement on the Clinical Global Impression scale) was higher on the combination treatment (55%) than lithium (33%) or carbamazepine (31%) monotherapy, this difference was not statistically significant, possibly due to the small sample sizes. Statistically significant benefit to combination therapy, however, was clearly present in patients with rapid-cycling bipolar disorder (56% combination therapy response versus 28% lithium response and 19% carbamazepine response) (Denicoff *et al.*, 1997). The most rigorous evidence basis for combination prophylaxis treatment supports primary use of standard mood stabilizers (lithium, valproate, or carbamazepine), with adjunctive use of atypical neuroleptic and novel anticonvulsant classes. Ineffective polypharmacy can result from a reversal of these emphases, with less aggressive long-term use of mood-stabilizing agents, and chronic neuroleptic or antidepressant pharmacotherapy.

Early treatment guidelines were limited to literature derived largely from lithium, traditional neuroleptic, and TCA studies. As these studies are limited, early guidelines were broad in their recommendations, often including the use of lithium in all phases of the illnesses, along with neuroleptics for manic symptoms and antidepressants for depressive symptoms. In the last decade, greater attention was placed in the USA on the lack of evidence of efficacy for traditional neuroleptic and antidepressants (Sachs, 1996; Ghaemi *et al.*, 2002a). Along with evidence from small observational studies of potential risks with those agents, recent US-based guidelines have tended to be more conservative (Sachs *et al.*, 2000; Hirschfeld *et al.*, 2002). These guidelines, in general, suggest limiting the use of typical neuroleptics in favor of atypical neuroleptics (especially olanzapine), and utilizing novel anticonvulsants such as lamotrigine. While these guidelines have engendered criticism in some quarters in Europe (Moller and Grunze, 2000), this review of evidence-based treatment of bipolar disorder tends to provide support for the recent trends in treatment guidelines from the USA, with overall emphasis on use of lithium and anticonvulsants as primary mood stabilizers, with frequent use of atypical neuroleptic and novel anticonvulsant agents, mainly as adjuncts. In Figure 2.1, we provide a visual representation of an interpretation of this literature which can be conceptualized for clinical use.

Acknowledgments

This work was supported by National Institute of Mental Health Research Career Award (MH-64189) (SNG).

REFERENCES

Abrams, R. and Taylor, M. (1974). Unipolar and bipolar depressive illness: phenomenology and response to electroconvulsive therapy. *Archives of General Psychiatry*, **30**, 320–1.

Ahlfors, U. G., Baastrup, P. C., and Dencker, S. J. (1981). Flupenthixol decanoate in recurrent manic depressive illness. A comparison with lithium. *Acta Psychiatrica Scandinavica*, **64**, 226–37.

Altshuler, L., Kiriakos, L., Calcagno, J., *et al.* (2001). The impact of antidepressant discontinuation versus antidepressant continuation on 1-year risk for relapse of bipolar depression: a retrospective chart review. *Journal of Clinical Psychiatry*, **62**, 612–16.

Amsterdam, J. D. and Garcia-Espana, F. (2000). Venlafaxine monotherapy in women with bipolar II and unipolar major depression. *Journal of Affective Disorders*, **59**, 225–9.

Amsterdam, J. D., Garcia-Espana, F., Fawcett, J., *et al.* (1998). Efficacy and safety of fluoxetine in treating bipolar II major depressive episode. *Journal of Clinical Psychopharmacology*, **18**, 435–40.

Anthony, J. C., Folstein, M., and Romanoski, A. J. (1985). Comparison of lay DIS and a standardized psychiatric diagnosis. *Archives of General Psychiatry*, **42**, 667–75.

Baastrup, P. C., Poulsen, J. C., Schou, M., Thomsen, K., and Amdisen, A. (1970). Prophylactic lithium: double blind discontinuation in manic-depressive and recurrent-depressive disorders. *Lancet*, **2**, 326–30.

Baldessarini, R. J. and Jamison, K. (1999). Effects of medical interventions on suicidal behavior: summary and conclusions. *Journal of Clinical Psychology*, **60** (suppl. 2), S117–22.

Baldessarini, R. J. and Tondo, L. (2000). Does lithium still work? Evidence of stable responses over three decades. *Archives of General Psychiatry*, **57**, 187–90.

Baldessarini, R. J., Tondo, L., Floris, G., and Hennen, J. (2000). Effects of rapid cycling on response to lithium maintenance treatment in 360 bipolar I and II disorder patients. *Journal of Affective Disorders*, **61**, 13–22.

Ballenger, J. C. and Post, R. M. (1978). Therapeutic effects of carbamazepine in affective illness: a preliminary report. *Community Psychopharmacology*, **2**, 159–75.

Barbini, C., Scherillo, P., Benedetti, F., *et al.* (1997). Response to clozapine in acute mania is more rapid than that of chlorpromazine. *International Clinical Psychopharmacology*, **12**, 109–12.

Baron, M., Gershon, E. S., Rudy, V., Jonas, W. Z., and Buchsbaum, M. (1975). Lithium carbonate response in depression. *Archives of General Psychiatry*, **32**, 1107–11.

Baumhackl, U., Biziere, K., Fischbach, R., *et al.* (1989). Efficacy and tolerability of moclobemide compared with imipramine in depressive disorder (DSM III): an Austrian double-blind, multicentre study. *British Journal of Psychiatry*, **155** (suppl.), 78–83.

Berk, M., Ichim, L., and Brook, S. (1999). Olanzapine compared to lithium in mania: a double-blind randomized controlled trial. *International Clinics in Psychopharmacology*, **14**, 339–43.

Berv, D., Klugman, J., Rosenquist, K. J., Hsu, D. J., and Ghaemi, S. N. (2002). Oxcarbazepine treatment of refractory bipolar depression (abstract). *Journal of Clinical Psychiatry*, **64**, 943–5.

Bowden, C. (2001). Novel treatments for bipolar disorder. *Expert Opinion of Investigational Drugs*, **10**, 661–71.

Bowden, C., Brugger, A., Swann, A., *et al.* (1994). Efficacy of divalproex vs lithium and placebo in the treatment of mania. *Journal of the American Medical Association*, **271**, 918–24.

Bowden, C., Calabrese, J., McElroy, S., *et al.* (2000). A randomized, placebo-controlled 12-month trial of divalproex and lithium in treatment of outpatients with bipolar I disorder. *Archives of General Psychiatry*, **57**, 481–9.

Bowden, C., Ghaemi, S. N., Gyulai, L., *et al.* (2002). Lamotrigine delays mood episodes in recently depressed bipolar I patients (abstract). In: *Annual Meeting of the American Psychiatric Association*, Philadelphia, PA.

Bradwejn, J., Shriqui Koszycki, D., and Meterissian, G. (1990). Double-blind comparison of the effects of clonazepam and lorazepam in mania. *Journal of Clinical Psychopharmacology*, **10**, 403–8.

Burgess, S., Geddes, J., Hawton, K., *et al.* (2002). Lithium maintenance treatment of mood disorders (Cochrane Review). In: *The Cochrane Library*, issue 4. Oxford: Update Software.

Cabrera, J., Muehlbauer, H., Schley, J., Stoll, K., and Muller-Oerlinghausen, B. (1986). Long-term randomized clinical trial on oxcarbazepine vs lithium in bipolar and schizoaffective disorders: preliminary results. *Pharmacopsychiatry*, **19**, 282–3.

Calabrese, J. (2000). Topiramate versus placebo in mania (abstract). In: *153rd Annual Meeting of the American Psychiatric Association*, Chicago, IL.

Calabrese, J. and Delucchi, G. A. (1990). Spectrum of efficacy of valproate in 55 patients with rapid-cycling bipolar disorder. *American Journal of Psychiatry*, **147**, 431–4.

Calabrese, J. R., Woyshville, M. J., Kimmel, S. E., and Rapport, D. J. (1993). Predictors of valproate response in bipolar rapid cycling. *Journal of Clinical Psychopharmacology*, **13**, 280–3.

Calabrese, J., Bowden, C., Sachs, G., *et al.* (1999). A double-blind placebo-controlled study of lamotrigine monotherapy in outpatients with bipolar I depression. *Journal of Clinical Psychology*, **60**, 79–88.

Calabrese, J. R., Suppes, T., Bowden, C. L., *et al.* (2000). A double-blind, placebo-controlled, prophylaxis study of lamotrigine in rapid-cycling bipolar disorder. Lamictal 614 Study Group. *Journal of Clinical Psychiatry*, **61**, 841–50.

Calabrese, J. R., Shelton, M. D., Rapport, D. J., Kimmel, S. E., and Elnaj, O. (2002). Long-term treatment of bipolar disorder with Lamotrigine. *Journal of Clinical Psychiatry*, **63** (suppl. 10), 18–22.

Chouinard, G., Young, S. N., and Annable, L. (1983). Antimanic effect of clonazepam. *Biology and Psychiatry*, **18**, 451–66.

Chouinard, G., Annable, L., Turnier, L., Holobow, N., and Szkrumelak, N. (1993). A double-blind randomized clinical trial of rapid tranquilization with IM clonazepam and IM haloperidol in agitated psychotic patients with manic symptoms. *Canadian Journal of Psychiatry*, **38** (suppl. 4), S114–21.

Ciapparelli, A., Dell'Osso, L., Tundo, A., *et al.* (2001). Electroconvulsive therapy in medication-nonresponsive patients with mixed mania and bipolar depression. *Journal of Clinical Psychiatry*, **62**, 552–5.

Cohn, J. B., Collins, G., Ashbrook, E., and Wernick, J. F. (1989). A comparison of fluoxetine, imipramine and placebo in patients with bipolar depressive disorder. *International Clinics in Psychopharmacology*, **4**, 313–14.

Coppen, A., Noguera, R., Bailey, J. *et al.* (1971). Prophylactic lithium in affective disorders. Controlled trial. Lancet, **2**, 275–9.

Coppen, A., Peet, M., Bailey, J., *et al.* (1973). Double-blind and open prospective studies on lithium prophylaxis in affective disorders. *Psychiatrica Neurologica Neurochirurgica*, **76**, 501–10.

Coppen, A., Montgomery, S. A., Gupta, R. K., and Bailey, J. E. (1976). A double blind comparison of lithium carbonate and maprotiline in the prophylaxis of the affective disorders. *British Journal of Psychiatry*, **128**, 479–85.

Cosgrove, V., Ghaemi, S. N., Baldassano, C., Demopulos, C., and Sachs, G. (1999). A double-blind placebo-controlled study of clonazepam as an adjunct to lithium maintenance treatment of bipolar disorder (abstract). In: *152nd Annual Meeting of the American Psychiatric Association*. Washington, DC.

Cundall, R. L., Brooks, P. W., and Murray, L. G. (1972). A controlled evaluation of lithium prophylaxis in affective disorders. *Psychological Medicine*, **2**, 308–11.

Davis, L. L., Kabel, S., Patel, D., *et al.* (1996). Valproate as an antidepressant in major depressive disorder. *Psychopharmacology Bulletin*, **32**, 647–52.

De Leon, O. A. (2001). Antiepileptic drugs for the acute and maintenance treatment of bipolar disorder. *Harvard Review of Psychiatry*, **9**, 209–22.

Delbello, M., Schwiers, M., Rosenberg, H., and Strakowski, S. (2002). A double-blind, randomized, placebo-controlled study of quetiapine as adjunctive treatment for adolescent mania. *Journal of the American Academy of Child and Adolescent Psychiatry*, **41**, 1216–23.

Denicoff, K., Smith-Jackson, E., Disney, E., *et al.* (1997). Comparative prophylactic efficacy of lithium, carbamazepine, and the combination in bipolar disorder. *Journal of Clinical Psychology*, **58**, 470–8.

Dilsaver, S. C., Swann, S. C., Chen, Y. W., *et al.* (1996). Treatment of bipolar depression with carbamazepine: results of an open study. *Biology and Psychiatry*, **40**, 935–7.

Dunner, D. L., Stallone, F., and Fieve, R. R. (1976). Lithium carbonate and affective disorders. A double-blind study of prophylaxis of depression in bipolar illness. *Archives of General Psychiatry*, **33**, 117–20.

Edwards, R., Stephenson, U., and Flewett, T. (1991). Clonazepam in acute mania: a double blind trial. *Australian and New Zealand Journal of Psychiatry*, **25**, 238–42.

Emrich, H. M. (1990). Studies with oxcarbazepine (trileptal) in acute mania. *International Clinics in Psychopharmacology*, **5** (suppl. 1), 83–8.

Emrich, H. M., Altmann, H., Dose, M., and von Zerssen, D. (1983). Therapeutic effects of GABA-ergic drugs in affective disorders. A preliminary report. *Pharmacology, Biochemistry and Behavior*, **19**, 369–72.

Esparon, J., Kolloori, J., Naylor, G. J., *et al.* (1986). Comparison of the prophylactic action of flupenthixol with placebo in lithium treated manic-depressive patients. *British Journal of Psychiatry*, **148**, 723–5.

Fieve, R. R., Platman, S. R., and Plutchik, R. R. (1968). The use of lithium in affective disorders: I. Acute endogenous depression. *American Journal of Psychiatry*, **125**, 487–91.

Fieve, R. R., Kumbaraci, T., and Dunner, D. L. (1976). Lithium prophylaxis of depression in bipolar I, bipolar II, and unipolar patients. *American Journal of Psychiatry*, **133**, 925–9.

Freeman, T., Clothier, J., Pazzaglia, P., Lesem, M., and Swann, A. (1992). A double-blind comparison of valproate and lithium in the treatment of acute mania. *American Journal of Psychiatry*, **149**, 108–11.

Frye, M. A., Ketter, T. A., Kimbrell, T. A., *et al.* (2000). A placebo-controlled study of lamotrigine and gabapentin monotherapy in refractory mood disorders. *Journal of Clinical Psychopharmacology*, **20**, 607–14.

Gagne, G. G., Jr., Furman, M. J., Carpenter, L. L., and Price, L. H. (2000). Efficacy of continuation ECT and antidepressant drugs compared to long-term antidepressants alone in depressed patients. *American Journal of Psychiatry*, **157**, 1960–5.

Ghaemi, S. N. (2002). *Polypharmacy in Psychiatry*. New York: Marcel Dekker.

Ghaemi, S. N. and Goodwin, F. K. (2001a). Gabapentin treatment of the non-refractory bipolar spectrum: an open case series. *Journal of Affective Disorders*, **65**, 167–71.

Ghaemi, S. N. and Goodwin, F. K. (2001b). Long-term naturalistic treatment of depressive symptoms in bipolar illness with divalproex vs. lithium in the setting of minimal antidepressant use. *Journal of Affective Disorders*, **65**, 281–7.

Ghaemi, S. N., Katzow, J. J., Desai, S. P., and Goodwin, F. K. (1998). Gabapentin treatment of mood disorders: a preliminary study. *Journal of Clinical Psychiatry*, **59**, 426–9.

Ghaemi, S. N., Lenox, M., and Baldessarini, R. (2001a). Effectiveness and safety of long-term antidepressant treatment in bipolar disorder. *Journal of Clinical Psychiatry*, **62**, 565–9.

Ghaemi, S. N., Manwani, S. G., Katzow, J. J., Ko, J. Y., and Goodwin, F. K. (2001b). Topiramate treatment of bipolar spectrum disorders: a retrospective chart review. *Annals of Clinical Psychiatry*, **13**, 185–9.

Ghaemi, S. N., Ko, J. Y., and Goodwin, F. K. (2002a). "Cade's disease" and beyond: misdiagnosis, antidepressant use, and a proposed definition for bipolar spectrum disorder. *Canadian Journal of Psychiatry*, **47**, 125–34.

Ghaemi, S. N., Ko, J. Y., and Katzow, J. J. (2002b). Oxcarbazepine treatment of refractory bipolar disorder: a retrospective chart review. *Bipolar Disorders*, **4**, 70–4.

Glen, A. I. M. (1985). Lithium prophylaxis of recurrent affective disorders. *Journal of Affective Disorders*, **8**, 259–65.

Goldberg, J. and Harrow, M. (1999). *Bipolar Disorders: Clinical Course and Outcome*. Washington, DC: American Psychiatric Press.

Goldberg, J. F., Harrow, M., and Grossman, L. S. (1995). Course and outcome in bipolar affective disorder: a longitudinal follow-up study. *American Journal of Psychiatry*, **152**, 379–84.

Goldberg, J. F., Burdick, K. E., and Endick, C. J. (2004). Preliminary randomized, double-blind, placebo-controlled trial of pramipexole added to mood stabilizers for treatment-resistant bipolar depression. *American Journal of Psychiatry*, **161**, 564–6.

Goodwin, F. and Jamison, K. (1990). *Manic Depressive Illness*. New York: Oxford University Press.

Goodwin, F. K., Murphy, D. L., and Bunney, W. E. Jr. (1969). Lithium-carbonate treatment in depression and mania: a longitudinal double-blind study. *Archives of General Psychiatry*, **21**, 486–96.

Goodwin, F. K., Murphy, D. L., Dunner, D. L., and Bunney, W. E. Jr. (1972). Lithium response in unipolar versus bipolar depression. *American Journal of Psychiatry*, **129**, 44–7.

Grossi, E., Sacchetti, E., Vita, A., *et al.* (1984). Carbamazepine versus chlorpromazine in mania: a double-blind trial. In: *Anticonvulsants in Affective Disorders*, ed. H. M. Emrich, T. Okuma, and A. A. Muller. Amsterdam: Excerpta Medica, pp. 177–87.

Grossman, F., Potter, W. Z., Brown, E. A., and Maislin, G. (1999). A double-blind study comparing idazoxan and bupropion in bipolar depressed patients. *Journal of Affective Disorders*, **56**, 237–43.

Harrow, M., Goldberg, J. F., Grossman, L. S., and Meltzer, H. Y. (1990). Outcome in manic disorders. *Archives of General Psychiatry*, **47**, 665–71.

Helzer, J., Robins, L., McEnvoy, L., *et al.* (1985). A comparison of clinical and diagnostic interview schedule diagnoses: physician reexamination of lay-interviewed cases in the general population. *Archives of General Psychiatry*, **42**, 657–66.

Himmelhoch, J. M., Thase, M. E., Mallinger, A. G., and Houck, P. (1991). Tranylcypromine versus imipramine in anergic bipolar depression. *American Journal of Psychiatry*, **148**, 910–16.

Hirschfeld, R. M., Allen, M. H., McEvoy, J. P., Keck, P. E., Jr., and Russell, J. M. (1999). Safety and tolerability of oral loading divalproex sodium in acutely manic bipolar patients. *Journal of Clinical Psychiatry*, **60**, 815–18.

Hirschfeld, R. M., Bowden, C., Gitlin, M., *et al.* (2002). American Psychiatric Association practice guideline for the treatment of patients with bipolar disorder (revision). *American Journal of Psychiatry*, **159** (suppl.), 1–50.

Janicak, P., Sharma, R., Pandey, G., and Davis, J. (1998). Verapamil for the treatment of acute mania: a double-blind placebo controlled trial. *American Journal of Psychiatry*, **155**, 972–3.

Johnson, G., Gershon, S., Burdock, E., Floyd, A., and Hekimian, L. (1971). Comparative effects of lithium and chlorpromazine in the treatment of acute manic states. *British Journal of Psychiatry*, **119**, 267–76.

Kane, J. M., Quitkin, F. M., Rifkin, A., *et al.* (1982). Lithium carbonate and imipramine in the prophylaxis of unipolar and bipolar II illness: a prospective, placebo-controlled comparison. *Archives of General Psychiatry*, **39**, 1065–9.

Kaplan, B. J., Simpson, J. S., Ferre, R. C., *et al.* (2001). Effective mood stabilization with a chelated mineral supplement: an open-label trial in bipolar disorder. *Journal of Clinical Psychiatry*, **62**, 936–44.

Keck, P. E., Jr., Versiani, M., Potkin, S., *et al.* (2003). Ziprasidone in the treatment of acute bipolar mania: a three-week, placebo-controlled, double-blind randomized trial. *American Journal of Psychiatry*, **160**, 741–8.

Keck, P. J., Jr., Saha, A., Iwamoto, T., *et al.* (2002). Aripiprazole versus placebo in acute mania (abstract). In: *Annual Meeting of the American Psychiatric Association*. Philadelphia, PA.

Klein, D. (1967). Importance of psychiatric diagnosis in prediction of clinical drug effects. *Archives of General Psychiatry*, **16**, 118–26.

Klein, E., Bental, E., Lerer, B., and Belmaker, R. H. (1984). Carbamazepine and haloperidol v placebo and haloperidol in excited psychoses: a controlled study. *Archives of General Psychiatry*, **41**, 165–70.

Koukopoulos, A., Sni, G., Koukopoulos, A., and Girardi, P. (2000). Cyclicity and manic-depressive illness. In: *Bipolar Disorders: 100 Years after Manic-Depressive Insanity*, ed. A. Marneros and J. Angst. London: Kluwer Academic, pp. 315–34.

Kramlinger, K. G. and Post, R. M. (1989). The addition of lithium to carbamazepine. Antidepressant efficacy in treatment-resistant depression. *Archives of General Psychiatry*, **46**, 794–800.

Lambert, P. and Venaud, G. (1992). Comparative study of valpromide vs lithium in treatment of affective disorders. *Nervure*, **5**, 57–65.

Laurell, B. and Ottosson, J. (1968). Prophylactic lithium? *Lancet*, **7**, 1245–6.

Lerer, B., Moore, N., Meyendorff Cho, S. R., and Gershon, S. (1987). Carbamazepine versus lithium in mania: a double-blind study. *Journal of Clinical Psychiatry*, **48**, 88–93.

Lindenmayer, J., Czobor, P., Volavka, J., *et al.* (2002). Changes in glucose and cholesterol levels in patients with schizophrenia treated with typical or atypical antipsychotics. *American Journal of Psychiatry*, **160**, 290–6.

Lusznat, R., Murphy, D., and Nunn, C. (1988). Carbamazepine vs. lithium in the treatment and prophylaxis of mania. *British Journal of Psychiatry*, **153**, 198–204.

Maggs, R. (1963). Treatment of manic illness with lithium carbonate. *British Journal of Psychiatry*, **109**, 56–65.

Marcotte, D. (1998). Use of topiramate, a new anti-epileptic as a mood stabilizer. *Journal of Affective Disorders*, **50**, 245–51.

McIntyre, R., McCann, S., and Kennedy, S. (2001). Antipsychotic metabolic effects: weight gain, diabetes mellitus, and lipid abnormalities. *Canadian Journal of Psychiatry*, **46**, 273–81.

McIntyre, R., Mancini, D., McCann, S., *et al.* (2002). Topiramate versus bupropion SR when added to mood stabilizer therapy for the depressive phase of bipolar disorder: a preliminary single-blind study. *Bipolar Disorders*, **4**, 207–13.

Melia, P. I. (1970). Prophylactic lithium: a double-blind trial in recurrent affective disorders. *British Journal of Psychiatry*, **116**, 621–4.

Mendels, J. (1976). Lithium in the treatment of depression. *American Journal of Psychiatry*, **133**, 373–8.

Mendels, J., Secunda, S. K., and Dyson, W. L. (1972). A controlled study of the antidepressant effects of lithium carbonate. *Archives of General Psychiatry*, **26**, 154–7.

Mishory, A., Yaroslavsky, Y., Bersudsky, Y., and Belmaker, R. (2000). Phenytoin as an antimanic anticonvulsant: a controlled study. *American Journal of Psychiatry*, **157**, 463–5.

Moller, H. J. and Grunze, H. (2000). Have some guidelines for the treatment of acute bipolar depression gone too far in the restriction of antidepressants? *European Archives of Psychiatry and Clinical Neuroscience*, **250**, 57–68.

Moller, H. J., Kissling, W., Riehl, T., *et al.* (1989). Doubleblind evaluation of the antimanic properties of carbamazepine as a comedication to haloperidol. *Progress in Neuro-Psychopharmacology and Biological Psychiatry*, **13**, 127–36.

Muller, A. A. and Stoll, K. D. (1984). Carbamazepine and oxcarbamazepine in the treatment of manic syndromes: studies in Germany. In: *Anticonvulsants in Affective Disorders*, ed. H. M. Emrich, T. Okuma, and A. A. Muller. Amsterdam: Excerpta Medica, pp. 139–47.

Muller-Oerlinghausen, B., Retzow, A., Henn, F. A., Giedke, H., and Walden, J. (2000). Valproate as an adjunct to neuroleptic medication for the treatment of acute episodes of mania: a prospective, randomized, double-blind, placebo-controlled, multicenter study. European Valproate Mania Study Group. *Journal of Clinical Psychopharmacology*, **20**, 195–203.

Nemeroff, C. B., Evans, D. L., Gyulai, L., *et al.* (2001). Double-blind, placebo-controlled comparison of imipramine and paroxetine in the treatment of bipolar depression. *American Journal of Psychiatry*, **158**, 906–12.

Normann, C., Hummel, B., Scharer, L. O., *et al.* (2002). Lamotrigine as adjunct to paroxetine in acute depression: a placebo-controlled, double-blind study. *Journal of Clinical Psychiatry*, **63**, 337–44.

Noyes, R., Dempsey, G. M., Blum, A., and Cavanaugh, G. L. (1974). Lithium treatment of depression. *Comprehensive Psychiatry*, **15**, 187–93.

Okuma, T., Inanaga, K., Otsuki, S., *et al.* (1979). Comparison of the antimanic efficacy of carbamazepine and chlorpromazine: a double-blind controlled study. *Psychopharmacology*, **66**, 211–17.

Okuma, T., Inanaga, K., Otsuki, S., *et al.* (1981). A preliminary double-blind study on the the efficacy of carbamazepine in prophylaxis of manic-depressive illness. *Psychopharmacology*, **73**, 95–6.

Pande, A. C., Crockatt, J. G., Janney, C. A., Werth, J. L., and Tsaroucha, G. (2000). Gabapentin in bipolar disorder: a placebo-controlled trial of adjunctive therapy. Gabapentin Bipolar Disorder Study Group. *Bipolar Disorders*, **2**, 249–55.

Peet, M. (1994). Induction of mania with selective serotonin reuptake inhibitors and tricyclic antidepressants. *British Journal of Psychiatry*, **164**, 549–50.

Platman, S. (1970). A comparison of lithium carbonate and chlorpromazine in mania. *American Journal of Psychiatry*, **127**, 351–3.

Pope, J. G., McElroy, S. L., Keck, P. E., Jr., and Hudson, J. I. (1991). Valproate in the treatment of acute mania. A placebo-controlled study. *Archives of General Psychiatry*, **48**, 62–8.

Popper, C. W. (2001). Do vitamins or minerals (apart from lithium) have mood-stabilizing effects? *Journal of Clinical Psychiatry*, **62**, 933–5.

Post, R. M., Uhde, T. W., Ballenger, J. C., *et al.* (1983). Carbamazepine and its -10,11-epoxide metabolite in plasma and CSF. Relationship to antidepressant response. *Archives of General Psychiatry*, **40**, 673–6.

Post, R., Uhde, T., Roy-Bryne, P., and Joffe, R. (1987). Correlates of antimanic responses to carbamazepine. *Psychiatry Research*, **21**, 71–83.

Post, R., Altshuler, L., Frye, M., *et al.* (2001). Rate of switch in bipolar patients prospectively treated with second-generation antidepressants as augmentation to mood stabilizers. *Bipolar Disorders*, **3**, 259–65.

Prien, R. F., Caffey, E. M., Jr., and Klett, C. J. (1972). Comparison of lithium carbonate and chlorpromazine in the treatment of mania: report of the Veterans Administration and National Institute of Mental Health Collaborative Study Group. *Archives of General Psychiatry*, **26**, 146–53.

Prien, R. F., Klett, C. J., and Caffey, E. M., Jr. (1973a). Lithium carbonate and imipramine in prevention of affective episodes: a comparison in recurrent affective illness. *Archives of General Psychiatry*, **29**, 420–5.

Prien, R. F., Point, P., Caffey, E. M., Jr., and Klett, C. J. (1973b). Prophylactic efficacy of lithium carbonate in manic-depressive illness: report of the Veterans Administration and National Institute of Mental Health collaborative study group. *Archives of General Psychiatry*, **28**, 337–41.

Prien, R. F., Kupfer, D. J., Mansky, P. A., *et al.* (1984). Drug therapy in the prevention of recurrences in unipolar and bipolar affective disorders: a report of the NIMH Collaborative Study

Group comparing lithium carbonate, imipramine, and a lithium carbonate–imipramine combination. *Archives of General Psychiatry*, **41**, 1096–104.

Quitkin, F. M., Kane, J., Rifkin, A., Ramos-Lorenzi, J. R., and Nayak, D. V. (1981). Prophylactic lithium carbonate with and without imipramine for bipolar 1 patients. *Archives of General Psychiatry*, **38**, 902–7.

Regier, D., Boyd, J., Burke, J. J., *et al.* (1988). One-month prevalence of mental disorders in the United States: based on five Epidemiologic Catchment Area sites. *Archives of General Psychiatry*, **45**, 977–86.

Reinstein, M., Sonnenberg, J., Chasanov, M., *et al.* (2002). Oxcarbazepine and divalproex sodium: a comparison of efficacy and side effects for mania (abstract). In: *Annual Meeting of the American Psychiatric Association*. Philadelphia, PA.

Sachs, G. S. (1996). Bipolar mood disorder: practical strategies for acute and maintenance phase treatment. *Journal of Clinical Psychopharmacology*, **16** (suppl. 1), 32S–47S.

Sachs, G. S., Lafer, B., Truman, C. J., Noeth, M., and Thibault, A. B. (1994a). Lithium monotherapy: miracle, myth and misunderstanding. *Psychiatric Annals*, **24**, 299–306.

Sachs, G. S., Lafer, B., Stoll, A. L., *et al.* (1994b). A double-blind trial of bupropion versus desipramine for bipolar depression. *Journal of Clinical Psychiatry*, **55**, 391–3.

Sachs, G. S., Printz, D., Kahn, D., Carpenter, D., and Docherty, J. (2000). The expert consensus guideline series: medication treatment of bipolar disorder 2000. *Postgraduate Medicine*, April, 1–104.

Sachs, G. S., Altshuler, L., Kelter, T., *et al.* (2001). Divalproex versus placebo for the treatment of bipolar depression (abstract). In: *Annual Meeting of the American College of Neuropsychopharmacology*. Puerto Rico.

Sachs, G. S., Mullen, J., Devine, N., and Sweitzer, D. (2002a). Quetiapine vs placebo as adjunct to mood stabilizer for the treatment of acute mania (abstract). In: *15th Congress of the European College of Neuropsychopharmacology*. Barcelona, Spain.

Sachs, G. S., Grossman, F., Ghaemi, S. N., Okamoto, A., and Bowden, C. L. (2002b). Combination of a mood stabilizer with risperidone or haloperidol for treatment of acute mania: a double-blind, placebo-controlled comparison of efficacy and safety. *American Journal of Psychiatry*, **159**, 1146–54.

Sanger, T. M., Grundy, S. L., Gibson, P. J., *et al.* (2001). Long-term olanzapine therapy in the treatment of bipolar I disorder: an open-label continuation phase study. *Journal of Clinical Psychiatry*, **62**, 273–81.

Schaffer, C. B. and Schaffer, L. C. (1999). Open maintenance treatment of bipolar disorder spectrum patients who responded to gabapentin augmentation in the acute phase of treatment. *Journal of Affective Disorders*, **55**, 237–40.

Schou, M., Juel-Nielsen, N., Stromgren, E., and Voldby, H. (1954). The treatment of manic psychosis by the administration of lithium salts. *Journal of Neurological Psychiatry*, **17**, 250–60.

Segal, J., Berk, M., and Brook, S. (1998). Risperidone compared with both lithium and haloperidol in mania: a double-blind randomized controlled trial. *Clinical Neuropharmacology*, **21**, 176–80.

Shelton, R. (2001). Risperidone in bipolar depression (abstract). In: *Annual Meeting of the American Psychiatric Association*. New Orleans, LA.

Shopsin, B., Gershon, S., Thompson, H., and Collins, P. (1975). Psychoactive drugs in mania. A controlled comparison of lithium carbonate, chlorpromazine, and haloperidol. *Archives of General Psychiatry*, **32**, 34–42.

Sikdar, S., Kulhara, P., Avasthi, A., and Singh, H. (1994). Combined chlorpromazine and electroconvulsive therapy in mania. *British Journal of Psychiatry*, **164**, 806–10.

Silverstone, T. (2001). Moclobemide vs. imipramine in bipolar depression: a multicentre double-blind clinical trial. *Acta Psychiatrica Scandinavica*, **104**, 104–9.

Small, J. G., Klapper, M. H., Kellams, J. J., *et al.* (1988). Electroconvulsive therapy compared with lithium in the management of manic states. *Archives of General Psychiatry*, **45**, 727–32.

Small, J., Klapper, M., Milstein, V., *et al.* (1991). Carbamazepine compared with lithium in the treatment of mania. *Archives of General Psychiatry*, **48**, 915–21.

Solomon, D. A., Ryan, C. E., Keitner, G. I., *et al.* (1997). A pilot study of lithium carbonate plus divalproex sodium for the continuation and maintenance treatment of patients with bipolar I disorder. *Journal of Clinical Psychiatry*, **58**, 95–9.

Spring, G., Schweid, D., Gray, C., Steinberg, J., and Horwitz, M. (1970). A double-blind comparison of lithium and chlorpromazine in the treatment of manic states. *American Journal of Psychiatry*, **126**, 1306–10.

Stallone, F., Shelley, E., Mendlewicz, J., and Fieve, R. R. (1973). The use of lithium in affective disorders, III: a double-blind study of prophylaxis in bipolar illness. *American Journal of Psychiatry*, **130**, 1006–10.

Stokes, P., Samoian, C., Stoll, P., and Patton, M. (1971). Efficacy of lithium as acute treatment of manic-depressive illness. *Lancet*, **1**, 1319–25.

Stoll, A. L., Severus, W. E., Freeman, M. P., *et al.* (1999). Omega 3 fatty acids in bipolar disorder: a preliminary double-blind, placebo-controlled trial. *Archives of General Psychiatry*, **56**, 407–12.

Suppes, T., Baldessarini, R. J., Faedda, G. L., and Tohen, M. (1991). Risk of reoccurrence following discontinuation of lithium treatment in bipolar disorder. *Archives of General Psychiatry*, **48**, 1082–8.

Suppes, T., Webb, A., Paul, B., *et al.* (1999). Clinical outcome in a randomized 1-year trial of clozapine versus treatment as usual for patients with treatment-resistant illness and a history of mania. *American Journal of Psychiatry*, **156**, 1164–9.

Takahashi, R., Sakuma, A., Itoh, K., and Kurihara, M. (1975). Comparison of efficacy of lithium carbonate and chlorpromazine in mania: report of collaborative study group on treatment of mania in Japan. *Archives of General Psychiatry*, **32**, 1310–18.

Thase, M., Mallinger, A. G., McKnight, D., and Himmelhoch, J. M. (1992). Treatment of imipramine-resistant recurrent depression IV: a double-blind crossover study of tranylcypromine for anergic bipolar depression. *American Journal of Psychiatry*, **149**, 195 –8.

Theis-Flechtner, K., Muller-Oerlinghausen, B., Seibert, W., Walther, A., and Greil, W. (1996). Effect of prophylactic treatment on suicide risk in patients with major affective disorders: data from a prospective randomized trial. *Pharmacopsychiatry*, **29**, 103–7.

Tohen, M., Sanger, T., McElroy, S., *et al.* (1999). Olanzapine versus placebo in the treatment of acute mania. Olanzapine HGEH study group. *American Journal of Psychiatry*, **156**, 702–9.

Tohen, M., Jacobs, T. G., Grundy, S. L., *et al.* (2000). Efficacy of olanzapine in acute bipolar mania: a double-blind, placebo-controlled study. The olanzapine HGGW study group. *Archives of General Psychiatry*, **57**, 841–9.

Tohen, M., Zhang, F., Feldman, P., Evans, A., and Breier, A. (2003). A 12-week, double-blind comparison of olanzapine vs. haloperidol in the treatment of acute mania. *Archives of General Psychiatry*, **60**, 1218–26.

Tohen, M., Baker, R. W., Altshuler, L. L., *et al.* (2002a). Olanzapine versus divalproex in the treatment of acute mania. *American Journal of Psychiatry*, **159**, 1011–17.

Tohen, M., Chengappa, K. N., Suppes, T., *et al.* (2002b). Efficacy of olanzapine in combination with valproate or lithium in the treatment of mania in patients partially nonresponsive to valproate or lithium monotherapy. *Archives of General Psychiatry*, **59**, 62–9.

Tohen, M., Marneros, A., Bowden, C., *et al.* (2002c). Olanzapine versus lithium in relapse prevention in bipolar disorder: a randomized double-blind controlled 12-month clinical trial (abstract). In: *Third European Stanley Foundation Conference on Bipolar Disorder*. Freiburg, Germany.

Tohen, M., Risser, R., Baker, R., *et al.* (2002d). Olanzapine in the treatment of bipolar depression (abstract). In: *Annual Meeting of the American Psychiatric Association*. Philadelphia, PA.

Tohen, M., Chengappa, K., Suppes, T., *et al.* (2004). Relapse prevention in bipolar I disorder: 18-month comparison of olanzapine plus mood stabiliser v. mood stabiliser alone. *British Journal of Psychiatry*, **184**, 337–45.

Tondo, L. and Baldessarini, R. J. (2000). Reduced suicide risk during lithium maintenance treatment. *Journal of Clinical Psychiatry*, **61** (suppl. 9), 97–104.

Tondo, L., Baldessarini, R., Hennen, J., *et al.* (1998a). Lithium treatment and risk of suicidal behavior in bipolar disorder patients. *Journal of Clinical Psychiatry*, **59**, 405–14.

Tondo, L., Baldessarini, R. J., Hennen, J., and Floris, G. (1998b). Lithium maintenance treatment: depression and mania in bipolar I and II disorders. *American Journal of Psychiatry*, **155**, 638–45.

Tondo, L., Hennen, J., and Baldessarini, R. J. (2001). Lower suicide risk with long-term lithium treatment in major affective illness: a meta-analysis. *Acta Psychiatrica Scandinavica*, **104**, 163–72.

Turvey, C. L., Coryell, W. H., Arndt, S., *et al.* (1999). Polarity sequence, depression, and chronicity in bipolar I disorder. *Journal of Nervous and Mental Disease*, **187**, 181–7.

Vieta, E., Goikolea, J. M., Corbella, B., *et al.* (2001a). Risperidone safety and efficacy in the treatment of bipolar and schizoaffective disorders: results from a 6-month, multicenter, open study. *Journal of Clinical Psychiatry*, **62**, 818–25.

Vieta, E., Reinares, M., Corbella, B., *et al.* (2001b). Olanzapine as long-term adjunctive therapy in treatment-resistant bipolar disorder. *Journal of Clinical Psychopharmacology*, **21**, 469–73.

Vieta, E., Martinez-Aran, A., Goikolea, J. M., *et al.* (2002). A randomized trial comparing paroxetine and venlafaxine in the treatment of bipolar depressed patients taking mood stabilizers. *Journal of Clinical Psychiatry*, **63**, 508–12.

Vinar, O., Dvorak, A., Obrovska, V., Kriskova, M., and Turcek, K. (1989). Does sodium valproate increase clinical effects of antidepressants? *Activitas Nervosa Superior (Praha)*, **31**, 103–5.

Watanabe, S., Ishino, H., and Otsuki, S. (1975). Double-blind comparison of lithium carbonate and imipramine in the treatment of depression. *Archives of General Psychiatry*, **32**, 659–68.

Watkins, S. E., Callender, K., Thomas, D. R., Tidmarsh, S. F., and Shaw, D. M. (1987). The effect of carbamazepine and lithium on remission from affective illness. *British Journal of Psychiatry*, **150**, 180–2.

Wehr, T. and Goodwin, F. (1979). Rapid cycling in manic-depressives induced by tricyclic antidepressants. *Archives of General Psychiatry*, **36**, 555–9.

Wehr, T. A., Sack, D. A., Rosenthal, N. E., and Cowdry, R. W. (1988). Rapid cycling affective disorder: contributing factors and treatment responses in 51 patients. *American Journal of Psychiatry*, **145**, 179–84.

Weissman, M. M., Leaf, P. J., Tischler, G. L., *et al.* (1988). Affective disorders in five United States communities. *Psychological Medicine*, **18**, 141–53. [Published erratum appears in *Psychological Medicine* 1988; **18**, following 792.]

Worrall, E. P., Moody, J. P., Peet, M., *et al.* (1979). Controlled studies of the acute antidepressant effects of lithium. *British Journal of Psychiatry*, **135**, 255–62.

Yatham, L. N., Grossman, F., Augustyns, I., Vieta, E., and Ravindran, A. (2003). Mood stabilisers plus risperidone or placebo in the treatment of mania. International, double-blind, randomised controlled trial. *British Journal of Psychiatry*, **182**, 141–7.

Young, L., Joffe, R., Robb, J., *et al.* (2000). Double-blind comparison of addition of a second mood stabilizer versus an antidepressant to an initial mood stabilizer for treatment of patients with bipolar depression. *American Journal of Psychiatry*, **157**, 124–6.

Zajecka, J., Weisler, R., Sachs, G., *et al.* (2002). A comparison of the efficacy, safety, and tolerability of divalproex sodium and olanzapine in the treatment of bipolar disorder. *Journal of Clinical Psychiatry*, **63**, 1148–55.

Zornberg, G. and Pope, H. J. (1993). Treatment of depression in bipolar disorder: new directions for research. *Journal of Clinical Psychopharmacology*, **13**, 397–408.

3

Evidence-based pharmacotherapy of schizophrenia

Robin Emsley and Piet Oosthuizen

University of Cape Town, South Africa

The introduction of the new atypical antipsychotics has changed the way we treat patients with schizophrenia. A number of agents are now available, providing new treatment options and producing heightened optimism for improved clinical outcomes. While commonly lumped together as a class, important differences are emerging among these compounds, particularly regarding their side-effect profiles. A great deal has been published on these agents and new important studies regularly appear in the literature. However, many questions remain unanswered regarding their safety and efficacy, and a great deal more remains to be learnt in order to place them in their correct perspective.

For antipsychotic trials, demonstration of superiority over placebo is still a requirement of most regulatory authorities (Laughren, 2001). Most of the earlier randomized controlled trials (RCTs) for the atypical antipsychotics used haloperidol as a comparator. However, a recent Cochrane meta-analysis of haloperidol versus placebo in clinical trials highlighted the neurotoxicity of the compound. The authors recommended that, for countries where haloperidol is not widely used, it should not be a control drug of choice for randomized trials of new antipsychotics (Joy et al., 2001). Most studies undertaken these days compare one atypical antipsychotic with another.

This chapter evaluates the evidence for efficacy, tolerability, and safety of the new atypical antipsychotics risperidone, olanzapine, quetiapine, ziprasidone, sertindole, amisulpride, and aripiprazole. In order to avoid the potential pitfalls of uncontrolled studies, we have focused mainly on published RCTs and meta-analytical reviews. The agents are discussed under the following headings: acute treatment; maintenance treatment; side-effect profiles; prodromal, first-episode, and refractory schizophrenia. Finally the following specific focuses of current clinical interest are dealt with: conventional versus atypical antipsychotics, head-to-head comparisons of atypical antipsychotics, and side-effect profiles.

Table 3.1 Acute-phase randomized controlled trials for risperidone

Comparator	Authors	n	Duration of trial	Dose of risperidone (mg/day)	Efficacy (overall, positive and negative symptoms)
Placebo	Chouinard et al. (1993)	135	8 weeks	2, 6, 10, 16	6–16 mg superior overall and positive, 6 mg superior negative symptoms
Placebo	Marder and Meibach (1994)	388	8 weeks	2, 6, 10, 16	6–16 mg superior overall and positive, 6 and 16 mg superior negative symptoms
Placebo	Kane et al. (2003)	400	12 weeks	25, 50, 75 mg IM_2-weekly	Superior overall, positive and negative symptoms
Haloperidol	Chouinard et al. (1993)	135	8 weeks	2, 6, 10, 16	6 mg superior overall
Haloperidol	Marder and Meibach (1994)	388	8 weeks	2, 6, 10, 16	6 and 16 mg superior overall
Haloperidol	Peuskens (1995)	1362	8 weeks	1, 4, 8, 12, 16	Equal
Haloperidol	Huttunen et al. (1995)	98	6 weeks	Mean 8	Equal
Haloperidol	Emsley (1999)	183	6 weeks	6	Equal
Olanzapine	Tran et al. (1997b)	339	28 weeks	4–12	Olanzapine superior for negative symptoms
Olanzapine	Conley and Mahmoud (2001)	377	8 weeks	2–6	Equal
Clozapine	Klieser et al. (1995)	59	4 weeks	4 and 8	Equal
Amisulpride	Peuskens et al. (1999)	228	8 weeks	8	Equal
Amisulpride	Sechter et al. (2002)	309	6 months	4–10	Equal
Amisulpride	Hwang et al. (2003)	48	6 weeks	4–8	Equal

IM, intramuscularly.

What is the first-line pharmacotherapy of schizophrenia?

Risperidone
Acute-phase trials (Table 3.1)

Risperidone versus placebo

The efficacy of oral risperidone has been demonstrated in two placebo-controlled trials. A dose-ranging study found risperidone 6–16 mg/day to be superior to placebo in overall and positive symptom improvement, while only 6 mg/day was better than placebo on negative symptom improvement (Chouinard *et al.*, 1993). A similar study reported significant improvements for 6 and 16 mg/day for overall clinical improvement, positive and negative symptoms, and 10 mg/day for positive symptoms only. The incidence of extrapyramidal symptoms (EPS) was significantly higher in patients treated with 16 mg of risperidone and 20 mg of haloperidol (Marder and Meibach, 1994).

Risperidone versus conventional antipsychotics

In one dose-ranging study, risperidone 6 mg/day was significantly better than haloperidol in reducing the Positive and Negative Symptom Scale (PANSS) total and general psychopathology scores. Haloperidol produced significantly more EPS than risperidone or placebo (Chouinard *et al.*, 1993). In another dose-ranging study, risperidone 6 and 16 mg/day were significantly better than haloperidol 20 mg/day in reducing overall symptoms. Significantly more subjects responded to risperidone 6 mg/day. The incidence of EPS was significantly higher in patients treated with 16 mg of risperidone and 20 mg of haloperidol (Marder and Meibach, 1994). A large multinational study compared risperidone 1, 4, 8, 12, and 16 mg/day with haloperidol 10 mg/day. The optimum risperidone doses were 4 and 8 mg/day, but no significant efficacy advantages over haloperidol were reported. Total EPS were greater in the haloperidol-treated patients than in the risperidone 1, 4, 8, and 12 mg groups (Peuskens, 1995). However, a later subanalysis of patients from Germany, Austria, and Switzerland reported significant advantages for risperidone over haloperidol according to PANSS total and subscale scores (Moller *et al.*, 1997a). Further post-hoc subanalyses reported that patients receiving risperidone 4 mg/day improved more rapidly than those receiving haloperidol (Rabinowitz *et al.*, 2001), and those hospitalized for >60 days (i.e., probably the more refractory patients) who received risperidone 4 mg/day improved significantly more than those treated with haloperidol (Rabinowitz and Davidson, 2001).

Flexible doses of risperidone (mean dose 8 mg/day) and flupenthixol (mean dose 38 mg/day) displayed comparable efficacy, and fewer patients experienced EPS with risperidone (Huttunen *et al.*, 1995). A small RCT (*n* = 35) compared risperidone to haloperidol and reported no differences in outcome, with risperidone causing fewer side-effects (Min *et al.*, 1993).

Long-acting risperidone injection

The first long-acting atypical antipsychotic has recently been introduced. An RCT comparing long-acting injectable risperidone (25, 50, or 75 mg 2-weekly) to placebo in 400 patients over 12 weeks reported it to be effective and well tolerated. No efficacy advantages were reported for 75 mg compared to 25 or 50 mg 2-weekly (Kane *et al.*, 2003).

Risperidone versus other atypical antipsychotics

Risperidone has been compared to other atypical antipsychotics in several studies. Two RCTs have been reported comparing risperidone with olanzapine. In the first, 339 subjects were evaluated over 28 weeks. Both olanzapine (10–20 mg/day) and risperidone (4–12 mg/day) were found to be effective, with olanzapine demonstrating superiority over risperidone in reducing negative symptoms, overall response rate, and maintenance of response at 28 weeks. A greater proportion of olanzapine subjects maintained their response at 28 weeks. The incidence of EPS, hyperprolactinemia, and sexual dysfunction was greater in the risperidone-treated patients (Tran *et al.*, 1997b). The second study, this time with a lower dose of risperidone, investigated 377 subjects with schizophrenia over 8 weeks. Once again, both olanzapine (5–20 mg/day, mean 12.4 mg/day) and risperidone (2–6 mg/day, mean 4.8 mg/day) were found to be effective. There were no differences in efficacy between the groups according to the last-observation carried-forward analysis, although the completers analysis reported significant advantages for risperidone in treating both positive and anxiety/depression symptoms. EPS were similar in the two groups. Greater weight gain was associated with olanzapine treatment (Conley and Mahmoud, 2001).

In a small RCT, risperidone 4 mg/day ($n = 20$), 8 mg/day ($n = 19$) and clozapine 400 mg/day ($n = 20$) were compared over 28 days in a non-refractory sample of patients with schizophrenia. No differences in efficacy were reported and risperidone appeared to be better tolerated (Klieser *et al.*, 1995). Three studies have compared risperidone and amisulpride. Risperidone (8 mg/day) was compared with amisulpride (800 mg/day) over 8 weeks in 228 patients with acute exacerbation of schizophrenia. The drugs showed equal efficacy, with both demonstrating good safety profiles. EPS did not differ between the two groups (Peuskens *et al.*, 1999). A 6-month trial in 309 subjects comparing amisulpride (400–1000 mg/day) and risperidone (4–10 mg/day) reported a superior response rate for amisulpride, similar incidence of EPS, and less weight gain and endocrine/sexual symptoms with amisulpride (Sechter *et al.*, 2002). A small ($n = 48$) trial reported similar efficacy and EPS for amisulpride (400–800 mg/day) and risperidone (4–8 mg/day), with greater weight gain for risperidone (Hwang *et al.*, 2003).

The efficacy and safety of clozapine, olanzapine, risperidone, and haloperidol were compared over 14 weeks in 150 patients with a suboptimal treatment response. Clozapine, risperidone, and olanzapine (but not haloperidol) treatment resulted in significant PANSS total score improvements. Negative symptoms improved significantly more for clozapine and olanzapine than haloperidol-treated patients. Olanzapine and clozapine were associated with weight gain (Volavka *et al.*, 2002). In a separate report of the neurocognitive effects of treatment in the same sample, global cognitive function improved significantly more with olanzapine and risperidone than with haloperidol (Bilder *et al.*, 2002).

Maintenance treatment

Until recently, very few RCTs had evaluated the efficacy and safety of the atypical antipsychotics in the maintenance treatment of schizophrenia. However, there are now a few studies suggesting advantages for atypical antipsychotics over their predecessors.

An RCT compared relapse rates in 365 clinically stable adult outpatients with schizophrenia or schizoaffective disorder receiving flexible doses of risperidone or haloperidol for a minimum of 1 year. Risk of relapse at the end of the study was significantly lower for the risperidone group (34%) than for the haloperidol group (60%). Early discontinuation of treatment was more frequent among the haloperidol patients. Risperidone patients had greater reductions in EPS scores (Csernansky *et al.*, 2002). In a 2-year maintenance trial comparing risperidone 6 mg/day with haloperidol 6 mg/day in 63 stable patients, both groups experienced similar improvements in symptoms and similar risks of psychotic exacerbations. However, risperidone-treated patients appeared to feel subjectively better, as indicated by less anxiety and depression and fewer extrapyramidal side-effects (Marder *et al.*, 2003a).

Meta-analyses

A meta-analysis of 11 RCTs comparing risperidone to conventional antipsychotics concluded that the short-term efficacy of risperidone is comparable to that of other antipsychotics. Risperidone patients showed slightly greater clinical improvement and lower overall dropout rate. Weight gain and tachycardia were more common in risperidone. There were significantly fewer EPS with risperidone (Song, 1997). Another meta-analysis of six trials comparing risperidone with haloperidol in subjects with chronic schizophrenia treated for at least 4 weeks in RCTs reported significantly higher response rates with risperidone and lower dropout rates. There was also significantly less prescribing of anticholinergic medication with risperidone patients (Davies *et al.*, 1998). A Cochrane review reported that in both the short and long term risperidone was more likely to produce improvement in symptoms, and to reduce the relapse rate at 12 months. Risperidone was

Table 3.2 Acute-phase randomized controlled trials for olanzapine

Comparator	Authors	n	Duration of trial	Dose of olanzapine (mg/day)	Efficacy (overall, positive and negative symptoms)
Placebo	Beasley et al. (1996a)	152	6 weeks	1 and 10	10 mg superior overall, positive, and negative
Placebo	Beasley et al. (1996b)	335	6 weeks	5 ± 2.5; 10 ± 2.5 and 15 ± 2.5	Medium and high dose superior overall and positive, low, and high dose superior negative
Haloperidol	Beasley et al. (1996b)	335	6 weeks	5 ± 2.5; 10 ± 2.5 and 15 ± 2.5	All doses equal overall and positive, 15 ± 2.5 mg superior for negative
Haloperidol	Beasley et al. (1997)	431	6 weeks	5 ± 2.5; 10 ± 2.5 and 15 ± 2.5	Equal
Haloperidol	Tollefson et al. (1997)	1996	6 weeks	5–20	Superior overall, positive, and negative
Haloperidol	Ishigooka et al. (2001)	182	8 weeks	5–15	Equal
Haloperidol	Lieberman et al. (2003)	263	12 weeks	Mean 9.1	Superior overall and negative, equal positive
Risperidone	Tran et al. (1997b)	339	28 weeks	10–20	Olanzapine superior negative
Risperidone	Conley and Mahmoud (2001)	377	8 weeks	5–20	Equal
Amisulpride	Martin et al. (2002)	377	8 weeks	5–20	Equal

less likely to cause motor disorders, but more likely to cause weight gain (Hunter et al., 2003).

Olanzapine
Acute-phase trials (Table 3.2)
Olanzapine versus placebo

Two pivotal dose-ranging studies found olanzapine to be significantly better than placebo in overall symptom improvement, as well as improvement in positive and negative symptoms (Beasley et al., 1996a, 1997). The most common treatment-emergent adverse events were somnolence, agitation, asthenia, and nervousness

(Beasley *et al.*, 1996a). Plasma prolactin elevation did not differ from placebo (Beasley *et al.*, 1996a).

Olanzapine versus conventional antipsychotics

Three RCTs have compared olanzapine with haloperidol (Beasley *et al.*, 1996b; Danion *et al.*, 1999; Tollefson *et al.*, 1997). Olanzapine demonstrated some efficacy advantages over haloperidol in these studies. In the first ($n = 335$), olanzapine 15 ± 2.5 mg/day was significantly better than haloperidol 15 ± 5 mg/day in reducing negative symptoms after 6 weeks (Beasley *et al.*, 1996b) while in the second study ($n = 431$), olanzapine 15 ± 2.5 mg/day over 6 weeks was equal to haloperidol 15 ± 5 mg/day on all efficacy measures (Beasley *et al.*, 1997). In a very large study ($n = 1996$) olanzapine 5–20 mg/day (mean 13.2 mg/day) was significantly better than haloperidol 5–20 mg/day (mean 11.8 mg/day) over 6 weeks in reducing overall psychopathology (Beasley *et al.*, 1997), positive symptoms (Beasley *et al.*, 1997), negative symptoms (Beasley *et al.*, 1996b; Wyatt *et al.*, 1998), and depressive symptoms (Tollefson *et al.*, 1997). Significant advantages for olanzapine over haloperidol treatment were found for EPS (Beasley *et al.*, 1996b, 1997; Tollefson *et al.*, 1997).

An RCT compared olanzapine with haloperidol in a sample of 182 Asian patients with schizophrenia. Olanzapine was as effective as haloperidol in treating overall symptomatology, and significantly superior in treating negative symptoms and EPS (Ishigooka *et al.*, 2001). In a recently reported non-industry-sponsored multisite RCT the long-term (12 month) effectiveness of olanzapine 5–20 mg/day versus haloperidol 5–20 mg/day (with prophylactic benztropine) was evaluated in 309 subjects with serious symptoms, and serious dysfunction for the previous 2 years. There were no significant differences between groups in study retention; positive, negative, or total symptoms; quality of life; or overall EPS. Olanzapine was associated with reduced akathisia, possibly less tardive dyskinesia and slight cognitive advantages, but more frequent reports of weight gain (Rosenheck *et al.*, 2003).

Intramuscular (IM) olanzapine

IM olanzapine was compared to IM haloperidol and IM placebo in treating acute agitation over a 24-h period in hospitalized patients with schizophrenia. Olanzapine showed superiority over haloperidol at 15, 30, and 45 min following the first injection. Both olanzapine and haloperidol reduced agitation significantly more than placebo at 2 and 24 h following the first injection. No patients treated with olanzapine experienced acute dystonia, compared with 7% of those treated with haloperidol (Wright *et al.*, 2001). In a similar study in 270 acutely agitated patients with schizophrenia, olanzapine (2.5, 5, 7.5, or 10 mg) showed a dose–response relationship in reduction of agitation. All doses of olanzapine, except 2.5 mg, were more effective than placebo at 30 min after injection, although not more effective than haloperidol. The lower doses of olanzapine (2.5, 5, and 7.5 mg) produced less treatment-emergent parkinsonism than haloperidol (Breier *et al.*, 2002).

Olanzapine versus other atypical antipsychotics

Two studies comparing olanzapine and risperidone are reported above. An RCT comparing amisulpride (200–800 mg/day) and olanzapine (5–20 mg/day) in 377 subjects reported similar efficacy and low EPS in both groups. Weight gain was significantly greater in the olanzapine-treated patients (Martin *et al.*, 2002).

Maintenance treatment

The efficacy of a standard dose of oral olanzapine (5–15 mg/day) was compared with placebo and with an ineffective dose of olanzapine (1 mg/day) in mainten-ance therapy of 120 subjects with schizophrenia. The standard-dose olanzapine-treated patients experienced significantly lower relapse risk over 1 year compared to patients treated with placebo or ineffective-dose olanzapine (Dellva *et al.*, 1997). Data from three double-blind extensions of acute studies (Beasley *et al.*, 1996b, 1997; Meltzer, 1999) comparing olanzapine and haloperidol in maintenance treat-ment were pooled and reported together. Fewer subjects experienced relapse at 1 year with olanzapine (19.7%) than with haloperidol (28%) (Tran *et al.*, 1998). Olanzapine has also been compared with risperidone for the prevention of relapse in an RCT conducted over 28 weeks. Survival analysis revealed that significantly more olanzapine patients maintained their response at endpoint. The incidence of EPS, hyperprolactinemia, and sexual dysfunction was significantly lower in the olanzapine-treated patients (Tran *et al.*, 1997a).

Meta-analyses

A Cochrane review included 21 RCTs comparing olanzapine to placebo or any antipsychotic treatment in subjects with schizophrenia or schizophreniform psy-chosis. Olanzapine was found to be superior to placebo (although results were equi-vocal for negative symptoms), and equally as effective as conventional antipsy-chotics. There were fewer EPS with olanzapine than with haloperidol. Weight change data were not conclusive (Duggan *et al.*, 2003).

Quetiapine
Acute-phase trials (Table 3.3)
Quetiapine versus placebo

High-dose (750 mg/day) and low-dose (250 mg/day) quetiapine were compared to placebo over 6 weeks in 286 hospitalized subjects. High withdrawal rates

Table 3.3 Acute-phase randomized controlled trials for quetiapine

Comparator	Authors	n	Duration of trial	Dose of quetiapine (mg/day)	Efficacy (overall, positive, and negative symptoms)
Placebo	Small *et al.* (1997)	286	6 weeks	250 and 750	750 mg superior overall, positive, and negative
Placebo	Arvanitis and Miller (1997)	361	6 weeks	75, 150, 300, 600, and 750	150–750 mg superior overall and positive, 300 mg superior negative
Haloperidol	Arvanitis and Miller (1997)	361	6 weeks	75, 150, 300, 600, and 750	Equal
Haloperidol	Copolov *et al.* (2000)	448	6 weeks	Mean 455	Equal
Chlorpromazine	Peuskens and Link (1997)	201	6 weeks	Mean 407	Equal

were recorded in all three treatment groups (42%, 57%, and 59%), primarily because of treatment failure. High-dose quetiapine was significantly better than placebo in reducing overall and positive scores. Reduction of negative symptoms was less consistent. Quetiapine was well tolerated, and did not induce EPS, sustained elevations of prolactin, or clinically significant hematological changes (Small *et al.*, 1997). A multiple fixed-dose study of quetiapine (75, 150, 300, 600, and 750 mg/day), haloperidol (12 mg/day) and placebo reported significant differences between the four highest doses of quetiapine and placebo for overall and positive symptoms, and between quetiapine 300 mg/day and placebo for negative scores. Across the dose range, quetiapine was no different from placebo regarding the incidence of EPS or change in prolactin concentrations (Arvanitis and Miller, 1997).

Quetiapine versus conventional antipsychotics

In the above dose-ranging study, there were no differences between quetiapine and haloperidol regarding the efficacy measures (Arvanitis and Miller, 1997). In a study comparing flexible doses of quetiapine (mean 455 mg/day) and haloperidol (mean 8 mg/day), both compounds produced clear reductions in symptoms. At endpoint, the mean PANSS total score was reduced by -18.7 in the quetiapine group, and -22.1 in the haloperidol group ($P = 0.13$, between treatment). Significantly fewer EPS and reduced prolactin levels were reported at endpoint for the quetiapine-treated patients (Copolov *et al.*, 2000). Flexible doses of quetiapine (mean endpoint dose 407 mg/day) and chlorpromazine (mean dose 384 mg/day) were equally

Table 3.4 Acute-phase randomized controlled trials for ziprasidone

Comparator	Authors	n	Duration of trial	Dose of ziprasidone (mg/day)	Efficacy (overall, positive and negative symptoms)
Placebo	Keck *et al.* (1998)	139	4 weeks	40 and 120	120 mg superior overall
Placebo	Daniel *et al.* (1999)	302	6 weeks	80 and 120	Both doses superior overall, positive and negative
Haloperidol	Goff *et al.* (1998)	90	4 weeks	4, 10, 40, and 160	160 mg equal

effective in the treatment of positive and negative symptoms. The quetiapine group had a lower incidence of adverse events and EPS than the chlorpromazine group (Peuskens and Link, 1997).

Quetiapine versus other atypical antipsychotics

No RCTs were found comparing quetiapine to other atypical antipsychotics.

Meta-analyses

A Cochrane systems review included 11 RCTs comparing quetiapine to placebo and other antipsychotic agents, and found that, compared to placebo, people treated with quetiapine showed greater symptom reduction and were less likely to leave the study early, particularly for treatment failure. Compared to conventional antipsychotics, the proportion of people leaving the studies early was marginally, but significantly, less for the quetiapine group. Symptom reduction was significantly greater in the high-dose range of quetiapine. Less anticholinergic medication was required in the quetiapine-treated patients. It was noted that most data are very short-term (Srisurapanont *et al.*, 2000).

Maintenance studies

No blinded maintenance studies were found for quetiapine.

Ziprasidone

Acute-phase trials (Table 3.4)

Ziprasidone versus placebo

A study comparing ziprasidone 40 or 120 mg/day and placebo found 120 mg/day to be significantly more effective than placebo in improving the overall, depressive, and anergia scores, and had significantly more responders than placebo. The most frequently reported adverse events were dyspepsia, constipation, nausea, and abdominal pain. There were no differences between ziprasidone and placebo regarding EPS (Keck *et al.*, 1998). In another placebo-controlled trial comparing ziprasidone

80 or 160 mg/day, both doses of ziprasidone were significantly more effective than placebo in reducing overall, core-item, and negative symptom scores. Ziprasidone had a very low liability for inducing movement disorders and weight gain (Daniel *et al.*, 1999).

Ziprasidone versus conventional antipsychotics

A dose-finding RCT comparing ziprasidone 4, 10, 40, and 160 mg/day and haloperidol 15 mg/day found ziprasidone 160 mg/day to be comparable to haloperidol in reducing overall psychopathology and positive symptoms, as well as overall response rate. In ziprasidone patients, only transient elevations in prolactin were recorded, and fewer required benzatropine to treat EPS (Goff *et al.*, 1998).

IM ziprasidone

An RCT evaluated IM ziprasidone (2 and 10 mg) injections in acutely agitated psychotic patients. The 10 mg dose was significantly more effective in reducing agitation up to 4 h after the first injection. No acute dystonia was reported (Lesem *et al.*, 2001). In another similar study, ziprasidone 2 and 20 mg injections were compared. The 20 mg dose substantially and significantly reduced symptoms of acute agitation. Both doses were well tolerated, and were not associated with EPS (Daniel *et al.*, 2001).

Maintenance studies

Patients with stable, chronic schizophrenia were treated with ziprasidone 40, 80, or 160 mg/day or placebo for 1 year. All the ziprasidone groups showed a lower probability of relapse than placebo. Discontinuation due to adverse events was similar for ziprasidone and placebo. Ziprasidone treatment was not associated with increased risk of movement disorders, weight gain, or cardiovascular abnormalities (Arato *et al.*, 2002). Another study compared ziprasidone (modal dose 80 mg/day) with haloperidol (modal dose 5 mg/day) in stable patients over 28 weeks. Similar reductions in all mean efficacy variables were observed. More ziprasidone-treated patients were negative symptom responders. Despite the low dose of haloperidol, ziprasidone had clear advantages in all evaluations of movement disorders. Changes in body weight were negligible with both treatments. No significant laboratory or cardiovascular changes were observed (Hirsch *et al.*, 2002).

Meta-analyses

A Cochrane review of available RCTs reported that, in studies ranging from 1 week (IM preparation) to over 6 months, ziprasidone seemed more effective than placebo and as effective as haloperidol. There were fewer EPS in the

Table 3.5 Acute-phase randomized controlled trials for sertindole

Comparator	Authors	n	Duration of trial	Dose of sertindole (mg/day)	Efficacy (overall, positive and negative symptoms)
Placebo	Van Kammen et al. (1996)	205	40 days	4, 8, 12, 20	20 mg superior overall
Placebo	Zimbroff et al. (1997)	497	8 weeks	12, 20, 24	All doses superior overall, 20 and 24 mg superior positive, 20 mg superior negative
Haloperidol	Zimbroff et al. (1997)	497	8 weeks	12, 20, 24	Equal

ziprasidone-treated patients. The authors noted that data for ziprasidone were limited at that stage (Bagnall et al., 2000).

Sertindole
Acute-phase trials (Table 3.5)
Sertindole versus placebo

An RCT compared sertindole 4, 8, 12 and 20 mg/day and placebo. A dose-related improvement was observed for total scores, with significant differences being recorded between sertindole 20 mg/day and placebo. EPS-related events were comparable in the placebo and sertindole groups (van Kammen et al., 1996). Another RCT compared sertindole 12, 20, and 24 mg/day with haloperidol 4, 8, and 16 mg/day, and placebo. All doses were more effective than placebo. For treating negative symptoms, only sertindole 20 mg/day was superior to placebo (Zimbroff et al., 1997).

Sertindole versus conventional antipsychotics

In two dose-ranging studies, sertindole and haloperidol were comparably effective. For EPS measures, sertindole was indistinguishable from placebo, and rates of EPS were not dose-related. All dose levels of haloperidol produced significantly more EPS than placebo or sertindole. Adverse events associated with sertindole treatment were mild in severity (van Kammen et al., 1996; Zimbroff et al., 1997).

Maintenance studies

Long-term efficacy and time to treatment failure were assessed in 282 clinically stable treatment-responsive outpatients with schizophrenia treated up to 1 year with sertindole or haloperidol. Time to treatment failure was not significantly different between the groups, but sertindole patients remained free of hospitalization for exacerbation of schizophrenia and remained compliant significantly longer than

Table 3.6 Acute-phase randomized controlled trials for amisulpride

Comparator	Authors	n	Duration of trial	Dose of amisulpride (mg/day)	Efficacy (overall, positive and negative symptoms)
Placebo	Paillere-Martinot et al. (1995)	27	6 weeks	50 to 100	Superior for negative symptoms
Placebo	Boyer et al. (1995)	104	6 weeks	100 and 300	Both doses superior for negative symptoms
Placebo	Danion et al. (1999)	243	12 weeks	50 and 100	Both doses superior for negative symptoms
Haloperidol	Delcker et al. (1990)	41	6 weeks	Flexible	Equal
Haloperidol	Puech et al. (1998)	319	4 weeks	100, 400, 800, 1200	400 and 800 mg equal
Haloperidol	Moller et al. (1997b)	191	6 weeks	800	Superior for negative symptoms
Haloperidol	Carriere et al. (2000)	199	4 months	400–1200	Superior for negative symptoms
Haloperidol	Wetzel et al. (1998)	132	6 weeks	1000	Superior for positive symptoms
Risperidone	Peuskens et al. (1999)	228	8 weeks	800	Equal
Risperidone	Sechter et al. (2002)	309	6 months	400–1000	Equal
Risperidone	Hwang et al. (2003)	48	6 weeks	400–800	Equal
Olanzapine	Martin et al. (2002)	377	8 weeks	200–800	Equal

did the haloperidol-treated patients. There were also significantly fewer reports of EPS in the sertindole patients (Daniel *et al.*, 1998).

Meta-analyses

A Cochrane review of sertindole versus placebo and other antipsychotics in schizophrenia included only two RCTs, as data on two others were incomplete. The evidence suggested that sertindole was more effective than placebo. Sertindole was associated with fewer EPS than haloperidol, but caused more weight gain. The authors expressed reservations about its use in clinical practice because of cardiac problems that arose in the trials (Lewis *et al.*, 2000).

Amisulpride

Acute-phase trials (Table 3.6)

Amisulpride versus placebo

The efficacy of low doses (50–300 mg/day) of amisulpride versus placebo for negative symptoms has been assessed in three RCTs (Boyer *et al.*, 1995; Paillere-Martinot *et al.*, 1995; Danion *et al.*, 1999). Amisulpride was consistently better than placebo in these studies, and the effect on negative symptoms was apparently unrelated to any changes in positive symptoms (Danion *et al.*, 1999). No controlled studies were found comparing high-dose amisulpride with placebo.

Amisulpride versus conventional antipsychotics

Fixed doses of amisulpride (400, 800, and 1200 mg/day) and haloperidol 16 mg/day were compared with a subtherapeutic dose of amisulpride (100mg/day). Total score reductions were greatest in the groups taking 400 or 800 mg amisulpride/day. Symptoms of parkinsonism did not increase for the amisulpride groups, whereas with haloperidol they did (Puech *et al.*, 1998). In a small flexible-dose study ($n = 41$) both amisulpride or haloperidol groups showed similar symptom reduction, with amisulpride doing significantly better regarding reduction of depressive symptoms. Significantly fewer EPS were recorded in the amisulpride group (Delcker *et al.*, 1990). In another study, amisulpride 800 mg/day was as effective as haloperidol 20 mg/day for positive symptoms, and significantly more effective for negative symptoms. The amisulpride patients exhibited significantly fewer EPS (Moller *et al.*, 1997b).

In a flexible-dose study comparing amisulpride 400–1200 mg/day to haloperidol 10–30 mg/day, overall and positive scores were equally reduced, while negative score reduction and percentage of responders were significantly greater with amisulpride. Haloperidol was associated with a greater incidence of EPS (Carriere *et al.*, 2000). Amisulpride (1000 mg/day) was compared with flupenthixol (25 mg/day) in a fixed-dose RCT. Efficacy results were similar for both drugs, except that amisulpride was significantly better in reducing positive symptoms. There were fewer EPS in the amisulpride group (Wetzel *et al.*, 1998).

Amisulpride versus other atypical antipsychotics

Three studies comparing amisulpride with risperidone, and one with olanzapine, are reported above.

Maintenance studies

Low-dose amisulpride (100 mg/day) and placebo were compared in patients with predominantly negative symptoms over 6 months. Significantly more amisulpride patients completed the study. Dropout rates were 27% with amisulpride and 47% with placebo. The incidence of EPS was similar in both groups (Loo *et al.*, 1997).

Table 3.7 Acute-phase randomized controlled trials for aripiprazole

Comparator	Authors	n	Duration of trial	Dose of aripiprazole (mg/day)	Efficacy (overall, positive and negative symptoms)
Placebo	Kane *et al.* (2002)	414	4 weeks	15 and 30	Both doses superior overall and positive, 30 mg superior negative
Placebo	Potkin *et al.* (2003)	404	4 weeks	20 and 30	Superior
Haloperidol	Kane *et al.* (2002)	414	4 weeks	15 and 30	Equal
Risperidone	Potkin *et al.* (2003)	404	4 weeks	20 and 30	Equal

Meta-analyses

A meta-analysis of 11 RCTs, comparing amisulpiride to conventional antipsychotics, concluded that amisulpiride was more effective than conventional antipsychotics for both global schizophrenic symptoms and negative symptoms. Amisulpiride was associated with significantly lower use of antiparkinsonian medication and fewer dropouts due to adverse events (Leucht *et al.*, 2002). Another meta-analysis specifically assessed the evidence for negative symptom efficacy. The overall analysis reported improvement of negative symptoms that could probably not be accounted for by improvement of positive symptoms, depressive symptoms, or EPS (Storosum *et al.*, 2002). A Cochrane review of 19 randomized studies with a total of 2443 participants found that, compared to typical antipsychotics, amisulpride was more effective in improving global state, and the negative symptoms of schizophrenia. Regarding positive symptoms, amisulpride was as effective as typical antipsychotics. Amisulpride was less prone to cause EPS or to require the use of antiparkinson medication, and also seemed to be more acceptable to patients than conventional drugs (Mota *et al.*, 2002).

Aripiprazole
Acute-phase trials (Table 3.7)
Aripiprazole versus placebo and conventional agents

An RCT comparing aripiprazole 15 and 30 mg/day to placebo and haloperidol 10 mg/day found that both doses of aripiprazole and haloperidol produced significant improvements in total and positive scores. Aripiprazole 15 mg and haloperidol 10 mg significantly improved negative scores. Unlike haloperidol, aripiprazole was not associated with significant EPS or prolactin elevation. There were no significant changes in body weight, and no clinically significant increases in QTc interval (Kane *et al.*, 2002).

In another study, aripiprazole 20 or 30 mg/day and risperidone 6 mg/day were significantly better than placebo on all efficacy measures. There were no significant differences between aripiprazole and placebo in EPS. Mean prolactin levels decreased with aripiprazole but significantly increased five-fold with risperidone. Mean change in QTc interval did not differ significantly from placebo with any active treatment group. Both aripiprazole and risperidone groups showed similar low incidence of weight gain (Potkin *et al.*, 2003).

A pooled analysis reported data from five acute-phase RCTs involving patients treated with aripiprazole ($n = 932$), placebo ($n = 416$), or haloperidol ($n = 201$). Aripiprazole was well tolerated, with similar adverse-event incidence rates to placebo, and lower rates than haloperidol for EPS and somnolence. There was minimal mean weight change with aripiprazole and haloperidol, and no QTc prolongation. Serum prolactin increased with haloperidol, but not with aripiprazole (Marder *et al.*, 2003b).

Maintenance treatment

In a 26-week RCT stable patients received fixed doses of aripiprazole 15 mg, or placebo. Time to relapse was significantly longer for aripiprazole compared with placebo. More patients relapsed with placebo (57%) than aripiprazole (34%). Aripiprazole was significantly superior to placebo from baseline to endpoint in PANSS total and positive scores. Aripiprazole was well tolerated, with no evidence of marked sedation and no evidence of hyperprolactinemia or prolonged QTc. EPS were comparable with placebo. There was a slight mean weight loss at endpoint in both groups (Pigott *et al.*, 2003). The prospectively pooled results of two 52-week RCTs evaluating aripiprazole 30 mg/day versus haloperidol 10 mg/day in 1294 patients were recently reported. Aripiprazole demonstrated efficacy comparable to haloperidol across most symptom measures, and greater improvements for negative and depressive scores. The time to discontinuation was significantly greater with aripiprazole than with haloperidol. Aripiprazole was associated with significantly lower scores than haloperidol on all EPS assessments (Kasper *et al.*, 2003).

Special populations of schizophrenia
Prepsychotic period

An RCT compared low-dose risperidone (mean dose 1.3 mg/day) and cognitive-behavioral therapy (CBT) with need-based intervention in 59 subjects at incipient risk of progression to first-episode psychosis. Both risperidone and CBT reduced the risk of early transition to psychosis (McGorry *et al.*, 2002). Another RCT evaluated the short-term efficacy (8 weeks) of olanzapine 5–15 mg/day versus placebo in 60 patients with prodromal schizophrenia. Results suggest that olanzapine is associated with significantly greater symptom improvement, but also significantly greater weight gain than placebo (Woods *et al.*, 2003).

First-episode schizophrenia

In spite of increasing attention focusing on early intervention, few RCTs have evaluated the efficacy and safety of atypical antipsychotic medications directly in patients with a first episode of psychosis. An international RCT compared flexible doses of risperidone (mean 6.1 mg/day) and haloperidol (mean 5.6 mg/day) over 8 weeks. The two compounds showed similar efficacy, with response rates for risperidone and haloperidol being 63% and 56% respectively. Both groups experienced considerable EPS, although this was significantly lower in the risperidone group. A post-hoc analysis showed that lower doses (<6 mg/day) were efficacious, and associated with far fewer EPS (Emsley, 1999).

A post-hoc analysis was conducted in a subpopulation of patients experiencing their first epsiode of psychosis from a larger RCT (Tollefson *et al.*, 1997). A greater reduction in total, positive, and negative scores, as well as a significantly higher response rate, was found for the olanzapine subjects compared to the haloperidol subjects. Olanzapine-treated patients showed a significant reduction in EPS, while haloperidol-treated patients showed an increase in EPS (Sanger *et al.*, 1999). A large (*n* = 263) prospective RCT compared olanzapine with haloperidol in first-episode psychosis. Twelve-week results reported similar symptom reduction for the two treatments with last-observation-carried-forward analyses, but greater decreases in PANSS total, negative, and general psychopathology scales for olanzapine with a mixed-model analysis. Significantly more olanzapine-treated subjects than haloperidol-treated subjects completed the acute phase of the study. Olanzapine-treated patients experienced a lower rate of treatment-emergent parkinsonism and akathisia but had significantly more weight gain (Lieberman *et al.*, 2003).

What is the best pharmacotherapy approach to resistant schizophrenia?

Clozapine is the most effective treatment in patients with severe refractory schizophrenia and remains the treatment of choice (Kane *et al.*, 1988). However, the benefits of clozapine are limited, and many patients tolerate the drug poorly (Kane *et al.*, 1988). The new atypical antipsychotics have raised expectations in the treatment of patients who are refractory to conventional agents, although studies to date have not been entirely convincing.

Risperidone

An RCT compared risperidone (mean dose 6.4 mg/day) to clozapine (mean dose 291.2 mg/day) over 8 weeks in 86 subjects with chronic schizophrenia who were either resistant or intolerant to conventional antipsychotics. Both drugs were found to be essentially similar, with a more rapid onset of action reported for risperidone. EPS and other adverse events were scarce and mild in both groups (Bondolfi *et al.*, 1998). This study does not represent a purely refractory sample, and has been criticized because the sample was not well defined, the sample size was relatively small, clozapine dosing was relatively low, and the treatment period was possibly too brief (Dunayevich and Chatterjee, 1999; Meltzer, 1999; Rubin, 1999). In a small RCT ($n = 29$) of subjects showing only a partial response to conventional antipsychotics, risperidone (mean 5.9 mg/day) was compared to clozapine (mean 403.6 mg/day) over 6 weeks. Clozapine was superior to risperidone for positive symptoms, while total symptoms, negative symptoms, and depression did not differ between the groups (Breier *et al.*, 1999).

Another RCT compared flexible doses of risperidone and clozapine over 8 weeks in 273 subjects with severe chronic schizophrenia. Improvement in mean Brief Psychiatric Rating Scale, Clinical Global Impression scores, and most of the secondary efficacy measures was significantly greater in the clozapine group (Azorin *et al.*, 2001). An RCT investigated the effects of risperidone versus haloperidol in a severely refractory sample of subjects with schizophrenia. Risperidone was significantly better than haloperidol in reducing overall symptomatology at 4 weeks, but not at endpoint (Wirshing *et al.*, 1999).

Olanzapine

An RCT compared the efficacy of olanzapine (25 mg/day) versus chlorpromazine (1200 mg/day) in treatment-resistant schizophrenia (Conley *et al.*, 1998). No differences in efficacy were demonstrated between the two drugs. Seven percent of the olanzapine-treated patients and none of the chlorpromazine patients met *a priori* criteria for clinical response. There were also no differences in dropout rates. Olanzapine was significantly better tolerated than chlorpromazine. The olanzapine-treated patients had fewer motor and cardiovascular side-effects. No antiparkinsonian drugs were necessary in the olanzapine group.

Quetiapine

An RCT was conducted to assess the efficacy of quetiapine in patients who were partially responsive to conventional antipsychotic treatment. Subjects were randomized to quetiapine 600 mg/day and haloperidol 20 mg/day for 8 weeks. Treatments were equally effective in symptom reduction, while quetiapine patients had a significantly greater response rate (Emsley *et al.*, 2000) and significantly greater reduction of depressive symptoms (Emsley *et al.*, 2003b). The quetiapine-treated patients experienced fewer EPS and had lower serum prolactin levels.

In a recently reported RCT, clozapine, olanzapine, risperidone, and haloperidol were compared in inpatients with chronic schizophrenia who had not responded adequately to other antipsychotic medications. Respective mean endpoint doses for clozapine, olanzapine, risperidone, and haloperidol were 526.6, 30.4, 11.6, and 25.7 mg/day. Compared to haloperidol, there were significant advantages for clozapine and olanzapine regarding overall improvement, and general psychopathology, and for clozapine, risperidone, and olanzapine regarding negative symptoms (Volavka *et al.*, 2002). A review and meta-analysis of 12 studies comparing typical and atypical antipsychotics in subjects with refractory schizophrenia reported that clozapine exhibits superiority over conventional antipsychotics in terms of both efficacy and tolerability. However, the magnitude of the advantage for clozapine was not consistently robust. Efficacy data for other atypical antipsychotics in the treatment of refractory schizophrenia were inconclusive (Chakos *et al.*, 2001).

Conventional versus atypical antipsychotics: the ongoing debate

The most robust difference between the conventional and atypical antipsychotics has been the reduced propensity of the latter to produce EPS. However, it could be argued that this difference is spurious, and may be explained on the basis that the dose of the conventional comparators (usually haloperidol) was too high. In fact, by employing strategies to reduce the EPS risk with conventional antipsychotics, differences between the conventional and atypical agents are less obvious. Three strategies have been adopted to reduce EPS with conventional antipsychotics: (1) the use of low-doses; (2) the addition of prophylactic anticholinergic agents; and (3) the use of low-potency conventional antipsychotics.

First, the use of low doses of haloperidol has been shown to be effective and well tolerated (Oosthuizen *et al.*, 2001), and haloperidol 2 mg/day was at least as effective, with significantly fewer EPS than 8 mg/day in the acute treatment of first-episode schizophrenia (Oosthuizen *et al.*, 2004). Second, the addition of prophylactic benztropine to reduce the risk of EPS with haloperidol in an RCT comparing it with olanzapine reported no significant differences between groups in study retention; positive, negative, or total symptoms of schizophrenia; quality of life; or EPS. While olanzapine showed benefits in reducing akathisia and improving cognition, the authors pointed out that this has to be balanced with the problems of weight gain and higher cost (Rosenheck *et al.*, 2003). Third, a recent meta-analysis of studies comparing atypical antipsychotics to low-potency conventional agents reported that mean doses less than 600 mg/day of chlorpromazine or its equivalent had no higher risk of EPS than atypical antipsychotics (Leucht *et al.*, 2003). However, even when utilizing these strategies, important differences exist between conventional and atypical agents. Thus, even at very low doses conventional agents are associated with some acute EPS (Oosthuizen *et al.*, 2004), and importantly, no reduction in the incidence of tardive dyskinesia (Oosthuizen *et al.*, 2003). Also, studies of conventional versus atypical agents in which more appropriately low doses of haloperidol were used showed significant differences in EPS in favor of the atypical antipsychotics (Emsley, 1999; Hirsch *et al.*, 2002; Lieberman *et al.*, 2003; Marder *et al.*, 2003a; Zimbroff *et al.*, 1997). Finally, although low-potency antipsychotics did not cause more EPS, they were found to be moderately less effective than atypical antipsychotics (Leucht *et al.*, 2003).

A meta-regression analysis of 52 RCTs comparing atypical antipsychotics (clozapine, risperidone, olanzapine, quetiapine, amisulpride, and sertindole) with conventional antipsychotics or alternative atypical antipsychotics found that the dose of conventional antipsychotics was a confounding factor. When compared to ≤6 mg/day haloperidol, atypical antipsychotics had no benefits in terms of efficacy or overall tolerability, although they still caused fewer EPS (Geddes *et al.*, 2000). A recent meta-analysis of RCTs comparing atypical antipsychotics with conventional agents or other atypicals reported that, compared to conventional agents, clozapine, amisulpride, risperidone, and olanzapine had significantly greater effect sizes (0.49, 0.29, 0.25, and 0.21, respectively). Unlike Geddes *et al.* (2000), these authors found no evidence that haloperidol dose affected the results (Davis *et al.*, 2003).

Head-to-head comparisons of atypical antipsychotics

A number of direct comparisons of atypical antipsychotics have now been published, allowing some comparison between these agents (Table 3.8). It can be seen that few, if any, efficacy differences have been demonstrated between these agents. However, side-effect profiles differ considerably.

Focusing on side-effect profiles

As can be seen from the above, to date no conclusive evidence exists for efficacy superiority of any of the atypical antipsychotics other than clozapine. However, the clear-cut differences in side-effect profiles have become a critical focus area for clinicians when choosing an antipsychotic. The most important side-effects to consider are EPS, weight gain, hyperprolactinemia, and cardiotoxicity.

Extrapyramidal symptoms

By definition, atypical antipsychotics are effective at doses below those that would normally cause EPS. However, there are significant intraclass differences in the EPS risk between the atypical antipsychotics. Risperidone and amisulpride, while not differing from placebo at the lower end of their therapeutic range, cause EPS in a dose-dependent manner. On the other hand, clozapine and quetiapine have a very low risk of inducing EPS (Seeman, 2002).

Table 3.8 Head-to-head randomized controlled trials of atypical antipsychotics

	Authors	n	Duration of trial	Efficacy	Tolerability
Risperidone versus olanzapine	Tran et al. (1997b)	339	28 weeks	Olanzapine superior for negative symptoms	Risperidone > EPS, hyperprolactinemia, sexual dysfunction
Risperidone versus olanzapine	Conley and Mahmoud (2001)	377	8 weeks	Similar	Olanzapine > weight gain
Risperidone versus clozapine	Klieser et al. (1995)	59	4 weeks	Similar	Risperidone better tolerated
Risperidone versus amisulpride	Peuskens et al. (1999)	228	8 weeks	Similar	Equal EPS
Risperidone versus amisulpride	Sechter et al. (2002)	309	6 months	Similar	Equal EPS. Risperidone > weight gain, sexual dysfunction
Risperidone versus amisulpride	Hwang et al. (2003)	48	6 weeks	Similar	Equal EPS. Risperidone > weight gain
Olanzapine versus amisulpride	Martin et al. (2002)	377	8 weeks	Similar	Equal EPS. Olanzapine > weight gain
Risperidone versus aripiprazole	Potkin et al. (2003)	404	4 weeks	Similar	Equal EPS. Risperidone > prolactin

EPS, extrapyramidal symptoms.

Weight gain

Whereas the treatment of schizophrenia previously focused mainly on the control of acute psychotic symptoms and strategies to minimize EPS, the substantially increased risk of medical morbidity and mortality in these patients has more recently become an area of attention. It has become apparent that atypical antipsychotics may contribute to this risk. Weight gain has been consistently associated with some of these agents, particularly clozapine and olanzapine. Risperidone appears to be associated with a modest risk, with ziprasidone, amisulpride, and aripiprazole having a low risk of weight gain (Bobes et al., 2003; Nasrallah, 2003). A meta-analysis and random-effects meta-regression that estimated the weight change after 10 weeks of treatment with a standard dose of each of the atypical antipsychotics showed the following mean increases in weight: clozapine, 4.45 kg; olanzapine, 4.15 kg; sertindole, 2.19 kg; risperidone, 2.10 kg and ziprasidone, 0.04 kg (Allison et al., 1999).

The possible metabolic concomitants of obesity, namely diabetes and hyper-triglyceridemia, have raised concern, and psychiatrists are now having to develop a better understanding of these conditions. Clozapine, olanzapine, and possibly risperidone have been significantly associated with glucose intolerance (Hedenmalm *et al.*, 2002; Wirshing *et al.*, 2002) and there appears to be an increased risk of diabetes mellitus in patients receiving atypical antipsychotics (Citrome and Jaffe, 2003). In an RCT conducted over 14 weeks, the effects of clozapine, olanzapine, risperidone, and haloperidol on glucose and cholesterol levels were assessed. Clozapine, olanzapine, and haloperidol were associated with an increase of plasma glucose, and clozapine and olanzapine were associated with an increase in cholesterol levels (Lindenmayer *et al.*, 2003). The combined risk factors of weight gain and elevated blood glucose and triglyceride levels increase the risk for coronary artery disease. For this reason, it has been recommended that routine monitoring of glucose and lipid levels should be undertaken during treatment with atypical antipsychotics (Wirshing *et al.*, 2002).

Hyperprolactinemia

Prolactin secretion is controlled by complex mechanisms, of which dopamine is the principal inhibitory component (Petty, 1999). Hyperprolactinemia may be a concern in the treatment of patients with schizophrenia, although correlations between prolactin elevations and clinical symptoms have not been well established. Elevated levels of prolactin in females cause menstrual disturbances and galactorrhea, are associated with reduced bone density (Sauer and Howard, 2002), have been linked with disturbed sexual function in terms of desire, erection, and orgasm in the male, and may even cause hypogonadism (Wilson, 1993).

Treatment with conventional antipsychotics has a profound effect on prolactin levels, producing increases of around two to three times above normal in most patients (Green and Brown, 1988). The majority of the atypical antipsychotics have much less of an effect on prolactin, although there are considerable differences between compounds. At one end of the spectrum, clozapine and quetiapine produce minimal sustained increases in prolactin levels that are no different from placebo, while olanzapine produces a transient increase in prolactin levels (Hamner, 2002). With risperidone and amisulpiride, the effect is largely dose-dependent, with higher doses causing a marked increase in prolactin levels (Peuskens, 1995; Peuskens *et al.*, 1999). There is evidence that with risperidone, the risk of hyperprolactinemia is even greater than that with conventional antipsychotics (Yasui-Furukori *et al.*, 2002; Kinon *et al.*, 2003). Risperidone has been associated with decreases in bone mineral density in premenopausal females (Becker *et al.*, 2003), as well as high levels of sexual dysfunction (Knegtering *et al.*, 2003).

QT interval prolongation

QTc prolongation by antipsychotic drugs has become a major concern, as it appears to be linked to an increased risk of sudden death (Zareba and Lin, 2003). Among antipsychotics available in the UK, droperidol was withdrawn, sertindole was voluntarily suspended, and restricted labeling was introduced for thioridazine and pimozide. The degree of QTc prolongation is dose-dependent, and varies amongst agents (Haddad and Anderson, 2002). Ziprasidone prolongs QTc to a moderate degree, though to a greater extent than quetiapine, risperidone, olanzapine, and haloperidol (Taylor, 2003).

Arrhythmias are more likely to occur if associated with other risk factors, such as another drug prolonging the QTc interval, electrolyte imbalance, congenital long QT syndromes, heart failure, bradycardia, female sex, restraint, old age, hepatic or renal impairment, and slow metabolizer status (Haddad and Anderson, 2002).

Conclusions

The atypical antipsychotics discussed here are at least as effective as the conventional antipsychotics in the treatment of positive symptoms. Furthermore, there is some evidence of superiority in the treatment of specific symptom domains, particularly negative symptoms (Carman et al., 1995; Moller et al., 1997b), mood symptoms (Tollefson et al., 1998, 1999; Peuskens et al., 2000; Emsley et al., 2003a), and cognitive symptoms (Green et al., 1997; Kern et al., 1998, 1999; Purdon et al., 2000, 2001) as well as advantages in maintaining or enhancing quality of life (Hamilton et al., 1998; Revicki et al., 1999). There is also a small, but growing literature on the pharmacoeconomic advantages of the atypical antipsychotics (Edgell et al., 2000; Revicki, 2000). But the most marked advantage of the atypical antipsychotics is their superiority over traditional antipsychotics in terms of EPS. This is of great importance, since EPS have been shown to be the principal cause of non-adherence to medication (Van Putten, 1974; Hoge et al., 1990). Taken together, there is extensive evidence to support the use of the atypical antipsychotics (excluding clozapine) as first-line treatment agents for schizophrenia. However, it needs to be borne in mind that these agents are not free of side-effects and appropriate caution should be exercised when prescribing them.

Statement of interest

Robin Emsley has participated in speakers/advisory boards and received honoraria from AstraZeneca, Bristol-Myers Squibb, Janssen, Lundbeck, Organon, and

Pfizer. Piet Oosthuizen has participated in speakers/advisory boards and received honoraria from AstraZeneca and Eli-Lilly.

REFERENCES

Allison, D. B., Mentore, J. L., Heo, M., *et al.* (1999). Antipsychotic-induced weight gain: a comprehensive research synthesis. *American Journal of Psychiatry*, **156**, 1686–96.

Arato, M., O'Connor, R., and Meltzer, H. Y. (2002). A 1-year, double-blind, placebo-controlled trial of ziprasidone 40, 80 and 160 mg/day in chronic schizophrenia: the Ziprasidone Extended Use in Schizophrenia (ZEUS) study. *International Clinics in Psychopharmacology*, **17**, 207–15.

Arvanitis, L. A. and Miller, B. G. (1997). Multiple fixed doses of "Seroquel" (quetiapine) in patients with acute exacerbation of schizophrenia: a comparison with haloperidol and placebo. The Seroquel Trial 13 Study Group. *Biological Psychiatry*, **42**, 233–46.

Azorin, J. M., Spiegel, R., Remington, G., *et al.* (2001). A double-blind comparative study of clozapine and risperidone in the management of severe chronic schizophrenia. *American Journal of Psychiatry*, **158**, 1305–13.

Bagnall, A., Lewis, R. A., and Leitner, M. L. (2000). Ziprasidone for schizophrenia and severe mental illness. *Cochrane Database Systematic Review* CD001945. Oxford: Update Software.

Beasley, C. M., Jr., Sanger, T., Satterlee, W., *et al.* (1996a). Olanzapine versus placebo: results of a double-blind, fixed-dose olanzapine trial. *Psychopharmacology (Berlin)*, **124**, 159–67.

Beasley, C. M., Jr., Tollefson, G., Tran, P., *et al.* (1996b). Olanzapine versus placebo and haloperidol: acute phase results of the North American double-blind olanzapine trial. *Neuropsychopharmacology*, **14**, 111–23.

Beasley, C. M., Jr., Hamilton, S. H., Crawford, A. M., *et al.* (1997). Olanzapine versus haloperidol: acute phase results of the international double-blind olanzapine trial. *European Neuropsychopharmacology*, **7**, 125–37.

Becker, D., Liver, O., Mester, R., *et al.* (2003). Risperidone, but not olanzapine, decreases bone mineral density in female postmenopausal schizophrenia patients. *Journal of Clinical Psychiatry*, **64**, 761–6.

Bilder, R. M., Goldman, R. S., Volavka, J., *et al.* (2002). Neurocognitive effects of clozapine, olanzapine, risperidone, and haloperidol in patients with chronic schizophrenia or schizoaffective disorder. *American Journal of Psychiatry*, **159**, 1018–28.

Bobes, J., Rejas, J., Garcia-Garcia, M., *et al.* (2003). Weight gain in patients with schizophrenia treated with risperidone, olanzapine, quetiapine or haloperidol: results of the EIRE study. *Schizophrenia Research*, **62**, 77–88.

Bondolfi, G., Dufour, H., Patris, M., *et al.* (1998). Risperidone versus clozapine in treatment-resistant chronic schizophrenia: a randomized double-blind study. The Risperidone Study Group. *American Journal of Psychiatry*, **155**, 499–504.

Boyer, P., Lecrubier, Y., Puech, A. J., Dewailly, J., and Aubin, F. (1995). Treatment of negative symptoms in schizophrenia with amisulpride. *British Journal of Psychiatry*, **166**, 68–72.

Breier, A. F., Malhotra, A. K., Su, T. P., *et al.* (1999). Clozapine and risperidone in chronic schizophrenia: effects on symptoms, parkinsonian side effects, and neuroendocrine response. *American Journal of Psychiatry*, **156**, 294–8.

Breier, A., Meehan, K., Birkett, M., *et al.* (2002). A double-blind, placebo-controlled dose–response comparison of intramuscular olanzapine and haloperidol in the treatment of acute agitation in schizophrenia. *Archives of General Psychiatry*, **59**, 441–8.

Carman, J., Peuskens, J., and Vangeneugden, A. (1995). Risperidone in the treatment of negative symptoms of schizophrenia: a meta-analysis. *International Clinics in Psychopharmacology*, **10**, 207–13.

Carriere, P., Bonhomme, D., and Lemperiere, T. (2000). Amisulpride has a superior benefit/risk profile to haloperidol in schizophrenia: results of a multicentre, double-blind study (the Amisulpride Study Group). *European Psychiatry*, **15**, 321–9.

Chakos, M., Lieberman, J., Hoffman, E., Bradford, D., and Sheitman, B. (2001). Effectiveness of second-generation antipsychotics in patients with treatment-resistant schizophrenia: a review and meta-analysis of randomized trials. *American Journal of Psychiatry*, **158**, 518–26.

Chouinard, G., Jones, B., Remington, G., *et al.* (1993). A Canadian multicenter placebo-controlled study of fixed doses of risperidone and haloperidol in the treatment of chronic schizophrenic patients. *Journal of Clinical Psychopharmacology*, **13**, 25–40.

Citrome, L. L. and Jaffe, A. B. (2003). Relationship of atypical antipsychotics with development of diabetes mellitus. *Annals of Pharmacotherapy*, **37**, 1849–57.

Conley, R. R. and Mahmoud, R. (2001). A randomized double-blind study of risperidone and olanzapine in the treatment of schizophrenia or schizoaffective disorder. *American Journal of Psychiatry*, **158**, 765–74.

Conley, R. R., Tamminga, C. A., Bartko, J. J., *et al.* (1998). Olanzapine compared with chlorpromazine in treatment-resistant schizophrenia. *American Journal of Psychiatry*, **155**, 914–20.

Copolov, D. L., Link, C. G., and Kowalcyk, B. (2000). A multicentre, double-blind, randomized comparison of quetiapine (ICI 204,636, 'Seroquel') and haloperidol in schizophrenia. *Psychological Medicine*, **30**, 95–105.

Csernansky, J. G., Mahmoud, R., and Brenner, R. (2002). A comparison of risperidone and haloperidol for the prevention of relapse in patients with schizophrenia. *New England Journal of Medicine*, **346**, 16–22.

Daniel, D. G., Wozniak, P., Mack, R. J., and McCarthy, B. G. (1998). Long-term efficacy and safety comparison of sertindole and haloperidol in the treatment of schizophrenia. The Sertindole Study Group. *Psychopharmacology Bulletin*, **34**, 61–9.

Daniel, D. G., Zimbroff, D. L., Potkin, S. G., *et al.* (1999). Ziprasidone 80 mg/day and 160 mg/day in the acute exacerbation of schizophrenia and schizoaffective disorder: a 6-week placebo-controlled trial. Ziprasidone Study Group. *Neuropsychopharmacology*, **20**, 491–505.

Daniel, D. G., Potkin, S. G., Reeves, K. R., Swift, R. H., and Harrigan, E. P. (2001). Intramuscular (IM) ziprasidone 20 mg is effective in reducing acute agitation associated with psychosis: a double-blind, randomised trial. *Psychopharmacology (Berlin)*, **155**, 128–34.

Danion, J. M., Rein, W., and Fleurot, O. (1999). Improvement of schizophrenic patients with primary negative symptoms treated with amisulpride. Amisulpride Study Group. *American Journal of Psychiatry*, **156**, 610–16.

Davies, A., Adena, M. A., Keks, N. A., *et al.* (1998). Risperidone versus haloperidol: I. Meta-analysis of efficacy and safety. *Clinical Therapy*, **20**, 58–71.

Davis, J. M., Chen, N., and Glick, I. D. (2003). A meta-analysis of the efficacy of second-generation antipsychotics. *Archives of General Psychiatry*, **60**, 553–64.

Delcker, A., Schoon, M. L., Oczkowski, B., and Gaertner, H. J. (1990). Amisulpride versus haloperidol in treatment of schizophrenic patients – results of a double-blind study. *Pharmacopsychiatry*, **23**, 125–30.

Dellva, M. A., Tran, P., Tollefson, G. D., Wentley, A. L., and Beasley, C. M., Jr. (1997). Standard olanzapine versus placebo and ineffective-dose olanzapine in the maintenance treatment of schizophrenia. *Psychiatric Services*, **48**, 1571–7.

Duggan, L., Fenton, M., Dardennes, R. M., El Dosoky, A., and Indran, S. (2003). Olanzapine for schizophrenia. *Cochrane Database Systematic Review* CD001359. Oxford: Update Software.

Dunayevich, E. and Chatterjee, A. (1999). Risperidone and clozapine for treatment-resistant schizophrenia (letter). *American Journal of Psychiatry*, **156**, 1127.

Edgell, E. T., Andersen, S. W., Johnstone, B. M., *et al.* (2000). Olanzapine versus risperidone. A prospective comparison of clinical and economic outcomes in schizophrenia. *Pharmacoeconomics*, **18**, 567–79.

Emsley, R. A. (1999). Risperidone in the treatment of first-episode psychotic patients: a double-blind multicenter study. Risperidone Working Group. *Schizophrenia Bulletin*, **25**, 721–9.

Emsley, R. A., Raniwalla, J., Bailey, P. J., and Jones, A. M. (2000). A comparison of the effects of quetiapine ('seroquel') and haloperidol in schizophrenic patients with a history of and a demonstrated, partial response to conventional antipsychotic treatment. PRIZE study group. *International Clinics in Psychopharmacology*, **15**, 121–31.

Emsley, R. A., Buckley, P., Jones, A. M., and Greenwood, M. R. (2003a). Differential effect of quetiapine on depressive symptoms in patients with partially responsive schizophrenia. *Journal of Psychopharmacology*, **17**, 210–15.

Emsley, R. A., Buckley, P., Jones, A. M., and Greenwood, M. R. (2003b). Differential effect of quetiapine on depressive symptoms in patients with partially responsive schizophrenia. *Journal of Psychopharmacology*, **17**, 210–15.

Geddes, J., Freemantle, N., Harrison, P., and Bebbington, P. (2000). Atypical antipsychotics in the treatment of schizophrenia: systematic overview and meta-regression analysis. *British Medical Journal*, **321**, 1371–6.

Goff, D. C., Posever, T., Herz, L., *et al.* (1998). An exploratory haloperidol-controlled dose-finding study of ziprasidone in hospitalized patients with schizophrenia or schizoaffective disorder. *Journal of Clinical Psychopharmacology*, **18**, 296–304.

Green, A. I. and Brown, W. A. (1988). Prolactin and neuroleptic drugs. *Endocrinological and Metabolic Clinics of North America*, **17**, 213–23.

Green, M. F., Marshall, B. D., Jr., Wirshing, W. C., *et al.* (1997). Does risperidone improve verbal working memory in treatment-resistant schizophrenia? *American Journal of Psychiatry*, **154**, 799–804.

Haddad, P. M. and Anderson, I. M. (2002). Antipsychotic-related QTc prolongation, torsade de pointes and sudden death. *Drugs*, **62**, 1649–71.

Hamilton, S. H., Revicki, D. A., Genduso, L. A., and Beasley, C. M., Jr. (1998). Olanzapine versus placebo and haloperidol: quality of life and efficacy results of the North American double-blind trial. *Neuropsychopharmacology*, **18**, 41–9.

Hamner, M. (2002). The effects of atypical antipsychotics on serum prolactin levels. *Annals of Clinical Psychiatry*, **14**, 163–73.

Hedenmalm, K., Hagg, S., Stahl, M., Mortimer, O., and Spigset, O. (2002). Glucose intolerance with atypical antipsychotics. *Drug Safety*, **25**, 1107–16.

Hirsch, S. R., Kissling, W., Bauml, J., Power, A., and O'Connor, R. (2002). A 28-week comparison of ziprasidone and haloperidol in outpatients with stable schizophrenia. *Journal of Clinical Psychiatry*, **63**, 516–23.

Hoge, S. K., Appelbaum, P. S., Lawlor, T., *et al.* (1990). A prospective, multicenter study of patients' refusal of antipsychotic medication. *Archives of General Psychiatry*, **47**, 949–56.

Hunter, R. H., Joy, C. B., Kennedy, E., Gilbody, S. M., and Song, F. (2003). Risperidone versus typical antipsychotic medication for schizophrenia. *Cochrane Database Systematic Review* CD000440. Oxford: Update Software.

Huttunen, M. O., Piepponen, T., Rantanen, H., *et al.* (1995). Risperidone versus zuclopenthixol in the treatment of acute schizophrenic episodes: a double-blind parallel-group trial. *Acta Psychiatrica Scandinavica*, **91**, 271–7.

Hwang, T. J., Lee, S. M., Sun, H. J., *et al.* (2003). Amisulpride versus risperidone in the treatment of schizophrenic patients: a double-blind pilot study in Taiwan. *Journal of the Formosan Medical Association*, **102**, 30–6.

Ishigooka, J., Inada, T., and Miura, S. (2001). Olanzapine versus haloperidol in the treatment of patients with chronic schizophrenia: results of the Japan multicenter, double-blind olanzapine trial. *Psychiatry Clinics of Neuroscience*, **55**, 403–14.

Joy, C. B., Adams, C. E., and Lawrie, S. M. (2001). Haloperidol versus placebo for schizophrenia. *Cochrane Database Systematic Review* CD003082. Oxford: Update Software.

Kane, J., Honigfeld, G., Singer, J., and Meltzer, H. (1988). Clozapine for the treatment-resistant schizophrenic. A double-blind comparison with chlorpromazine. *Archives of General Psychiatry*, **45**, 789–96.

Kane, J. M., Carson, W. H., Saha, A. R., *et al.* (2002). Efficacy and safety of aripiprazole and haloperidol versus placebo in patients with schizophrenia and schizoaffective disorder. *Journal of Clinical Psychiatry*, **63**, 763–71.

Kane, J. M., Eerdekens, M., Lindenmayer, J. P., *et al.* (2003). Long-acting injectable risperidone: efficacy and safety of the first long-acting atypical antipsychotic. *American Journal of Psychiatry*, **160**, 1125–32.

Kasper, S., Lerman, M. N., McQuade, R. D., *et al.* (2003). Efficacy and safety of aripiprazole vs. haloperidol for long-term maintenance treatment following acute relapse of schizophrenia. *International Journal of Neuropsychopharmacology*, **6**, 325–37.

Keck, P., Jr., Buffenstein, A., Ferguson, J., *et al.* (1998). Ziprasidone 40 and 120 mg/day in the acute exacerbation of schizophrenia and schizoaffective disorder: a 4-week placebo-controlled trial. *Psychopharmacology (Berlin)*, **140**, 173–84.

Kern, R. S., Green, M. F., Marshall, B. D., Jr., *et al.* (1998). Risperidone vs. haloperidol on reaction time, manual dexterity, and motor learning in treatment-resistant schizophrenia patients. *Biological Psychiatry*, **44**, 726–32.

Kern, R. S., Green, M. F., Marshall, B. D., Jr., *et al.* (1999). Risperidone versus haloperidol on secondary memory: can newer medications aid learning? *Schizophrenia Bulletin*, **25**, 223–32.

Kinon, B. J., Gilmore, J. A., Liu, H., and Halbreich, U. M. (2003). Prevalence of hyperprolactinemia in schizophrenic patients treated with conventional antipsychotic medications or risperidone. *Psychoneuroendocrinology*, **28** (suppl. 2), 55–68.

Klieser, E., Lehmann, E., Kinzler, E., Wurthmann, C., and Heinrich, K. (1995). Randomized, double-blind, controlled trial of risperidone versus clozapine in patients with chronic schizophrenia. *Journal of Clinical Psychopharmacology*, **15**, 45S–51S.

Knegtering, H., van der Moolen, A. E., Castelein, S., Kluiter, H., and van den Bosch, R. J. (2003). What are the effects of antipsychotics on sexual dysfunctions and endocrine functioning? *Psychoneuroendocrinology*, **28** (suppl. 2), 109–23.

Laughren, T. P. (2001). The scientific and ethical basis for placebo-controlled trials in depression and schizophrenia: an FDA perspective. *European Psychiatry*, **16**, 418–23.

Lesem, M. D., Zajecka, J. M., Swift, R. H., Reeves, K. R., and Harrigan, E. P. (2001). Intramuscular ziprasidone, 2 mg versus 10 mg, in the short-term management of agitated psychotic patients. *Journal of Clinical Psychiatry*, **62**, 12–18.

Leucht, S., Pitschel-Walz, G., Engel, R. R., and Kissling, W. (2002). Amisulpride, an unusual "atypical" antipsychotic: a meta-analysis of randomized controlled trials. *American Journal of Psychiatry*, **159**, 180–90.

Leucht, S., Wahlbeck, K., Hamann, J., and Kissling, W. (2003). New generation antipsychotics versus low-potency conventional antipsychotics: a systematic review and meta-analysis. *Lancet*, **361**, 1581–9.

Lewis, R., Bagnall, A., and Leitner, M. (2000). Sertindole for schizophrenia. *Cochrane Database Systematic Review* CD001715. Oxford: Update Software.

Lieberman, J. A., Tollefson, G., Tohen, M., *et al.* (2003). Comparative efficacy and safety of atypical and conventional antipsychotic drugs in first-episode psychosis: a randomized, double-blind trial of olanzapine versus haloperidol. *American Journal of Psychiatry*, **160**, 1396–404.

Lindenmayer, J. P., Czobor, P., Volavka, J., *et al.* (2003). Changes in glucose and cholesterol levels in patients with schizophrenia treated with typical or atypical antipsychotics. *American Journal of Psychiatry*, **160**, 290–6.

Loo, H., Poirier-Littre, M. F., Theron, M., Rein, W., and Fleurot, O. (1997). Amisulpride versus placebo in the medium-term treatment of the negative symptoms of schizophrenia. *British Journal of Psychiatry*, **170**, 18–22.

Marder, S. R. and Meibach, R. C. (1994). Risperidone in the treatment of schizophrenia. *American Journal of Psychiatry*, **151**, 825–35.

Marder, S. R., Glynn, S. M., Wirshing, W. C., *et al.* (2003a). Maintenance treatment of schizophrenia with risperidone or haloperidol: 2-year outcomes. *American Journal of Psychiatry*, **160**, 1405–12.

Marder, S. R., McQuade, R. D., Stock, E., *et al.* (2003b). Aripiprazole in the treatment of schizophrenia: safety and tolerability in short-term, placebo-controlled trials. *Schizophrenia Research*, **61**, 123–36.

Martin, S., Ljo, H., Peuskens, J., *et al.* (2002). A double-blind, randomised comparative trial of amisulpride versus olanzapine in the treatment of schizophrenia: short-term results at two months. *Current Medical Research Opinion*, **18**, 355–62.

McGorry, P. D., Yung, A. R., Phillips, L. J., *et al.* (2002). Randomized controlled trial of interventions designed to reduce the risk of progression to first-episode psychosis in a clinical sample with subthreshold symptoms. *Archives of General Psychiatry*, **59**, 921–8.

Meltzer, H. Y. (1999). Risperidone and clozapine for treatment-resistant schizophrenia. *American Journal of Psychiatry*, **156**, 1126–7.

Min, S. K., Rhee, C. S., Kim, C. E., and Kang, D. Y. (1993). Risperidone versus haloperidol in the treatment of chronic schizophrenic patients: a parallel group double-blind comparative trial. *Yonsei Medical Journal*, **34**, 179–90.

Moller, H. J., Bauml, J., Ferrero, F., *et al.* (1997a). Risperidone in the treatment of schizophrenia: results of a study of patients from Germany, Austria, and Switzerland. *European Archives of Psychiatry and Clinical Neuroscience*, **247**, 291–6.

Moller, H. J., Boyer, P., Fleurot, O., and Rein, W. (1997b). Improvement of acute exacerbations of schizophrenia with amisulpride: a comparison with haloperidol. PROD-ASLP study group. *Psychopharmacology (Berlin)*, **132**, 396–401.

Mota, N. E., Lima, M. S., and Soares, B. G. (2002). Amisulpride for schizophrenia. *Cochrane Database Systematic Review* CD001357. Oxford: Update Software.

Nasrallah, H. (2003). A review of the effect of atypical antipsychotics on weight. *Psychoneuroendocrinology*, **28** (suppl. 1), 83–96.

Oosthuizen, P., Emsley, R. A., Turner, J., and Keyter, N. (2001). Determining the optimal dose of haloperidol in first-episode psychosis. *Journal of Psychopharmacology*, **15**, 251–5.

Oosthuizen, P., Emsley, R., Maritz, J., Turner, J., and Keyter, N. (2003). Incidence of tardive dyskinesia in first-episode psychosis treated with low-dose haloperidol. *Journal of Clinical Psychiatry*, **64**, 1075–80.

Oosthuizen, P., Emsley, R., Turner, J., and Keyter, N. (2004). A randomized, controlled comparison of the efficacy and tolerability of low and high dose haloperidol in the treatment of first-episode psychosis. *International Journal of Neuropsychopharmacology*, **7**, 125–32.

Paillere-Martinot, M. L., Lecrubier, Y., Martinot, J. L., and Aubin, F. (1995). Improvement of some schizophrenic deficit symptoms with low doses of amisulpride. *American Journal of Psychiatry*, **152**, 130–4.

Petty, R. G. (1999). Prolactin and antipsychotic medications: mechanism of action. *Schizophrenia Research*, **35**, S67–73.

Peuskens, J. (1995). Risperidone in the treatment of patients with chronic schizophrenia: a multinational, multi-centre, double-blind, parallel-group study versus haloperidol. Risperidone study group. *British Journal of Psychiatry*, **166**, 712–26.

Peuskens, J. and Link, C. G. (1997). A comparison of quetiapine and chlorpromazine in the treatment of schizophrenia. *Acta Psychiatrica Scandinavica*, **96**, 265–73.

Peuskens, J., Bech, P., Moller, H. J., *et al.* (1999). Amisulpride vs. risperidone in the treatment of acute exacerbations of schizophrenia. Amisulpride study group. *Psychiatry Research*, **88**, 107–17.

Peuskens, J., van Baelen, B., De Smedt, C., and Lemmens, P. (2000). Effects of risperidone on affective symptoms in patients with schizophrenia. *International Clinical Psychopharmacology*, **15**, 343–9.

Pigott, T. A., Carson, W. H., Saha, A. R., *et al.* (2003). Aripiprazole for the prevention of relapse in stabilized patients with chronic schizophrenia: a placebo-controlled 26-week study. *Journal of Clinical Psychiatry*, **64**, 1048–56.

Potkin, S. G., Saha, A. R., Kujawa, M. J., *et al.* (2003). Aripiprazole, an antipsychotic with a novel mechanism of action, and risperidone vs placebo in patients with schizophrenia and schizoaffective disorder. *Archives of General Psychiatry*, **60**, 681–90.

Puech, A., Fleurot, O., and Rein, W. (1998). Amisulpride, and atypical antipsychotic, in the treatment of acute episodes of schizophrenia: a dose-ranging study vs. haloperidol. The amisulpride study group. *Acta Psychiatrica Scandinavica*, **98**, 65–72.

Purdon, S. E., Jones, B. D., Stip, E., *et al.* (2000). Neuropsychological change in early phase schizophrenia during 12 months of treatment with olanzapine, risperidone, or haloperidol. The Canadian collaborative group for research in schizophrenia. *Archives of General Psychiatry*, **57**, 249–58.

Purdon, S. E., Malla, A., LaBelle, A., and Lit, W. (2001). Neuropsychological change in patients with schizophrenia after treatment with quetiapine or haloperidol. *Journal of Psychiatry and Neuroscience*, **26**, 137–49.

Rabinowitz, J. and Davidson, M. (2001). Risperidone versus haloperidol in long-term hospitalized chronic patients in a double blind randomized trial: a post hoc analysis. *Schizophrenia Research*, **50**, 89–93.

Rabinowitz, J., Hornik, T., and Davidson, M. (2001). Rapid onset of therapeutic effect of risperidone versus haloperidol in a double-blind randomized trial. *Journal of Clinical Psychiatry*, **62**, 343–6.

Revicki, D. A. (2000). The new atypical antipsychotics: a review of pharmacoeconomic studies. *Expert Opinion in Pharmacotherapy*, **1**, 249–60.

Revicki, D. A., Genduso, L. A., Hamilton, S. H., Ganoczy, D., and Beasley, C. M., Jr. (1999). Olanzapine versus haloperidol in the treatment of schizophrenia and other psychotic disorders: quality of life and clinical outcomes of a randomized clinical trial. *Quality of Life Research*, **8**, 417–26.

Rosenheck, R., Perlick, D., Bingham, S., *et al.* (2003). Effectiveness and cost of olanzapine and haloperidol in the treatment of schizophrenia. A randomised controlled trial. *Journal of the American Medical Association*, **290**, 2693–702.

Rubin, E. (1999). Risperidone and clozapine for treatment-resistant schizophrenia (letter). *American Journal of Psychiatry*, **156**, 1127.

Sanger, T. M., Lieberman, J. A., Tohen, M., *et al.* (1999). Olanzapine versus haloperidol treatment in first-episode psychosis. *American Journal of Psychiatry*, **156**, 79–87.

Sauer, J. and Howard, R. (2002). The beef with atypical antipsychotics. *American Journal of Psychiatry*, **159**, 1249.

Sechter, D., Peuskens, J., Fleurot, O., *et al.* (2002). Amisulpride versus risperidone in chronic schizophrenia: results of a 6-month double-blind study. *Neuropsychopharmacology*, **27**, 1071–81.

Seeman, P. (2002). Atypical antipsychotics: mechanism of action. *Canadian Journal of Psychiatry*, **47**, 27–38.

Small, J. G., Hirsch, S. R., Arvanitis, L. A., Miller, B. G., and Link, C. G. (1997). Quetiapine in patients with schizophrenia. A high- and low-dose double-blind comparison with placebo. Seroquel study group. *Archives of General Psychiatry*, **54**, 549–57.

Song, F. (1997). Risperidone in the treatment of schizophrenia: a meta-analysis of randomized controlled trials. *Journal of Psychopharmacology*, **11**, 65–71.

Srisurapanont, M., Disayavanish, C., and Taimkaew, K. (2000). Quetiapine for schizophrenia. *Cochrane Database Systematic Review* CD000967. Oxford: Update Software.

Storosum, J. G., Elferink, A. J., van Zwieten, B. J., *et al.* (2002). Amisulpride: is there a treatment for negative symptoms in schizophrenia patients? *Schizophrenia Bulletin*, **28**, 193–201.

Taylor, D. (2003). Ziprasidone in the management of schizophrenia: the QT interval issue in context. *CNS Drugs*, **17**, 423–30.

Tollefson, G. D., Beasley, C. M., Jr., Tran, P. V., *et al.* (1997). Olanzapine versus haloperidol in the treatment of schizophrenia and schizoaffective and schizophreniform disorders: results of an international collaborative trial. *American Journal of Psychiatry*, **154**, 457–65.

Tollefson, G. D., Sanger, T. M., Lu, Y., and Thieme, M. E. (1998). Depressive signs and symptoms in schizophrenia: a prospective blinded trial of olanzapine and haloperidol. *Archives of General Psychiatry*, **55**, 250–8.

Tollefson, G. D., Andersen, S. W., and Tran, P. V. (1999). The course of depressive symptoms in predicting relapse in schizophrenia: a double-blind, randomized comparison of olanzapine and risperidone. *Biological Psychiatry*, **46**, 365–73.

Tran, P. V., Dellva, M. A., Tollefson, G. D., *et al.* (1997a). Extrapyramidal symptoms and tolerability of olanzapine versus haloperidol in the acute treatment of schizophrenia. *Journal of Clinical Psychiatry*, **58**, 205–11.

Tran, P. V., Hamilton, S. H., Kuntz, A. J., *et al.* (1997b). Double-blind comparison of olanzapine versus risperidone in the treatment of schizophrenia and other psychotic disorders. *Journal of Clinical Psychopharmacology*, **17**, 407–18.

Tran, P. V., Dellva, M. A., Tollefson, G. D., Wentley, A. L., and Beasley, C. M., Jr. (1998). Oral olanzapine versus oral haloperidol in the maintenance treatment of schizophrenia and related psychoses. *British Journal of Psychiatry*, **172**, 499–505.

van Kammen, D. P., McEvoy, J. P., Targum, S. D., Kardatzke, D., and Sebree, T. B. (1996). A randomized, controlled, dose-ranging trial of sertindole in patients with schizophrenia. *Psychopharmacology (Berlin)*, **124**, 168–75.

Van Putten, T. (1974). Why do schizophrenic patients refuse to take their drugs? *Archives of General Psychiatry*, **31**, 67–72.

Volavka, J., Czobor, P., Sheitman, B., *et al.* (2002). Clozapine, olanzapine, risperidone, and haloperidol in the treatment of patients with chronic schizophrenia and schizoaffective disorder. *American Journal of Psychiatry*, **159**, 255–62.

Wetzel, H., Grunder, G., Hillert, A., *et al.* (1998). Amisulpride versus flupentixol in schizophrenia with predominantly positive symptomatology – a double-blind controlled study comparing a selective D2-like antagonist to a mixed D1-/D2-like antagonist. The amisulpride study group. *Psychopharmacology (Berlin)*, **137**, 223–32.

Wilson, C. A. (1993). Pharmacological targets for the control of male and female sexual behaviour. In: *Sexual Pharmacology*, ed. Riley, A. J., Peet, M., Wilson, C. Oxford: Oxford Medical Publications, pp. 1–58.

Wirshing, D. A., Marshall, B. D., Jr., Green, M. F., *et al.* (1999). Risperidone in treatment-refractory schizophrenia. *American Journal of Psychiatry*, **156**, 1374–9.

Wirshing, D. A., Boyd, J. A., Meng, L. R., *et al.* (2002). The effects of novel antipsychotics on glucose and lipid levels. *Journal of Clinical Psychiatry*, **63**, 856–65.

Woods, S. W., Breier, A., Zipursky, R., *et al.* (2003). Randomised trial of olanzapine versus placebo in the symptomatic acute treatment of the schizophrenic prodrome. *Biological Psychiatry*, **54**, 453–64.

Wright, P., Birkett, M., David, S. R., *et al.* (2001). Double-blind, placebo-controlled comparison of intramuscular olanzapine and intramuscular haloperidol in the treatment of acute agitation in schizophrenia. *American Journal of Psychiatry*, **158**, 1149–51.

Wyatt, R. J., Damiani, L. M., and Henter, I. D. (1998). First-episode schizophrenia. Early intervention and medication discontinuation in the context of course and treatment. *British Journal of Psychiatry*, **172** (suppl.), 77–83.

Yasui-Furukori, N., Kondo, T., Suzuki, A., Mihara, K., and Kaneko, S. (2002). Comparison of prolactin concentrations between haloperidol and risperidone treatments in the same female patients with schizophrenia. *Psychopharmacology (Berlin)*, **162**, 63–6.

Zareba, W. and Lin, D. A. (2003). Antipsychotic drugs and QT interval prolongation. *Psychiatry Quarterly*, **74**, 291–306.

Zimbroff, D. L., Kane, J. M., Tamminga, C. A., *et al.* (1997). Controlled, dose–response study of sertindole and haloperidol in the treatment of schizophrenia. Sertindole study group. *American Journal of Psychiatry*, **154**, 782–91.

4

Evidence-based pharmacotherapy of generalized anxiety disorder

David S. Baldwin[1] and Claire Polkinghorn[2]

[1] University of Southampton, UK
[2] Royal South Hants Hospital, West Hampshire NHS Trust, Southampton, UK

Generalized anxiety disorder (GAD) is a common, typically chronic, and disabling mental disorder associated with substantial medical and psychiatric comorbidity and occupational impairment. It is characterized by inappropriate or excessive anxiety and worrying that persist over time and are not restricted to a particular set of circumstances. Common features include apprehension, with worries about future misfortune; inner tension and difficulty in concentrating; motor tension, with restlessness, tremor, and headache; and autonomic anxiety symptoms, with excessive perspiration, dry mouth, and epigastric discomfort. The last decade has seen major increases in understanding of the epidemiology and neurobiology of the condition, together with development and widespread availability of a range of treatment approaches.

The lifetime prevalence of GAD in the general population is around 5–6%, the 12-month prevalence varying according to diagnostic criteria – from 1.5% with *Diagnostic and Statistical Manual*, 4th edition (DSM-IV) to 3.1% with DSM-III-R criteria (Wittchen, 2002). The age of onset of GAD differs from that with other anxiety disorders: most cases present aged between 35 and 45 years (Wittchen *et al.*, 2000; Yonkers *et al.*, 2000; Carter *et al.*, 2001). It is probably the most common anxiety disorder among the older population (55–85 years) (Beekman *et al.*, 1998). Typically, symptoms fluctuate in intensity over time, but GAD is usually a chronic condition (Weiller *et al.*, 1998). The functional impairment associated with GAD is similar in severity to that seen with major depression (Kessler *et al.*, 1999; Wittchen *et al.*, 2000).

GAD is amongst the most common mental disorders seen in primary care. The point prevalence (defined according to *International Classification of Disease* (ICD-10) criteria) in European primary care settings was 4.8% for GAD without comorbid depressive or anxiety disorders, and 3.7% for GAD with depression: a further 4.1% had "sub-threshold" GAD (Weiller *et al.*, 1998). Comorbid GAD is associated with more severe symptoms, greater functional impairment, a more prolonged course, and decreased productivity (Weiller *et al.*, 1998; Kessler *et al.*, 1999) and higher use of health services (Greenberg *et al.*, 1999; Maier and Falkai, 1999). Comorbid depressive symptoms are associated with an improved chance of a patient being recognized as having a psychological problem, though not necessarily as having GAD (Weiller *et al.*, 1998).

The pathophysiology of GAD is uncertain, but disturbances in neurotransmission of serotonin (5-hydroxytryptamine, 5-HT), norepinephrine (noradrenaline), gamma-aminobutyric acid (GABA), cholecystokinin, and corticotropin-releasing factor may all be important. Serotonin is integrally involved in the mediation of anxiety, through serotonergic innervation of the limbic system, hypothalamus, and thalamus. Levels of the serotonin metabolite 5-hydroxyindoleacetic acid in cerebrospinal fluid in patients with GAD are low, and anxiety symptoms may be worsened by administration of the $5\text{-HT}_1/5\text{-HT}_2$-receptor agonist, *m*-chlorophenylpiperazine. In addition, patients with GAD show a reduction in binding of the selective serotonin reuptake inhibitor (SSRI) paroxetine to platelets (Connor and Davidson, 1998).

Disturbances of the noradrenergic system may also be important. The α_2-adrenoceptor antagonist yohimbine increases noradrenergic cell firing and induces anxiety, whereas the α_2-adrenoceptor agonist clonidine reduces firing rates and inhibits anxiety. In GAD patients, challenge with yohimbine is associated with a blunting of the increase in plasma 3-methoxy-4-hydroxyphenylglycol, compared to that seen in healthy controls (Charney *et al.*, 1989). In addition, ^{3}H-yohimbine binding to platelets is reduced, compared to controls or patients with major depression (Sevy *et al.*, 1989).

The GABA/benzodiazepine receptor system also appears implicated in the pathophysiology of GAD. Untreated patients have a reduced number of benzodiazepine binding sites on platelet membranes; the number increases after diazepam treatment (Weizman *et al.*, 1987); an investigation of lymphocyte membrane benzodiazepine binding sites has produced similar findings (Rocca *et al.*, 1991). The reduction in binding sites may explain the reduction in saccadic eye movement velocity seen in GAD, as this velocity has been used as a marker of functional integrity of the GABA/benzodiazepine system (Connor and Davidson, 1998).

The best evidence for a role of disturbances in these neurotransmitter systems in the pathophysiology of GAD comes from randomized placebo-controlled treatment studies involving certain SSRIs, the serotonin-(norepinephrine) reuptake inhibitor (SNRI) venlafaxine, certain benzodiazepine anxiolytics, and the novel anxiolytic pregabalin. The results of these studies are reviewed below, the focus being on addressing three fundamental questions:

1. What is the first-line treatment for GAD?
2. How long should treatment continue?
3. What is the best intervention after non-response to first-line and second-line treatments?

We conducted a computerized literature search of electronic databases (MEDLINE, Embase, and PsychInfo) for the years 1980–2003 using a strategy which combined the terms "generalised/generalized anxiety disorder" with "randomised/randomized controlled trial". In addition, we consulted with colleagues about other potential treatment studies, not identified by the search; examined published systematic reviews in the Cochrane Collaboration database; and attempted to identify recently completed treatment studies, currently only available as scientific conference abstracts.

What is the first-line pharmacotherapy of GAD?

Summary of published clinical trials of SSRIs and venlafaxine

Citalopram

No randomized controlled trials with citalopram in GAD have been published. A randomized controlled trial comparing two dose ranges of citalopram and imipramine in 472 primary care depressed patients found that the treatments were associated with a similar reduction in mean score on the Hamilton Rating Scale for Depression (HAM-D) (Hamilton, 1967) anxiety factor (Rosenberg *et al.*, 1994). Another study comparing citalopram and paroxetine in 104 patients with either DSM-IV major depression or mixed anxiety–depressive disorder (Jefferson and Greist, 2000) found that both treatments were associated with significant reductions in total score on the Hamilton Rating Scale for Anxiety (HAM-A) (Hamilton, 1959). By contrast, the results of a 24-week double-blind placebo-controlled treatment study comparing citalopram and sertraline in 323 patients with DSM-IV major depressive disorder indicate that citalopram, but not sertraline, was significantly more efficacious than placebo in reducing the mean score on the HAM-D anxiety cluster ($P < 0.01$) (Stahl, 2000).

Escitalopram

Citalopram is a racemic mixture of two enantiomers, of which only the S-isomer (escitalopram) has significant serotonin reuptake inhibitory properties (Hyttel *et al.*, 1992). Escitalopram is more selective and more potent than citalopram, and has been found to be significantly more efficacious than citalopram on some measures in a pooled analysis of randomized controlled trials in patients with major depressive disorder (Gorman *et al.*, 2002). The results of three 8-week randomized double-blind placebo-controlled parallel-group trials in patients with

DSM-IV GAD all indicate that escitalopram is significantly more efficacious than placebo, in reducing anxiety symptoms as measured by the HAM-A (Davidson *et al.*, 2002). Further investigations of the efficacy of fixed doses of escitalopram and paroxetine and of escitalopram in the prevention of relapse are currently underway.

Fluoxetine

There are no published controlled treatment studies in adults with DSM-IV GAD. An open pilot treatment study in 16 children and adolescents (aged between 9 and 18 years) with mixed anxiety disorders showed that fluoxetine was of only limited benefit (Fairbanks *et al.*, 1997). Double-blind treatment studies in depressed patients have indicated that fluoxetine is as efficacious as imipramine, clomipramine, or amitriptyline in relieving anxiety symptoms in depression, but the efficacy of fluoxetine in patients with comorbid depression and GAD is not proven (Hurst and Lamb, 2000).

Fluvoxamine

The efficacy of fluvoxamine as a treatment for GAD is not established. A small ($n = 30$) open study in patients with comorbid major depression and GAD showed that fluvoxamine treatment was associated with significant improvement in both anxiety and depressive symptoms (Sonawalla *et al.*, 1999), but this result needs to be replicated in patients with GAD before the efficacy of fluvoxamine in that disorder can be assumed.

Paroxetine

The efficacy of paroxetine in the short-term treatment of patients with GAD has been evaluated in four randomized double-blind placebo-controlled studies (Baldwin, 2001). The first evaluation was an 8-week comparator-controlled trial involving 81 patients with a DSM-IV diagnosis of GAD, in which paroxetine was compared to imipramine and the benzodiazepine 2'-chlorodesmethyl-diazepam. Paroxetine was superior to 2'-chlorodesmethyldiazepam and had similar efficacy to imipramine: in addition, paroxetine treatment differed significantly ($P < 0.05$) from 2'-chlorodesmethyl-diazepam from week 4 onwards, while imipramine only did so at the end of the study (Rocca *et al.*, 1997).

The second investigation was an 8-week, fixed-dose study involving 566 patients, performed in the USA (Rickels *et al.*, 2003). Paroxetine treatment (20 or 40 mg/day) was significantly superior to placebo ($P < 0.001$) in reducing both the mean HAM-A total score, and the mean scores on HAM-A items 1 (anxious mood) and 2 (tension), considered by some to reflect the most important symptoms of GAD. There was no dose–response relationship in the mean change in HAM-A scores, but overall response rates were 68% and 81% with paroxetine 20 and 40 mg/day respectively, compared with 52% of patients in the placebo group ($P < 0.001$). By the end of the study, the mean change from baseline on a health-related quality-of-life questionnaire (EuroQoL-5D) and visual analog scale was significantly greater for both paroxetine-treatment groups, indicating a significant improvement in quality of life.

The third randomized controlled trial was an 8-week, flexible-dose study conducted in 326 US patients with GAD. Paroxetine (20–50 mg/day) was significantly superior to placebo ($P < 0.05$) in reducing both the mean HAM-A total score and the mean scores on HAM-A items 1 and 2, and was generally well tolerated (Pollack *et al.*, 2001). A fourth study of similar design conducted in 372 patients in Europe has revealed similar reductions in HAM-A total score and HAM-A items 1 and 2.

The effects of paroxetine treatment appear to extend beyond simple symptom reduction or improved quality of life. A small ($n = 29$) uncontrolled study showed that paroxetine treatment was associated with a reduction in maladaptive personality traits, with significant decreases in harm avoidance ($P = 0.0001$) and novelty seeking ($P = 0.006$), and a significant increase in self-directedness ($P = 0.0004$) (Allgulander *et al.*, 1998). The placebo-controlled paroxetine treatment studies also show that as symptoms of GAD resolve there is an associated improvement in symptom-related disability, assessed using the patient-rated Sheehan Disability Scale (SDS) (Sheehan *et al.*, 1996), which covers symptom-related impairment in social, work, and family life. At endpoint in all three studies, there was a statistically significant difference between paroxetine and placebo in the SDS total score (flexible-dose study 1 difference = −1.8, $P = 0.037$; study 2 difference = −2.4, $P = 0.001$; fixed-dose study for 20 mg/day regimen, difference = −3.1, $P < 0.001$; for 40 mg/day regimen, difference = −3.6, $P < 0.001$) (Baldwin *et al.*, 2002).

Sertraline

Double-blind treatment studies indicate that sertraline is efficacious in relieving anxiety symptoms within depression and the symptoms and impairment associated with panic disorder, social phobia, posttraumatic disorder, and obsessive-compulsive disorder. The efficacy of sertraline in adult patients with GAD has been examined only recently, although a small ($n = 22$) randomized placebo-controlled 12-week trial in children and adolescents aged 5–16 years found significant advantages for sertraline over placebo on both the HAM-A and Clinical Global Impression (CGI) scales (Rynn *et al.*, 2001).

A preliminary report of a randomized placebo-controlled parallel-group flexible-dose (50–150 mg/day, mean dose 95.1 mg) 12-week study in 370 patients with

DSM-IV GAD found that sertraline was significantly more efficacious than placebo across a variety of measures, including the HAM-A and CGI (Morris *et al.*, 2003). The reduction in mean HAM-A score between baseline and endpoint was 11.7 with sertraline, compared to 8.0 with placebo; furthermore, 37% of sertraline-treated patients entered symptomatic remission (defined as a HAM-A score of 7 or less), compared to 23.0% with placebo (Sjodin *et al.*, 2003).

Venlafaxine

A preliminary study (Feighner *et al.*, 1998) in depressed outpatients indicated that once-daily treatment with the SNRI venlafaxine was efficacious in relieving anxiety symptoms, and suggested it might therefore have a role in the management of patients with GAD. The evidence for the efficacy of venlafaxine in the short-term and long-term treatment of GAD is now based upon the results of five randomized placebo-controlled trials, two of which involved an active comparator (diazepam or buspirone).

Pooled analysis of these five placebo-controlled trials, which includes 1839 patients with a DSM-IV diagnosis of GAD, provides good evidence for venlafaxine in short-term treatment. In these studies, the effect size for venlafaxine (i.e., difference from placebo in mean HAM-A score at study endpoint) ranges between 1.6 and 4.2, with a mean effect size from the pooled data of 2.78 (Gorman, 2002). In a further analysis, which examined the effects of age on treatment response, venlafaxine was superior to placebo in both younger ($P < 0.001$) and older ($P < 0.01$) subgroups of patients (Katz *et al.*, 2002).

In the first comparator-controlled study, which included 564 patients, there was no significant advantage for either active treatment (venlafaxine XL 75 mg/day, or diazepam 15 mg/day) over placebo in the intention-to-treat last observation carried-forward analysis. However, in a second analysis, which omitted those study centers that had been unable to distinguish diazepam from placebo (designated the "verum-sensitive population"), there were significant advantages for both venlafaxine and diazepam over placebo in the reduction of HAM-A total score and other efficacy measures (Hackett *et al.*, 2000).

In the second comparator-controlled study, with 405 participating patients, there were numerical advantages for venlafaxine XL (75 or 150 mg/day) over both placebo and buspirone (30 mg/day) across a range of primary efficacy variables, but none of these reached statistical significance. There were significant advantages ($P < 0.05$) for venlafaxine over placebo on both the HAM-A psychic anxiety item scores at study endpoint, and on the HAM-A anxious mood item at weeks 2, 4, 6, and 8 ($P < 0.05$). Venlafaxine was associated with significantly greater overall improvement, compared to buspirone, on the CGI scores at week 3 (CGI-S), week 4 (CGI-I and CGI-S), and week 8 (CGI-S) (Davidson *et al.*, 1999).

The dose–response relationship with venlafaxine was examined in two of the randomized placebo-controlled treatment studies. In the first, lasting 8 weeks, daily doses of 75, 150, and 225 mg all showed superior efficacy to placebo ($P < 0.05$), the most positive efficacy results being seen with the highest dosage (Rickels *et al.*, 2000). In the second, lasting 24 weeks, daily doses of 75 and 150 mg showed significantly greater improvement than patients allocated to placebo on all outcome measures ($P < 0.01$), whereas a daily dose of 37.5 mg was only superior on one measure at some time points. Furthermore, there were significant advantages for the two higher doses over the lowest dose on some outcome measures (Allgulander *et al.*, 2001).

Summary of published clinical trials of other psychotropic compounds
Benzodiazepines

A systematic review of the findings of randomized controlled trials has established that benzodiazepines are an effective and rapid treatment for many patients with GAD, having similar efficacy to cognitive therapy (Gould *et al.*, 1997). However, the benzodiazepines are far from ideal in the treatment of GAD, having limited efficacy against comorbid depressive symptoms. The unwanted effects of benzodiazepines include sedation, memory disruption, and psychomotor impairment, with an associated increased risk of traffic accidents. Other problems include the development of tolerance, abuse, or dependence, and distressing withdrawal symptoms on stopping the drug. Many authorities counsel that benzodiazepines should be reserved for short-term use (up to 4 weeks), and only prescribed at low dosage (Lader, 1999). Others have argued that benzodiazepines are clearly efficacious, and that withholding treatment from patients on the basis of a potential risk of dependence is unjustified and probably detrimental to overall well-being (Argyropoulos and Nutt, 1999).

Pregabalin

Pregabalin is a novel psychotropic drug with anticonvulsant, anxiolytic, and analgesic properties. The mechanism of action is largely unknown, although it binds to an auxiliary subunit ($\alpha_2\delta$) of voltage-gated calcium channels, thereby increasing whole-brain GABA. The results of a recently published placebo-controlled study indicate that pregabalin was superior to placebo in reducing mean HAM-A score from the first week of double-blind treatment (Feltner *et al.*, 2003). In three randomized double-blind placebo-controlled treatment studies (two involving an active comparator), pregabalin was significantly more efficacious in relieving symptoms than placebo and had similar overall efficacy to either alprazolam (Pande *et al.*, 2000) or venlafaxine (Rickels *et al.*, 2002). Further studies with pregabalin are complete, and demonstrate it has anxiolytic effects within 1 week (Montgomery, 2003).

Imipramine

The tricyclic antidepressant (TCA) imipramine has proven efficacy in the treatment of patients with GAD, defined according to DSM-III criteria. In a seminal 8-week, double-blind, placebo-controlled study involving 230 patients with symptoms lasting at least 4 months, a baseline HAM-A score of 18 or more, and no indication of current depression or panic disorder, subjects were randomized to treatment with imipramine, diazepam, trazodone, or placebo. During the first 2 weeks of treatment, diazepam was associated with most improvement in anxiety symptoms, but from the third week to the study endpoint imipramine had significantly greater anxiolytic efficacy, compared with diazepam (Rickels *et al.*, 1993). However, TCAs such as imipramine have a rather poor tolerability profile due to blockade of histamine H_1 receptors, α_1-adrenoceptors, and muscarinic receptors, and this limits their long-term use in treating patients with GAD.

5-HT$_{1a}$-agonists

Buspirone is an azapirone anxiolytic drug, with partial agonist properties at 5-HT$_{1a}$-receptors, which has proven efficacy in the treatment of patients with GAD (Goa and Ward, 1986). An early study (Goldberg and Finnerty, 1979) established that buspirone had comparable efficacy to diazepam in patients with generalized anxiety. Not all studies with buspirone have been positive (Ansseau *et al.*, 1990), but a meta-analysis of eight controlled treatment studies has indicated that buspirone has comparable efficacy to benzodiazepines in the management of GAD (Gammans *et al.*, 1992). Buspirone appears efficacious in reducing associated depressive symptoms in patients with GAD, but it is not an accepted treatment for patients with major depression, and therefore is not a suitable first-line treatment in patients with comorbid GAD and depression (Sramek *et al.*, 1996).

Flesinoxan is a related drug which acts as a full agonist at somatodendritic 5-HT$_{1a}$-receptors: it too has been found efficacious in the treatment of GAD. A five-arm study comparing three doses of flesinoxan, alprazolam, and placebo found that both the highest dose of flesinoxan and alprazolam were significantly more efficacious than placebo in reducing anxiety symptoms, rated by the HAM-A (Bradford and

Stevens, 1994), but there is little additional information on the efficacy of the drug, and its further development has been halted.

Hydroxyzine

The efficacy of the antihistamine hydroxyzine in acute treatment of patients with GAD has been examined in three randomized placebo-controlled trials. A preliminary French general practice study (using observed case analysis only) found some evidence for efficacy of hydroxyzine (Darcis *et al.*, 1995); this was supported by the findings of a UK primary care study involving 244 patients with DSM-IV GAD, with or without comorbid depressive symptoms. This study also included buspirone, although only hydroxyzine was superior to placebo ($P < 0.02$) on the primary outcome measure (HAM-A) (Lader and Scotto, 1998). In the third study, hydroxyzine had similar efficacy to the benzodiazepine bromazepam, and superior efficacy to placebo, with fewer patients experiencing discontinuation symptoms with hydroxyine (40.2%) than with placebo or bromazepam (each 51%) (Llorca *et al.*, 2002).

Propranolol

A double-blind randomized placebo- and comparator-controlled 3-week dose-ranging parallel-group study has examined the efficacy of the beta-blocker propranolol (80, 160, or 320 mg/day) and the benzodiazepine chlordiazepoxide (30 or 45 mg/day) in GAD. Both propranolol and the active comparator showed significantly greater efficacy than placebo after 1 week of double-blind treatment, but there were no advantages at study endpoint (Meibach *et al.*, 1987).

Trifluoperazine

The results of a randomized placebo-controlled flexible-dose acute treatment study indicate that the antipsychotic drug trifluoperazine had superior efficacy from the first week of double-blind treatment, although there were markedly more treatment-emergent adverse events with trifluoperazine (62%, compared to 46% with placebo) (Mendels *et al.*, 1986).

Taken together, the findings of the randomized placebo-controlled trials with escitalopram, paroxetine, sertraline, and venlafaxine indicate that SSRI or SNRI treatment can be efficacious in the acute management of patients with GAD. There is also some evidence for the efficacy of certain benzodiazepines, buspirone, imipramine, hydroxyzine, and trifluoperazine. Systematic reviews support these observations: a recent but already outdated Cochrane Collaboration review concluded that imipramine, paroxetine, and venlafaxine all had superior efficacy to placebo (Kapczinski *et al.*, 2003). Two comprehensive but similarly outdated reviews both inferred that the SSRI paroxetine offered advantages over comparator benzodiazepines, such as its efficacy in comorbid depression, and the now-disputed low risk of causing discontinuation symptoms (Davidson *et al.*, 2001; Wagstaff *et al.*, 2002). The most recent consensus statement and guidelines on treating anxiety disorders state that SSRIs are the preferred first-line drug treatment in patients with GAD (Bandelow *et al.*, 2002). There are of course many further research needs, such as establishing the comparative efficacy and acceptability of differing drugs in both short- and long-term treatment; examining the effects of combining drug treatment with psychological approaches such as cognitive-behavioral therapy; and evaluating the effectiveness of SSRI or SNRI treatment in patients with comorbid or resistant GAD.

How long should pharmacotherapy of GAD continue?

There have been few randomized controlled trials of the treatment of patients with GAD beyond early response to acute treatment, although the findings of studies with paroxetine, venlafaxine, and escitalopram all suggest that treatment should probably continue for at least a further 6 months. Two different approaches to assessing maintenance of effect have been utilized: (1) a relapse prevention design, in which responders to open-label acute treatment are randomly allocated to either continue with active treatment or to switch to placebo; or (2) a continuation treatment design, in which responders to double-blind acute treatment continue with double treatment for a further 6 months.

In a double-blind relapse prevention study, paroxetine was found efficacious in the long-term treatment of patients with GAD; there were significantly ($P < 0.001$) fewer relapses with paroxetine (10.9%) than with placebo (33.9%) (Stocchi *et al.*, 2003). By contrast, the placebo-controlled relapse prevention study with venlafaxine, over a period of 4 months, did not find greater efficacy than placebo in preventing relapse.

However, the long-term efficacy of venlafaxine extended-release capsules has been shown through the results of a pooled analysis of the results of two 6-month randomized double-blind placebo-controlled parallel-group studies. With venlafaxine, 61% of the patients who had responded but not remitted by week 8 showed remission by 6 months, whereas only 39% of non-remitting placebo-responders at 8 weeks were in symptomatic remission at study endpoint (Montgomery *et al.*, 2002a). The advantage for continuing with venlafaxine was also seen in a survival analysis of patients stopping treatment due to lack of efficacy, in which patients allocated to placebo stopped double-blind treatment at a fairly constant rate from the first month of treatment, whereas few venlafaxine-treated patients discontinued after the second month. After 6 months of double-blind treatment, discontinuation rates were 10% for venlafaxine and 21% for placebo (Montgomery *et al.*, 2002b).

A preliminary report of a relatively small ($n = 123$) randomized 24-week controlled flexible-dose comparison of escitalopram (10–20 mg/day) and paroxetine (20–50 mg/day) in GAD shows the two SSRIs had similar overall efficacy, at 8 and 24 weeks of double-blind treatment. The proportion of patients who responded to treatment increased in both groups over time (escitalopram, 52–70%; paroxetine, 46–61%), as did the proportion of patients entering symptomatic remission (escitalopram, 30–55%; paroxetine, 28–46%) (data on file, Lundbeck).

What is the best pharmacotherapy approach to resistant GAD?

Our literature search did not identify any placebo-controlled studies in patients who have not responded to first-line or second-line treatments. As such, the management of patients with resistant GAD is based largely on experience and anecdotal case reports. Approaches which could be employed include all those compounds described above for which there is evidence of efficacy from placebo-controlled studies, and various forms of psychological treatment, both alone and in combination with psychotropic drugs.

A systematic review of 35 randomized controlled trials has found that cognitive-behavioral therapy (CBT) (using a combination of approaches including exposure, cognitive restructuring, anxiety management, and relaxation) is more efficacious than anxiety management alone, non-directive therapy, or staying on a waiting list (Gould et al., 1997). In one long-term follow-up study, cognitive therapy appeared associated with better long-term outcomes than either placebo or drug treatment; in another, there was no difference in outcome between cognitive therapy, analytic psychotherapy, and anxiety management (Durham et al., 1999).

It is unclear whether it is more helpful to combine pharmacological and psychological approaches in the management of patients with GAD, compared to using single approaches alone (Lader and Bond, 1998). Concomitant treatment with benzodiazepines was associated with markedly reduced response rates, compared to cognitive or behavior therapy alone, in one small study (Durham and Turvey, 1987). However in another study performed in primary care, the combination of diazepam and CBT was more efficacious than either given alone, although the study was unable to detect a difference between diazepam and placebo (Power et al., 1990).

Conclusions

GAD is a common and disabling anxiety disorder: epidemiological studies indicate a lifetime prevalence of approximately 5%, and substantial associated social and occupational impairment, comparable to that with major depression. GAD has considerable comorbidity, with depression, other anxiety disorders, and physical illness. Many patients with GAD are not recognized as suffering from a potentially treatable anxiety disorder: others are recognized as having some form of mental disorder, but are either not treated or receive treatment with drugs of unproven efficacy. Whilst some TCAs and benzodiazepines have been found efficacious in patients with GAD, tolerability problems and other risks limit their use in clinical practice. By contrast, buspirone, the SSRIs escitalopram, paroxetine, and sertraline, the SNRI venlafaxine, and the novel anxiolytic pregabalin have all established efficacy in placebo-controlled trials. At present, SSRIs are probably the first-line treatment, with venlafaxine being used in those patients who do not respond.

REFERENCES

Allgulander, C., Cloninger, C. R., Przybeck, T. R., and Brandt, L. (1998). Changes on the temperament and character inventory after paroxetine treatment in volunteers with generalized anxiety disorder. *Psychopharmacology Bulletin*, **34**, 165–6.

Allgulander, C., Hackett, D., and Salinas, E. (2001). Venlafaxine extended release (ER) in the treatment of generalised anxiety disorder: twenty-four-week placebo-controlled dose-ranging study. *British Journal of Psychiatry*, **179**, 15–22.

Ansseau, M., Papart, P., Gerard, M. A. A., von Frenckell, R., and Franck, G. (1990). Controlled comparison of buspirone and oxazepam in generalised anxiety. *Neuropsychobiology*, **24**, 74–8.

Argyropoulos, S. V. and Nutt, D. J. (1999). The use of benzodiazepines in anxiety and other disorders. *European Neuropsychopharmacology*, **9** (suppl. 9), S407–12.

Baldwin, D. S. (2001). SSRIs in the treatment of generalised anxiety disorder. In: *SSRIs in Depression and Anxiety*, ed. Montgomery, S. A., and den Boer, J. A. Chichester: Wiley, pp. 193–209.

Baldwin, D. S., McCafferty, J., Bellew, K., *et al.* (2002). Improving the disability and impairment associated with generalised anxiety disorder with paroxetine treatment. *International Journal of Neuropsychopharmacology*, **5** (suppl. 1), S213.

Bandelow, B., Zohar, J., Hollander, E., *et al.* (2002). World Federation of Societies of Biological Psychiatry (WFSBP) guidelines for the pharmacological treatment of anxiety, obsessive compulsive and posttraumatic stress disorders. *World Journal of Biological Psychiatry*, **3**, 171–99.

Beekman, A. T., Bremmer, M. A., Deeg, D. J., *et al.* (1998). Anxiety disorders in later life: a report from the Longitudinal Aging Study Amsterdam. *International Journal of Geriatric Psychiatry*, **13**, 717–26.

Bradford, L. D. and Stevens, G. (1994). Double-blind, placebo-controlled fixed dose study of flesinoxan in generalized anxiety disorder. *American College of Neuropsychopharmacology*, 167.

Carter, R. M., Wittchen, H. U., Pfisster, H., and Kessler, R. C. (2001). One-year prevalence of sub-threshold and threshold DSM-IV generalised anxiety disorder in a nationally representative sample. *Depression and Anxiety*, **13**, 78–88.

Charney, D. S., Woods, S. W., and Heninger, G. R. (1989). Noradrenergic function in generalized anxiety disorder: effects of yohimbine in healthy subjects and patients with generalized anxiety disorder. *Psychiatry Research*, **27**, 173–82.

Connor, K. M. and Davidson, J. R. T. (1998). Generalized anxiety disorder: neurobiological and pharmacotherapeutic perspectives. *Biological Psychiatry*, **44**, 1286–94.

Darcis, T., Ferreri, M., Natens, J., *et al.* (1995). A multicentre double-blind placebo-controlled study investigating the anxiolytic efficacy of hydroxyzine in patients with generalized anxiety disorder. *Human Psychopharmacology*, **10**, 181–7.

Davidson, J. R., DuPont, R. L., Hedges, D., and Haskins, J. T. (1999). Efficacy, safety, and tolerability of venlafaxine extended release and buspirone in outpatients with generalised anxiety disorder. *Journal of Clinical Psychiatry*, **60**, 528–35.

Davidson, J. R. T., Ballenger, J. C., Lecrubier, Y., and Nutt, D. J. (2001). Pharmacotherapy of generalized anxiety disorder. *Journal of Clinical Psychiatry*, **62** (suppl. 11), 46–52.

Davidson, J., Bose, A., and Su, G. (2002). Escitalopram in the treatment of generalized anxiety disorder. *International Journal of Neuropsychopharmacology*, **5M** (suppl. 1), S214.

Durham, R. C. and Turvey, A. A. (1987). Cognitive therapy versus behaviour therapy in the treatment of chronic generalised anxiety. *Behavior Research and Therapy*, **25**, 229–34.

Durham, R. C., Fisher, P. L., and Trevling, L. R. (1999). One year follow-up of cognitive therapy, analytic psychotherapy and anxiety management training for generalised anxiety disorder: symptom change, medication usage and attitudes to treatment. *Behavioural and Consulting Psychotherapy*, **27**, 19–35.

Fairbanks, J. M., Pine, D. S., Tancer, N. K., *et al.* (1997). Open fluoxetine treatment of mixed anxiety disorders in children and adolescents. *Journal of Child and Adolescent Psychopharmacology*, **7**, 17–29.

Feighner, J. P., Entsuah, A. R., and McPherson, M. K., (1998). Efficacy of once-daily venlafaxine extended release (XR) for symptoms of anxiety in depressed outpatients. *Journal of Affective Disorders*, **47**, 55–62.

Feltner, D. E., Crockatt, J. G., Dubovsky, S. J., *et al.* (2003). A randomized, double-blind, placebo-controlled, fixed-dose, multicenter study of pregabalin in patients with generalized anxiety disorder. *Journal of Clinical Psychopharmacology*, **23**, 240–9.

Gammans, R. E., Stringfellow, J. C., Hvidzos, A. J., *et al.* (1992). Use of buspirone in patients with generalised anxiety disorder and coexisting depressive symptoms: a meta-analysis of eight randomised controlled trials. *Neuropsychobiology*, **25**, 193–201.

Goa, K. L. and Ward, A. (1986). Buspirone: a preliminary review of its pharmacological properties and therapeutic efficacy as an anxiolytic. *Drugs*, **32**, 114–29.

Goldberg, H. L. and Finnerty, R. J. (1979). The comparative efficacy of buspirone and diazepam in the treatment of anxiety. *American Journal of Psychiatry*, **136**, 1184–7.

Gorman, J. (2002). Treatment of generalised anxiety disorder. *Journal of Clinical Psychiatry*, **63** (suppl.), 17–23.

Gorman, J. M., Korotzer, A., and Su, G. (2002). Efficacy comparison of escitalopram and citalopram in the treatment of major depressive disorder: pooled analysis of placebo-controlled trials. *CNS Spectrums*, **7** (suppl. 1), S40–4.

Gould, R. A., Otto, M. W., Pollack, M. H., and Yap, L. (1997). Cognitive behavioural and pharmacological treatment of generalised anxiety disorder: a preliminary meta-analysis. *Behavior Therapy*, **28**, 285–305.

Greenberg, P. E., Sisitsky, T., Kessler, R. C., *et al.* (1999). The economic burden of anxiety disorders in the 1990s. *Journal of Clinical Psychiatry*, **60**, 427–35.

Hackett, D., Haudiquet, V., and Salinas, E. (2000). Controlling for the placebo response rate: a methodological approach to data from double-blind studies with a high placebo response. Presented at British Association for Psychopharmacology, Harrogate, 2000.

Hamilton, M. (1959). The assessment of anxiety states by rating. *British Journal of Medical Psychology*, **32**, 50–5.

Hamilton, M. (1967). Development of a rating scale for primary depressive illness. *British Journal of Social and Clinical Psychology*, **6**, 278–96.

Hurst, M. and Lamb, H. M. (2000). Fluoxetine: a review of its use in anxiety disorders and mixed anxiety and depression. *CNS Drugs*, **14**, 51–80.

Hyttel, J., Bsego, K. P., Perregard, J. A., and Sanchez, C. (1992). The pharmacological effect of citalopram resides in the (S)-(+)-enantiomer. *Journal of Neural Transmission General Section*, **88**, 157–60.

Jefferson, J. and Greist, J. (2000). A double-blind comparison of citalopram and paroxetine in the treatment of patients with depression and anxiety. Presented at ACNP, Puerto Rico.

Kapczinski, F., Schmitt, R., Lima, M. S. (2003). The use of antidepressants for generalized anxiety disorder. *Cochrane Database of Systematic Reviews* CD 003592.

Katz, I. R., Reynolds, C., Alexopoulos, G. S., and Hackett, D. (2002). Venlafaxine ER as treatment for generalized anxiety disorder in older adults: pooled analysis of five randomized placebo-controlled clinical trials. *Journal of the American Geriatric Society*, **50**, 18–25.

Kessler, R. C., DuPont, R. L., Berglund, P., and Wittchen, H. U. (1999). Impairment in pure and comorbid generalized anxiety disorder and major depression at 12 months in two national surveys. *American Journal of Psychiatry*, **156**, 1915–23.

Lader, M. H. (1999). Limitations on the use of benzodiazepines in anxiety and insomnia: are they justified? *European Neuropsychopharmacology*, **9** (suppl. 9), S399–405.

Lader, M. H. and Bond, A. J. (1998). Interaction of pharmacological and psychological treatments of anxiety. *British Journal of Psychiatry*, **173** (suppl. 34), 42–8.

Lader, M. and Scotto, J. C. (1998). A multicentre double-blind comparison of hydroxyzine, buspirone and placebo in patients with generalized anxiety disorder. *Psychopharmacology*, **139**, 402–6.

Llorca, P. M., Sapdone, C., Sol, O., *et al.* (2002). Efficacy and safety of hydroxyzine in the treatment of generalized anxiety disorder: a three-month double-blind study. *Journal of Clinical Psychiatry*, **63**, 1020–7.

Maier, W. and Falkai, P. (1999). The epidemiology of comorbidity between depression, anxiety disorders and somatic diseases. *International Clinical Psychopharmacology*, **14** (suppl. 2), 51–6.

Meibach, R. C., Dunner, D., Wilson, L. G., Ishiki, D., and Dager, S. R. (1987). Comparative efficacy of propranolol, chlordiazepoxide, and placebo in the treatment of anxiety: a double-blind trial. *Journal of Clinical Psychiatry*, **84**, 355–8.

Mendels, J., Krajewski, T. F., Huffer, V., *et al.* (1986). Effective short-term treatment of generalized anxiety with trifluoperazine. *Journal of Clinical Psychiatry*, **47**, 170–4.

Montgomery, S. A. (2003). Pregabalin in generalized anxiety disorder: speed of onset. *European Neuropsychopharmacology*, **13** (suppl. 4), S376.

Montgomery, S. A., Sheehan, D. V., Meoni, P., Haudiquet, V., and Hackett, D. (2002a). Characterization of the longitudinal course of improvement in generalized anxiety disorder during long-term treatment with venlafaxine XR. *Journal of Psychiatric Research*, **36**, 209–17.

Montgomery, S. A., Mahe, V., Haudiquet, V., and Hackett, D. (2002b). Effectiveness of venlafaxine, extended release formulation, in short-term and long-term treatment of generalized anxiety disorder: results of a survival analysis. *Journal of Clinical Psychopharmacology*, **22**, 561–7.

Morris, P. L. P., Dahl, A. A., Kutcher, S. P., *et al.* (2003). Efficacy of sertraline for the acute treatment of generalized anxiety disorder (GAD). *European Neuropsychopharmacology*, **13** (suppl. 4), S375.

Pande, A. C., Crockatt, J. G., Janney, C., *et al.* (2000). Pregabalin, a novel agent, in the treatment of generalized anxiety disorder. Presented at American Psychiatric Association, San Diego, May 2000.

Pollack, M. H., Zaninelli, R., Goddard, A., *et al.* (2001). Paroxetine in the treatment of generalized anxiety disorder: results of a placebo-controlled, flexible-dosage trial. *Journal of Clinical Psychiatry*, **62**, 350–7.

Power, K. G., Simpson, R. J., Swanson, V., and Wallace, L. A. (1990). Controlled comparison of pharmacological and psychological treatment of generalized anxiety disorder in primary care. *British Journal of General Practice*, **40**, 289–94.

Rickels, K., Downing, R., Schweizer, E., and Hassman, H. (1993). Antidepressants for the treatment of generalised anxiety disorder. A placebo-controlled comparison of imipramine, trazodone and diazepam. *Archives of General Psychiatry*, **50**, 884–98.

Rickels, K., Pollack, M. H., Sheehan, D. V., and Haskins, J. T. (2000). Efficacy of extended-release venlafaxine in non-depressed outpatients with generalized anxiety disorder. *American Journal of Psychiatry*, **157**, 968–74.

Rickels, K., Pollack, M. H., Lydiard, R. B., *et al.* (2002). Comparison of the efficacy and safety of pregabalin and alprazolam in generalised anxiety disorder. *International Journal of Neuropsychopharmacology*, **5** (suppl. 1), S213.

Rickels, K., Zaninelli, R., McCafferty, J. P., *et al.* (2003). Paroxetine treatment of generalized anxiety disorder: a double-blind, placebo-controlled study. *American Journal of Psychiatry*, **160**, 749–56.

Rocca, P., Ferrero, P., Gualerzi, A., *et al.* (1991). Peripheral-type benzodiazepine receptors in anxiety disorders. *Acta Psychiatrica Scandinavica*, **84**, 537–44.

Rocca, P., Fonzo, V., Scotta, M., Zanalda, E., and Ravizza, L. (1997). Paroxetine efficacy in the treatment of generalized anxiety disorder. *Acta Psychiatrica Scandinavica*, **95**, 444–50.

Rosenberg, C., Damsbo, N., Fuglum, E., Jacobsen, L. V., and Horsgard, S. (1994). Citalopram and imipramine in the treatment of depressive patients in general practice. A Nordic multicentre clinical study. *International Clinical Psychopharmacology*, **9** (suppl. 1), 41–8.

Rynn, M. A., Siqueland, L., and Rickels, K. (2001). Placebo-controlled trial of sertraline in the treatment of children with generalised anxiety disorder. *American Journal of Psychiatry*, **158**, 2008–14.

Sevy, S., Papadimitriou, G. N., Surmont, D. W., Goldman, S., and Mendlewicz, J. (1989). Noradrenergic function in generalized anxiety disorder, major depressive disorder, and healthy subjects. *Biological Psychiatry*, **25**, 141–52.

Sheehan, D. V., Harnett-Sheehan, K., and Raj, B. A. (1996). The measurement of disability. *International Clinical Psychopharmacology*, **11** (suppl. 3), 89–95.

Sjodin, I., Kutcher, S. P., Ravindran, A., and Burt, T. (2003). Efficacy of sertraline in improving quality of life and functioning in generalized anxiety disorder. *European Neuropsychopharmacology*, **13** (suppl. 4), S365.

Sonawalla, S. B., Spillmann, M. K., Kolsky, A. R., *et al.* (1999). Efficacy of fluvoxamine in the treatment of major depression with comorbid anxiety disorders. *Journal of Clinical Psychiatry*, **60**, 580–3.

Sramek, J. J., Tansman, M., Suri, A., *et al.* (1996). Efficacy of buspirone in generalised anxiety disorder with coexisting mild depressive symptoms. *Journal of Clinical Psychiatry*, **57**, 287–91.

Stahl, S. (2000). Placebo-controlled comparison of the selective serotonin reuptake inhibitors citalopram and sertraline. *Biological Psychiatry*, **48**, 894–901.

Stocchi, F. G., Nordera, G., Jokinen, R. H., *et al.* (2003). Efficacy and tolerability of paroxetine for the long-term treatment of generalised anxiety disorder. *Journal of Clinical Psychiatry*, **64**, 250–8.

Wagstaff, A. J., Cheer, S. M., Matheson, A. J., Ormrod, D., and Goa, K. L. (2002). Paroxetine – an update of its use in psychiatric disorders in adults. *Drugs*, **62**, 655–703.

Weiller, E., Bisserbe, J. C., Maier, W., and Lecrubier, Y. (1998). Prevalence and recognition of anxiety syndromes in five European primary care settings. A report from the WHO study on psychological problems in general health care. *British Journal of Psychiatry*, **173** (suppl. 34), 18–23.

Weizman, R., Tanne, Z., Granek, M., *et al.* (1987). Peripheral benzodiazepine binding sites on platelet membranes are increased during diazepam treatment of anxious patients. *European Journal of Pharmacology*, **138**, 289–92.

Wittchen, H. U. (2002). Generalized anxiety disorder: prevalence, burden and cost to society. *Depression and Anxiety*, **16**, 162–71.

Wittchen, H. U., Carter, R. M., Pfisster, H., Montgomery, S. A., and Kessler, R. C. (2000). Disabilities and quality of life in pure and comorbid generalized anxiety disorder and major depression in a national survey. *International Clinical Psychopharmacology*, **15**, 319–28.

Yonkers, K. A., Dyck, I. R., Warshaw, M., and Keller, M. B. (2000). Factors predicting the clinical course of generalised anxiety disorder. *British Journal of Psychiatry*, **176**, 544–9.

5

Evidence-based pharmacotherapy of panic disorder

Abraham Bakker,[1] Anton J. L. M. van Balkom,[2] and Dan J. Stein[3]

[1] Robert Fleury Stichting, Leidschendam, the Netherlands
[2] Vrije Universiteit Amsterdam, the Netherlands
[3] University of Cape Town, South Africa

Introduction

Panic disorder (PD) with or without agoraphobia is one of the most prevalent of the anxiety disorders. It is also accompanied by significant morbidity and comorbidity. Fortunately, a number of effective treatments for PD are available. This chapter focuses on pharmacotherapy, assessing the evidence base in order to address questions about: (1) the optimal first-line pharmacotherapy of PD; (2) the optimal duration of pharmacotherapy; and (3) the optimal approach to pharmacotherapy in the treatment-refractory patient. In order to ensure that all relevant randomized controlled trials were considered, a MEDLINE search (1966–2003) was undertaken using the key words "panic" and "treatment." In addition, recent meta-analyses of PD and treatment guidelines on PD were reviewed. We begin by briefly discussing the diagnosis and target symptoms of PD.

Diagnosis

Panic attacks and agoraphobic avoidance are defined in the *Diagnostic and Statistical Manual* (DSM-IV-TR: American Psychiatric Association, 2000) as follows: a panic attack is "a discrete period of intense fear or discomfort, in which four or more of the following symptoms develop abruptly and reach a peak within 10 minutes." The symptoms listed are: palpitations, sweating, trembling or shaking, sensations of shortness of breath or smothering, feeling of choking, chest pain or discomfort, nausea or abdominal distress, feeling dizzy or faint, derealization or depersonalization, feeling of losing control or going crazy, fear of dying, paresthesias, and chills or hot flushes. Agoraphobia is defined as:

anxiety about being in places or situations from which escape might be difficult or in which help may not be available in the event of an unexpected or situationally predisposed panic attack. Agoraphobic fears typically involve characteristic clusters of situations that include being outside the home alone, being in a crowd or standing in a line, being on a bridge, and traveling in a bus, train or automobile.

Given that panic attacks and agoraphobia occur in different anxiety disorders, a first issue in the assessment of panic symptoms is the accurate differentiation of PD from these other entities. DSM-IV-TR emphasizes that PD is diagnosed when the attacks experienced are unexpected and when at least one of the attacks has been followed by 1 month (or more) of persistent concern about having additional attacks, worry about the implications of the attacks or their consequences, or a significant change in behavior related to the attacks (American Psychiatric Assocation, 2000). When a patient with PD is also extremely afraid of going into public places like shopping malls, trains, cinemas, or other situations from which escape would be difficult or in which help would not be available in case of a panic attack, this person is said to have PD with agoraphobia.

A second important diagnostic issue is the differentiation of PD from general medical disorders. Given the high prevalence of PD and its frequent presentation in medical settings, it is important to have a high index of suspicion for this disorder. As many as 3.5% of the population are estimated to suffer from PD (Katerndahl and Realini, 1993; Eaton *et al.*, 1994), and 1-month prevalence rates are 0.7–2.2% for females and 0.4–0.8% for males (Eaton *et al.*, 1991; Bijl *et al.*, 1997). For agoraphobia, high prevalence rates are also found; 1-month prevalence rates for females are 4.4%, and for males 1.6% (Bourdon *et al.*, 1988). PD usually develops during the third decade of life, with a mean age of onset of 28 years (Marks, 1987). People with panic attacks may present to primary care practitioners or to a range of medical specialists. Unnecessary special investigations are frequently ordered.

Conversely, however, a comprehensive medical history and examination may be needed to exclude the presence of physical disorders that can cause the symptoms of a panic attack (Raj and Sheehan, 1987). Well-known causes of panic-like symptoms are hyperfunction of the thyroid, hypoglycemia, and pheochromocytoma. In general, any clinical condition that is associated with physical signs that can also occur during a panic attack has the potency to provoke anxiety. The most important mechanism for this is probably the cognitive misinterpretation of these bodily sensations (Clark, 1986). The use of psychoactive substances like caffeine, cannabis, or cocaine may also produce panic attacks. Withdrawal from benzodiazepines or alcohol is another cause of panic symptoms. In all these situations, the patient should be diagnosed not with PD, but rather with "anxiety disorder due to a general medical condition with panic attacks/phobic symptoms" or "substance-induced anxiety disorder with panic attacks/phobic symptoms." In some cases, substance abuse may be denied, and drug screening may be required before an accurate diagnosis is made.

Target symptoms in PD include not only panic attacks and agoraphobia, but also comorbid symptoms and associated impairment. PD is frequently associated with mood disorders, other anxiety disorders (e.g., social anxiety disorder), and substance-related disorders. The clinical relevance of diagnosing PD with or without comorbid disorders lies in the fact that patients with comorbidity are more severely and chronically ill, more disabled, utilize services more frequently, and are more difficult to treat (Roy-Byrne *et al.*, 2000). Formulated in other words, "comorbidity" points to a more severe subgroup of PD. PD is characterized by significant distress and functional impairment, and it is important these features are also targeted by treatment interventions.

Treatment options

Although the pathogenesis of PD remains incompletely understood, a range of effective pharmacological, non-pharmacological, and combination treatments have been developed in the past three decades. Pharmacological treatments mainly comprise treatment with high-potency benzodiazepines and antidepressants. Other medications that have been suggested for the treatment of PD include β-adrenergic blocking agents (e.g., propranolol), α_2-adrenergic receptor agonist (e.g., clonidine), mood stabilizers (e.g., carbamazepine, lithium), and antipsychotic agents. Propranolol has been found ineffective in controlled trials, while most of these other agents have not been studied systematically.

Behavioral and cognitive therapies have also been found effective for the treatment of PD. Questions remain about how best to sequence and combine pharmacotherapy and psychotherapy. In practice, they are frequently combined, with the rationale that this may lead not only to symptom improvement, but also to a more persistent recovery. Although psychodynamic psychotherapeutic intervention strategies have been developed (Milrod *et al.*, 1997), the efficacy of non-directive therapies has not been documented in controlled studies. Brief psychodynamic psychotherapy has, however, been reported to be helpful in reducing relapse rates following treatment with an antidepressant (Wiborg and Dahl, 1996).

In the treatment of PD, separate options for panic attacks and agoraphobic avoidance behavior can perhaps be distinguished. Pharmacological and cognitive-behavioral therapy for panic attacks diminish frequency and severity of panic attacks. With pharmacological treatments, the accompanying avoidance behavior improves as well, as do comorbid general anxiety symptoms, and, in case of treatment with an antidepressant, there is also reduction in comorbid depressive symptoms. Behavioral treatment strategies such as "exposure *in vivo*" may be particularly effective in treating agoraphobic avoidance behavior. In clinical practice, pharmacological panic management is therefore frequently combined with exposure *in vivo*. In the remainder of this chapter, we focus however on pharmacotherapy.

Table 5.1 Start, mean, and maximum dosage of drugs effective in panic disorder with or without agoraphobia

	Dosages (mg/day)		
	Start	Mean	Maximum
High-potency benzodiazepines			
Alprazolam	1.5	4–6	_[a]
Clonazepam	1	2–3	_[a]
Lorazepam	1	2–4	_[a]
Selective serotonin reuptake inhibitors			
Citalopram	10	20–30	60
Fluoxetine	20	20	60
Fluvoxamine	50	100–150	300
Paroxetine	10–20	20–40	60
Sertraline	50	100	200
Tricyclic antidepressants			
Clomipramine	25	100–150	250
Imipramine	25	100–150	300
Monoamine oxidase inhibitors			
Phenelzine	10	40–60	_[a]
Tranylcypromine	10	30–60	_[a]

[a] Only use mean dosage.

Pharmacotherapy of PD

High-potency benzodiazepines and antidepressants are the best-studied pharmacotherapy options for PD. The high-potency benzodiazepines (e.g., alprazolam and clonazepam) have been extensively researched, and appear to be more effective than placebo in the short-term treatment of this disorder (Beauclair *et al.*, 1994; Jonas and Cohon, 1993). Dosage of the high-potency benzodiazepines in PD is higher than the usual dosages used in generalized anxiety disorder (Table 5.1). Low-potency benzodiazepines like diazepam may also only have an antipanic effect at higher doses than normally prescribed for other disorders like generalized anxiety disorder. When such medication is effective, panic and phobia symptoms improve soon after administration of benzodiazepines (Burrows and Norman, 1999).

The majority of studies investigating medication therapy in PD have focused on treatment with antidepressants. Tricyclic antidepressants (TCAs), selective serotonin reuptake inhibitors (SSRIs), and irreversible monoamine oxidase inhibitors (MAOIs) have been proven to be effective in PD (Gorman, 1997; Bakker *et al.*,

2000). These agents have a slower onset of action than the benzodiazepines, and an initial trial of 6–8 weeks is required.

MAOIs such as phenelzine have shown efficacy in the treatment of PD, but are not used on a regular basis since patients need to be on low-tyramine diets to avoid hypertensive crises (Rosenberg, 1999). Within the TCAs, both imipramine and clomipramine have been studied (Papp *et al.*, 1997; Cross National Collaborative Panic Study, Second Phase Investigators, 1992). The currently available SSRIs citalopram, escitalopram, fluvoxamine, fluoxetine, paroxetine, and sertraline have all been proven more effective than pill-placebo in reducing symptomatology in PD (Black *et al.*, 1993; Hoehn-Saric *et al.*, 1993; Sharp *et al.*, 1996; Lecrubier *et al.*, 1997; Wade *et al.*, 1997; Ballenger *et al.*, 1998a; Michelson *et al.*, 1998; Rapaport *et al.*, 1998). The daily dosages of these antidepressants are similar to those used in the treatment of major depressive disorder (Table 5.1).

Indeed, antidepressants that influence the serotonergic system have consistently been shown to have efficacy in the treatment of PD. In contrast, data on norepinephrine (noradrenaline) reuptake inhibitors for PD has been less consistent. For example, in a double-blind comparison between the SSRI fluvoxamine and the norepinephrine uptake inhibitor maprotiline, only fluvoxamine demonstrated good antipanic properties (den Boer and Westenberg, 1988). Nevertheless, there are also some positive studies with norepinephrine reuptake inhibitors, such as reboxetine, in PD.

Side-effects that occur during the first weeks of treatment with antidepressants can easily be misinterpreted as symptoms of a panic attack, e.g., palpitations, sweating, and nausea. In patients unaware of the possibility that such side-effects may occur, an apparent increase in the frequency and intensity of panic attacks may be seen. The best way to prevent such an outcome is to provide patients with sufficient information about the working mechanisms and potential side-effects of antidepressants before treatment with these agents is initiated. Early dropout, noncompliance, and suboptimal treatment outcome can also be prevented with this strategy. Outcome can be evaluated properly only after 6 weeks of treatment.

Antidepressants versus benzodiazepines

A number of studies have compared different pharmacological therapies for PD, with the majority of these focusing on the comparison between antidepressants and benzodiazepines. These studies have consistently found similar efficacy. In the largest of these studies, both imipramine and alprazolam were superior to placebo for most outcome measures (Cross National Collaborative Panic Study, Second Phase Investigators, 1992). To date, a total of nine studies comparing imipramine with high-potency benzodiazepines (alprazolam, clonazepam) have been published (van Balkom *et al.*, 1995). Both classes of agent appear effective for panic and phobic symptoms. Differences were observed in the time to response (earlier with benzodiazepines) and dropout rate (lower with benzodiazepines). Despite these differences, intent-to-treat analyses revealed no significant differences in efficacy at endpoint.

TCAs versus SSRIs

Relatively few studies have compared different antidepressants in PD (den Boer *et al.*, 1987; Cassano *et al.*, 1988; den Boer and Westenberg, 1988; Modigh *et al.*, 1992; Nair *et al.*, 1996; Lecrubier *et al.*, 1997; Tiller *et al.*, 1997; Wade *et al.*, 1997; Bakker *et al.*, 1999; Seedat *et al.*, 2003). In most studies, different antidepressants have shown equal efficacy in reducing the total number of panic attacks. In particular, comparison of TCAs and SSRIs has not found differences in efficacy between these classes of medication (Lecrubier *et al.*, 1997; Wade *et al.*, 1997; Bakker *et al.*, 1999; Otto *et al.*, 2001). Some data suggest that SSRIs have a more rapid onset of action than TCAs (Lecrubier *et al.*, 1997), and that SSRIs are associated with a lower dropout rate (Bakker *et al.*, 2002).

Combination treatments

In everyday clinical practice combinations of different medications are frequently used, as well as combinations of pharmacotherapy and cognitive-behavioral therapy. However, the number of controlled studies that include combination treatments is disappointingly low.

The combination of an SSRI with a benzodiazepine is particularly widely used in clinical practice. Early coadministration of (high-potency) benzodiazepines like alprazolam and clonazepam may prevent the initial worsening of anxiety symptoms reported during the first weeks of treatment with a SSRI. The number of well-designed studies that have investigated this strategy is however limited. The most recent and important study was carried out by Goddard *et al.* (2001). They studied double-blind, placebo-controlled coadministration of clonazepam (0.5 mg three times daily) with open-label sertraline for the first 4 weeks of treatment. Fifty patients were randomized, and 34 completed the trial. There was no significant difference in dropout rate between the sertraline/clonazepam and the sertraline/placebo condition (25% versus 38%). The intent-to-treat analysis found a higher percentage of responders in the sertraline/clonazepam group at both the end of week 1 and week 3 of the trial (41% and 63%) in comparison to the sertraline/placebo-treated subjects (4% and 32%). The authors concluded that rapid stabilization of PD can be safely achieved with a sertraline/clonazepam combination, supporting the clinical utility of this type of regimen.

With respect to the combination of medication and psychotherapy, the distinction between benzodiazepines and antidepressants appears relevant. In a large

8-week study Marks *et al.* (1993) found no differences in efficacy between alprazolam and exposure, alprazolam and relaxation, placebo and exposure, and placebo and relaxation. However, there were longer-lasting gains with exposure alone than with alprazolam following withdrawal of the medication. In contrast, there is evidence that SSRIs plus cognitive-behavioral therapy appear more effective than SSRIs alone.

Thus, in early work (de Beurs *et al.*, 1995), using a double-blind, placebo-controlled design, fluvoxamine followed by exposure *in vivo* demonstrated efficacy superior to that of psychological panic management followed by exposure, and exposure *in vivo* alone. Similarly, a study by Sharp *et al.* (1996) included conditions with combinations of placebo with cognitive-behavioral therapy and of fluvoxamine with cognitive-behavioral therapy: the largest and most consistent treatment gains were found in the fluvoxamine with cognitive-behavioral therapy group. Oehrberg and coworkers (1995) investigated paroxetine plus standardized cognitive therapy (CT) versus pill-placebo plus CT; paroxetine with CT was significantly more effective than placebo with CT on nearly all efficacy measures.

Meta-analyses

Since comparisons within one study between different pharmacotherapies are relatively scarce, additional information on the differential efficacy of different agents on panic attacks and agoraphobic avoidance can arguably be derived from comparisons between studies. These comparisons can be performed in a quantitative manner by means of meta-analytic methods.

Several meta-analyses comparing different pharmacological treatments for PD have been published (Wilkinson *et al.*, 1991; Boyer, 1995; van Balkom *et al.*, 1997; Bakker *et al.*, 1998). More recently a number of meta-analyses focusing on the comparison of TCAs and SSRIs have been published (Otto *et al.*, 2001; Bakker *et al.*, 2002). The most relevant results of these studies are summarized here.

The meta-analysis of Wilkinson *et al.* (1991) included 19 double-blind placebo-controlled trials of antidepressants ($n = 13$) and benzodiazepines ($n = 6$) for patients with PD. It showed that active treatment had a 25% greater success rate than placebo over a mean duration of 14 weeks. There were no statistically significant differences observed between antidepressants and benzodiazepines.

The meta-analysis of Boyer (1995) reviewed 27 published or presented placebo-controlled, double-blind studies of PD. The serotonin reuptake inhibitors included clomipramine, fluvoxamine, paroxetine, and zimelidine. The comparison treatments were imipramine and alprazolam. All three treatments were significantly superior to placebo in alleviating panic. The serotonin reuptake inhibitors were also significantly superior to both imipramine and alprazolam. The superiority of the serotonin reuptake inhibitors remained, but was less pronounced, when they were compared to the studies which used higher doses of imipramine or alprazolam.

The meta-analysis of van Balkom *et al.* (1997) evaluated the short-term efficacy of benzodiazepines, antidepressants, psychological panic management, exposure *in vivo*, and combination treatments in PD with or without agoraphobia. Included were 52 treatment conditions with medication (28 high-potency benzodiazepines, 24 antidepressants), with 1653 patients at pretest and 1324 at posttest. Pre/posteffect sizes of Cohen's *d* were calculated *within* the treatment conditions. Seven large treatment conditions were used in the main analyses, including high-potency benzodiazepines and antidepressants. Both benzodiazepines and antidepressants were superior to a control condition, consisting of pill-placebo, attention placebo, and waiting list for both panic attacks and agoraphobic avoidance. A comparison between high-potency benzodiazepines and antidepressants found no differences in efficacy. In this meta-analysis the combination of antidepressants with exposure *in vivo* was found to be the most potent short-term treatment of PD with or without agoraphobia, especially with respect to agoraphobic avoidance.

Longer-term follow-up data in the studies included in the meta-analysis of van Balkom *et al.* (1997) were reported separately (Bakker *et al.*, 1998). Eight studies reported on high-potency benzodiazepines and five on antidepressants. The results were consistent with those of the short-term comparison.

A more recent meta-analysis exclusively focused on the short-term efficacy of SSRIs versus TCAs (Bakker *et al.*, 2002). Included were 43 studies, published prior to or during 1999 (34 randomized, nine open), including 53 treatment conditions, 2367 patients at pretest, and 1804 at posttest. Outcome was measured by the proportion of patients becoming panic-free, and with pre/post Cohen's *d*-effect sizes, calculated for four clinical variables: panic, agoraphobia, depression, and general anxiety. The results are summarized in Table 5.2, and indicated no differences between SSRIs and TCAs on any of the effect sizes, with both groups of antidepressants equally effective in reducing panic symptoms, agoraphobic avoidance, depressive symptoms, and general anxiety. Also the percentage of patients free of panic attacks at posttest did not differ across treatments. As mentioned earlier, the number of dropouts was significantly lower in the group of patients treated with SSRIs (18% versus TCAs 31%). The main conclusion was that SSRIs and TCAs have equal efficacy in the treatment of PD, but SSRIs are better tolerated.

First-line pharmacotherapy for PD

There are two categories of medication with sufficient evidence to support their use as a first-line treatment for PD: high-potency benzodiazepines and antidepressants. There are several reasons for choosing antidepressants rather than benzodiazepines.

Table 5.2 Characteristics of treatment conditions and effect sizes at posttest

	TCAs	N^a	SSRIs	N^a
Treatment conditions	30		23	
Male/female ratio	0.50	25	0.51	22
Age ($\pm$ SD)	34.4 ($\pm$ 4.1)	26	35.5 ($\pm$ 5.4)	22
Illness duration in years ($\pm$ SD)	8.4 ($\pm$ 2.8)	22	9.6 ($\pm$ 1.0)	13
Weeks of treatment ($\pm$ SD)	9.7 ($\pm$ 4.7)	30	9.6 ($\pm$ 2.7)	22
Number of patients				
Pretest	1059	30	1308	23
Dropout (%)	327 (31%[b])		236 (18%[b])	
Completer	732		1072	
Patients free of panic attacks	304/510 (60%)	16	539/985	18
at posttest (%)			(55%)	
Panic d ($\pm$ SD)	1.46 ($\pm$ 0.84)	20	1.26 ($\pm$ 0.41)	9
Agoraphobia d ($\pm$ SD)	1.15 ($\pm$ 0.50)	15	1.10 ($\pm$ 0.49)	11
Depression d ($\pm$ SD)	1.25 ($\pm$ 0.69)	13	1.41 ($\pm$ 0.99)	13
Anxiety d ($\pm$ SD)	1.27 ($\pm$ 0.58)	16	1.55 ($\pm$ 0.84)	16

d, Cohen's d-effect size; SD, standard deviation; TCAs, tricyclic antidepressants; SSRIs, selective serotonin reuptake inhibitors.
[a] Number of treatment conditions providing data with respect to this item.
[b] $Chi^2 = 32.8$, df $= 1$, $P < 0.001$.

Perhaps the most important is the adverse-effect profile of the benzodiazepines, including problems with withdrawal. Furthermore, in contrast to antidepressants, benzodiazepines are not effective in reducing the depressive symptomatology that often accompanies PD (van Balkom et al., 1997). Finally, the risk of relapse or recurrence of PD after discontinuation of the benzodiazepines is relatively high. It is not surprising therefore that antidepressants have become the first-line pharmacotherapy of choice in the treatment of PD.

The relative efficacy of different groups of antidepressants in the treatment of PD and related symptoms is, however, still a matter of debate (Otto et al., 2001; Bakker et al., 2002). To date, no differences in efficacy have been demonstrated between the two groups of antidepressants that are used most frequently, SSRIs and TCAs (Otto et al., 2001; Bakker et al., 2002). However, there are indications that the dropout rate differs significantly in favor of the SSRIs (Bakker et al., 2002). Dropouts may occur for different reasons, varying from ineffectiveness to serious side-effects. The lower dropout rate of SSRIs is most likely due to a more tolerable side-effect profile. Side-effects of TCAs may also prevent therapeutic doses of these drugs being given. Taken together, this has led to a preference for SSRIs over TCAs in both clinical practice and in consensus guidelines (Ballenger *et al.*, 1998b; Bandelow *et al.*, 2002).

There are no data that show clear advantages of one of the SSRIs over the others. All six that are currently available (citalopram, escitalopram, fluvoxamine, fluoxetine, paroxetine, and sertraline) have been found to be effective in the treatment of PD in double-blind, placebo-controlled trials.

During the first weeks of treatment with a SSRI it may be helpful to add a low dose of a high-potency benzodiazepine (alprazolam, clonazepam) as an additional medication (Goddard *et al.*, 2001). This may result in more rapid stabilization and higher response rates during the first weeks of treatment. The risk of an initial worsening of anxiety symptoms is probably reduced by this regimen as well. The main problem that may result from prescribing a benzodiazepine as a co-medication is that patients refuse to stop taking this agent. This may lead to dependence and other problems related to long-term use of benzodiazepines. In our clinical practice we mention the possibility of taking a benzodiazepine during the first 2–3 weeks of treatment with an antidepressant. We tell the patients that they can decide themselves whether they want this co-medication, but that the duration of the prescription is strictly limited to 3 weeks.

It has been suggested that treatment of PD requires a lower starting dose of the antidepressant compared with depression to prevent an initial worsening of symptoms and reduce the rate of dropout due to adverse effects. In patients who have previously been unable to tolerate a standard dose of antidepressant medication, this would certainly seem a rational approach. However, explaining to the patient that such a regimen may be associated with a delayed response may lead the patient to choose to start a therapeutic dose sooner. In such cases, patients should be made aware of the possibility of early transient side-effects, and the possibility of lowering the dose to help cope with these.

For how long should maintenance pharmacotherapy be continued?

As PD runs a chronic course, long-term treatment outcome may be more important than short-term efficacy. Cognitive-behavioral therapy appears to have long-term benefits, and generally the short-term results are maintained. Naturalistic follow-up studies of psychotherapy have been published as long as 9 years after short-term treatment (Emmelkamp *et al.*, 1992).

The long-term effect of psychopharmacological treatments for PD has received less attention. A major clinical problem is the fact that treatment gains may disappear after tapering off the medication. This is perhaps especially true for the high-potency benzodiazepines. Relapse rates up to 80% have been reported following complete withdrawal from alprazolam (Noyes *et al.*, 1991).

There are relatively few data that address the optimal duration of pharmacotherapy for PD. Mavissakalian and Perel (1992) reported that, when responders to a 6-month trial of imipramine were treated at half-dose for another 6 months, they maintained their improvement. This group of patients showed significantly lower relapse rates than a group of patients treated with imipramine for 6 months only. These data suggest that successful pharmacotherapy should be continued for at least 1 year. A number of consensus guidelines (Ballenger *et al.*, 1998b; Bandelow *et al.*, 2002) have reached a similar conclusion.

Nevertheless, a more recent paper by the same authors (Mavissakalian and Perel, 2002) concluded that neither the duration of treatment with imipramine nor the method of discontinuation were predictors of relapse. In this study, the rate of relapse after only 6 months of treatment was identical to the rate of relapse after 12–30 months of treatment. The main limitation of these findings is the limited sample size: only 51 patients were included in the analyses.

Relapse prevention for patients who want to discontinue their medication can potentially be enhanced by the addition of psychotherapy. An interesting study by Wiborg and Dahl (1996) reported that patients treated with clomipramine plus brief psychodynamic psychotherapy had significantly lower relapse rates 18 months after treatment than patients treated with clomipramine alone. Research on long-term treatment and discontinuation of therapies requires more attention, for pharmacotherapy as well as psychotherapy. The conflicting results of the limited data that are available with respect to the optimal duration of pharmacotherapy underline this need.

What is the optimal approach to the treatment-refractory patient?

Despite advances in the pharmacotherapy of PD, not all patients respond to the first trial of medication. Unfortunately, there are very little persuasive data with respect to this topic. We suggest that when an SSRI fails, irrespective of the reason, a second SSRI is a reasonable step to take next. Co-medication with a benzodiazepine, preferably a high-potency benzodiazepine like alprazolam or clonazepam, can also be considered on a case-by-case basis, depending on the clinician's judgment.

If a second SSRI is not effective, then a third choice of medication may be a TCA like clomipramine or imipramine. Such an agent can also be combined with a benzodiazepine. Subsequent options for pharmacological treatment of refractory patients include a high dose of high-potency benzodiazepines (up to 6 mg alprazolam or the equivalent), and treatment with an irreversible MAOI like phenelzine. The addition of cognitive-behavioral therapy to non- or partial medication responders should also be considered. Table 5.3 summarizes the strategies in case of non-response to first-line pharmacotherapy.

Table 5.3 Treatment options for refractory patients

Step 1[a]	SSRI (for at least 4 weeks in a therapeutic dosage)
Step 2[a]	Another SSRI
Step 3[a]	Tricyclic antidepressant (clomipramine or imipramine)
Step 4	High-potency benzodiazepine (in a high dosage)
Step 5[a]	MAOI

[a] Early co-administration of clonazepam or alprazolam may be considered.

SSRI, selective serotonin reuptake inhibitor; MAOI, monoamine oxidase inhibitor.

Conclusions

When untreated, PD may run a chronic course, with a waxing and waning of symptoms. The high prevalence and significant disability associated with PD, as well as the frequent co-occurrence of PD with mood disorders and substance abuse disorders, underline the importance of having effective treatments available. Fortunately, recent decades have witnessed the development of a number of effective treatments, including psychopharmacological interventions.

With regard to the short-term treatment of PD, several standard pharmacological and psychological interventions show equal efficacy in reducing panic, agoraphobia, and related complaints. Nevertheless, SSRIs are increasingly viewed as a pharmacotherapy of choice, partly because benzodiazepines have relatively little effect on the depressive symptoms that often complicate PD. Short-term co-medication with high-potency benzodiazepines may be a useful strategy in some cases.

For both pharmacotherapy and psychotherapy it is still unclear how long treatment should be continued, in what dose medication should optimally be continued after remission of symptoms has been achieved, and what the optimal approach to refractory patients is. After withdrawal of short-term benzodiazepine and antidepressant treatment there are relatively high percentages of relapse. Data for valid comparisons of the differences in relapse between different medication classes are not yet available.

With regard to the combination of different treatment strategies, there is some evidence that the combination of an antidepressant and exposure *in vivo* produces the largest treatment gains in PD. Agoraphobic behavior in particular may respond well to this combined strategy. It is, however, unclear how long and in which dosage the medication should be continued, and what the optimal duration and frequency of the exposure treatment are.

Another important issue that remains to be fully resolved is the costs that accompany different treatment strategies. Dropout due to adverse side-effects of medication, lack of efficacy, lack of compliance, and relapse after cessation of medication are important factors that increase the total cost of treatment with pharmacological agents. Psychotherapeutic interventions also have associated costs. Further work on the cost-efficacy of the treatment of PD is required.

In the interim, we suggest that when patients suffer from panic attacks with no or only limited avoidance, then the treatment of first choice is an SSRI. When patients suffer from agoraphobic avoidance due to their panic attacks, exposure should be added. Our advice is to give the antidepressant first, and start formal exposure after the first positive effects of the medication have occurred. The antidepressant should be continued at least 9 months after maximal efficacy has been attained. Psychotherapy should continue throughout this whole period, and can be stopped after patients have been free of medication for at least some months.

REFERENCES

American Psychiatric Association (2000). *Diagnostic and Statistical Manual of Mental Disorders,* 4th edn, text revision. Washington, DC: American Psychiatric Association.

Bakker, A., van Balkom, A. J. L. M., Spinhoven, Ph., *et al.* (1998). Follow-up on the treatment of panic disorder with or without agoraphobia: a quantitative review. *Journal of Nervous and Mental Disease,* **186**, 414–19.

Bakker, A., van Dyck, R., Spinhoven, Ph., *et al.* (1999). Paroxetine, clomipramine and cognitive therapy in the treatment of panic disorder. *Journal of Clinical Psychiatry,* **60**, 831–8.

Bakker, A., van Balkom, A. J. L. M., and van Dyck, R. (2000). Selective serotonin reuptake inhibitors in the treatment of panic disorder and agoraphobia. *International Clinical Psychopharmacology,* **15** (suppl. 2), S25–30.

Bakker, A., van Balkom, A. J. L. M., and Spinhoven, Ph. (2002). SSRIs versus TCAs in the treatment of panic disorder: a meta-analysis. *Acta Psychiatrica Scandinavica,* **106**, 163–7.

Ballenger, J. C., Wheadon, D. E., Steiner, M., *et al.* (1998a). Double-blind, fixed-dose, placebo-controlled study of paroxetine in the treatment of panic disorder. *American Journal of Psychiatry,* **155**, 36–42.

Ballenger, J. C., Davidson, J. R. T., Lecrubier, Y., *et al.* (1998b). Consensus statement on panic disorder from the international consensus group on depression and anxiety. *Journal of Clinical Psychiatry,* **59** (suppl. 8), 47–54.

Bandelow, B., Zohar, J., Hollander, E., *et al.* (2002). World Federation of Societies of Biological Psychiatry (WFSBP) guidelines for the pharmacological treatment of anxiety, obsessive-compulsive and posttraumatic stress disorders. *World Journal Biological Psychiatry,* **3**, 171–99.

Beauclair, L., Fontaine, R., Annable, L., *et al.* (1994). Clonazepam in the treatment of panic disorder: a double-blind, placebo-controlled trial investigating the correlation between clonazepam concentrations in plasma and clinical response. *Journal of Clinical Psychopharmacology*, **14**, 111–18.

Bijl, R. V., van Zessen, G., and Ravelli, A. (1997). Psychiatrische morbiditeit onder volwassenen in Nederland: het NEMESIS-onderzoek. II. Prevalentie van psychiatrische stoornissen. *Nederlands Tijdschrift voor Geneeskunde*, **141**, 2453–60.

Black, D. W., Wesner, R., Bowers, W., *et al.* (1993). A comparison of fluvoxamine, cognitive therapy, and placebo in the treatment of panic disorder. *Archives of General Psychiatry*, **50**, 44–50.

Bourdon, K. H., Boyd, J. H., Rae, D. S., *et al.* (1988). Gender differences in phobias: results of the ECA community survey. *Journal of Anxiety Disorders*, **2**, 227–41.

Boyer, W. (1995). Serotonin uptake inhibitors are superior to imipramine and alprazolam in alleviating panic attacks: a meta-analysis. *International Clinical Psychopharmacology*, **10**, 45–9.

Burrows, G. D. and Norman, T. R. (1999). The treatment of panic disorder with benzodiazepines. In: *Panic Disorder: Clinical Diagnosis, Management and Mechanisms*, ed. D. J. Nutt, J. C. Ballenger, and J. P. Lepine. London: Martin Dunitz, pp. 145–58.

Cassano, G. B., Petracca, A., Perugi, G., *et al.* (1988). Clomipramine for panic disorder, I: the first 10 weeks of a long-term comparison with imipramine. *Journal of Affective Disorders*, **14**, 123–7.

Clark, D. M. (1986). A cognitive approach to panic. *Behaviour Research and Therapy*, **24**, 461–70.

Cross National Collaborative Panic Study, Second Phase Investigators (1992). Drug treatment of panic disorder. *British Journal of Psychiatry*, **160**, 191–202.

de Beurs, E., van Balkom, A. J. L. M., Lange, A., *et al.* (1995). Treatment of panic disorder with agoraphobia: comparison of fluvoxamine, placebo, and psychological panic management combined with exposure and of exposure *in vivo* alone. *American Journal of Psychiatry*, **152**, 683–92.

den Boer, J. A. and Westenberg, H. G. M. (1988). Effect of a serotonin and noradrenaline uptake inhibitor in panic disorder; a double-blind comparative study with fluvoxamine and maprotiline. *International Clinical Psychopharmacology*, **3**, 59–74.

den Boer, J. A., Westenberg, H. G. M., and Kamerbeek, W. D. J. (1987). Effect of a serotonin uptake inhibitor in anxiety disorders: a double-blind comparison of clomipramine and fluvoxamine. *International Clinical Psychopharmacology*, **2**, 21–32.

Eaton, W. W., Dryman, A., and Weissman, M. M. (1991). Panic and phobia. In: *Psychiatric Disorders in America*, ed. L. N. Robins and D. A. Regier. New York: Free Press, pp. 155–79.

Eaton, W. W., Kessler, R. C., Wittchen, H. U., *et al.* (1994). Panic and panic disorder in the United States. *American Journal of Psychiatry*, **151**, 413–20.

Emmelkamp, P. M. G., Bouman, T., and Scholing, H. A. (1992). *Anxiety Disorders: A Practitioner's Guide*. Chichester: Wiley.

Goddard, A. W., Brouette, T., Almai, A., *et al.* (2001). Early coadministration of clonazepam with sertraline for panic disorder. *Archives of General Psychiatry*, **58**, 681–6.

Gorman, J. M. (1997). The use of newer antidepressants for panic disorder. *Journal of Clinical Psychiatry*, **58** (suppl. 14), 54–8.

Hoehn-Saric, R., McLeod, D., and Hipsley, P. A. (1993). Effect of fluvoxamine on panic disorder. *Journal of Clinical Psychopharmacology*, **13**, 321–6.

Jonas, J. M., and Cohon, M. S. (1993). A comparison of the safety and efficacy of alprazolam versus other agents in the treatment of anxiety, panic, and depression: a review of the literature. *Journal of Clinical Psychiatry*, **54** (suppl. 10), 25–45.

Katerndahl, D. A. and Realini, J. P. (1993). Lifetime prevalence of panic states. *American Journal of Psychiatry*, **150**, 246–9.

Lecrubier, Y., Bakker, A., Dunbar, G., *et al.* (1997). A comparison of paroxetine, clomipramine and placebo in the treatment of panic disorder. *Acta Psychiatrica Scandinavica*, **95**, 145–52.

Marks, I. M. (1987). *Fears, Phobias and Rituals.* Oxford: Oxford University Press.

Marks, I. M., Swinson, R. P., Basoglu, M., *et al.* (1993). Alprazolam and exposure alone and combined in panic disorder with agoraphobia. *British Journal of Psychiatry*, **162**, 776–87.

Mavissakalian, M. and Perel, J. M. (1992). Clinical experiments in maintenance and discontinuation of imipramine therapy in panic disorder with agoraphobia. *Archives of General Psychiatry*, **49**, 318–23.

(2002). Duration of imipramine therapy and relapse in panic disorder with agoraphobia. *Journal of Clinical Psychopharmacology*, **22**, 294–9.

Michelson, D., Lydiard, R. B., Pollack, M. H., *et al.* (1998). Outcome assessment and clinical improvement in panic disorder: evidence from a randomized controlled trial of fluoxetine and placebo. *American Journal of Psychiatry*, **155**, 1570–7.

Milrod, B. L., Busch, F. N., Cooper, A. M., *et al.* (1997). Washington, DC: *Manual of Panic-Focused Psychodynamic Psychotherapy.* American Psychiatric Association.

Modigh, K., Westberg, P., and Eriksson, E. (1992). Superiority of clomipramine over imipramine in the treatment of panic disorder: a placebo-controlled trial. *Journal of Clinical Psychopharmacology*, **12**, 251–61.

Nair, N. P. V., Bakish, D., Saxena, B., *et al.* (1996). Comparison of fluvoxamine, imipramine, and placebo in the treatment of outpatients with panic disorder. *Anxiety*, **2**, 192–8.

Noyes, R., Garvey, M. J., Cook, B., *et al.* (1991). Controlled discontinuation of benzodiazepine treatment for patients with panic disorder. *American Journal of Psychiatry*, **148**, 517–23.

Oehrberg, S., Christiansen, P. E., Behnke, K., *et al.* (1995). Paroxetine in the treatment of panic disorder. A randomised, double-blind, placebo-controlled study. *British Journal of Psychiatry*, **167**, 374–9.

Otto, M. W., Tuby, K. S., Gould, R. A., *et al.* (2001). An effect-size analysis of the relative efficacy and tolerability of serotonin selective reuptake inhibitors for panic disorder. *American Journal of Psychiatry*, **158**, 1989–92.

Papp, L. A., Schneier, F. R., Fyer, A. J., *et al.* (1997). Clomipramine treatment of panic disorder: pros and cons. *Journal of Clinical Psychiatry*, **58**, 423–5.

Raj, A. and Sheehan, D. V. (1987). Medical evaluation of panic attacks. *Journal of Clinical Psychiatry*, **48**, 309–13.

Rapaport, M. H., Wolkow, R. M., and Clary, C. M. (1998). Methodologies and outcomes from the sertraline multicenter flexible-dose trials. *Psychopharmacology Bulletin*, **34**, 183–9.

Rosenberg, R. (1999). Treatment of panic disorder with tricyclics and MAOIs. In: *Panic Disorder: Clinical Diagnosis, Management and Mechanisms.* London: Martin Dunitz, pp. 125–44.

Roy-Byrne, P. R., Stang, G., Wittchen, H. U., *et al.* (2000). Lifetime panic-depression co-morbidity in the National Comorbidity Survey. *British Journal of Psychiatry*, **176**, 229–35.

Seedat, S., van Rheede, Oudtshoorn, E., Muller, J. E., *et al.* (2003). Reboxetine and citalopram in panic disorder: a single-blind, cross-over, flexible-dose pilot study. *International Clinical Psychopharmacology*, **18**, 279–84.

Sharp, D. M., Power, K. G., Simpson, R. J., *et al.* (1996). Fluvoxamine, placebo, and cognitive behaviour therapy used alone and in combination in the treatment of panic disorder and agoraphobia. *Journal of Anxiety Disorders*, **10**, 219–42.

Tiller, J. W. G., Bouwer, C., and Behnke, K. (1997). Moclobemide for anxiety disorders: a focus on moclobemide for panic disorder. *International Clinical Psychopharmacology*, **12** (suppl. 6), S27–30.

van Balkom, A. J. L. M., Nauta, M. C. E., and Bakker, A. (1995). Meta-analysis on the treatment of panic disorder with agoraphobia: review and re-examination. *Clinical Psychology and Psychotherapy*, **2**, 1–14.

van Balkom, A. J. L. M., Bakker, A., Spinhoven, Ph., *et al.* (1997). A meta-analysis of the treatment of panic disorder with or without agoraphobia: a comparison of psychopharmacological, cognitive-behavioral, and combination treatments. *Journal of Nervous and Mental Disease*, **185**, 510–16.

Wade, A. G., Lepola, U., Koponen, H. J., *et al.* (1997). The effect of citalopram in panic disorder. *British Journal of Psychiatry*, **170**, 549–53.

Wiborg, I. M. and Dahl, A. A. (1996). Does brief dynamic psychotherapy reduce the relapse rate of panic disorder? *Archives of General Psychiatry*, **53**, 689–94.

Wilkinson, G., Balestrieri, M., Ruggeri, M., and Bellantuono, C. (1991). Meta-analysis of double-blind placebo controlled-trials of antidepressants and benzodiazepines for patients with panic disorders. *Psychological Medicine*, **21**, 991–8.

6

Evidence-based pharmacotherapy of posttraumatic stress disorder

C. Barbara Portier,[1] Abraham Bakker,[2] Anton J. L. M. van Balkom,[3] and Dan J. Stein[4]

[1] Sint Lucas Andreas Hospital, Amsterdam, the Netherlands
[2] Robert Fleury Stichting, Leidschendam, the Netherlands
[3] Vrije Universiteit Amsterdam, the Netherlands
[4] University of Cape Town, South Africa

Introduction

Although posttraumatic stress disorder (PTSD) has long been recognized as an important condition by clinicians (for instance, as "shell shock", "soldiers heart," "combat neurosis"), it was only recently recognized in the official nosology (*Diagnostic and Statistical Manual of Mental Disorders* (DSM-III): American Psychiatric Association, 1994). Epidemiological studies show that PTSD is one of the most prevalent and costly psychiatric disorders. Approximately one-third of all people are exposed to a traumatic event during their life, and a significant percentage (approximately 10–20%) develop PTSD (Brunello *et al.*, 2001). The lifetime prevalence of PTSD in the USA is estimated at 1.3–7.8% (Kessler *et al.*, 1995). PTSD is twice as common among women than men (Kessler *et al.*, 1995). Rates of comorbid psychiatric disorders in PTSD patients are relatively high, with data suggesting that approximately 80% of patients with PTSD meet criteria for at least one other DSM disorder (Kessler *et al.*, 1995; Kessler, 2000). Furthermore PTSD severely impacts on patients' functioning, and is associated with significant medical costs and economic loss (Kessler *et al.*, 1995; Solomon and Davidson, 1997). Unfortunately, underdiagnosis and undertreatment contribute to these costs.

PTSD is defined in DSM-IV as a condition that develops after exposure to a traumatic event, and that is characterized by persistent reexperiencing of the traumatic event, avoidance of stimuli associated with the trauma and numbing of general responsiveness, and symptoms of increased arousal. There are three subcategories of PTSD: (1) acute PTSD (symptoms last less than 3 months); (2) chronic PTSD (symptoms last 3 months or more); and (3) PTSD with delayed onset (symptoms begin at least 6 months after the traumatic event) (American Psychiatric Association, 1994). The diagnosis of PTSD can be established with a structured clinical interview such as the Structured Clinical Interview for DSM-IV disorders (SCID-IV), and symptoms can be rated with standardized scales such as the clinician-administered PTSD scale (CAPS) or the Davidson Trauma Scale (DTS) (Spitzer *et al.*, 1994; Davidson *et al.*, 1997; Wheaters *et al.*, 2001). It may also be useful to quantify disability using a scale such as the Sheehan Disability Scale (SDS) (Leon *et al.*, 1997).

A rationale for the use of medication in PTSD is supported by growing evidence for specific dysregulation of neurotransmitters (serotonin, norepinephrine (noradrenaline), and dopamine) and neuroendocrine (hypothalamus–pituitary–adrenal (HPA) axis) systems and for neuroanatomical abnormalities in PTSD. Several studies have pointed to the involvement of the serotonin system in PTSD, providing some rationale for the use of medications that act on this system. However, a range of other alterations are noted, including elevated levels of corticotrophin-releasing factor, decreased levels of circulating cortisol, increased concentration and responsiveness of glucocorticoid receptors, and increased sensitivity of the HPA negative feedback inhibition (Vermetten *et al.*, 2003). Reduced volume of the hippocampal region has been found in a number of structural imaging studies in PTSD, and may be increased after treatment with a selective serotonin reuptake inhibitor (SSRI). Functional neuroanatomical abnormalities may also be normalized by this class of agent (Vermetten *et al.*, 2003).

Pharmacotherapy of PTSD

The MEDLINE, PsychLit, and Cochrane databases were searched for publications with the following keywords: posttraumatic stress disorder, PTSD, treatment, and therapy. Articles were included up to and including 2003. Relevant publications from the reference sections of the articles that were found were also included. Meta-analyses and expert consensus articles were also reviewed. The evidence base was used to address three questions: (1) What is the first-line pharmacotherapy of choice for PTSD? (2) For how long should maintenance pharmacotherapy be continued? and (3) What is the optimal pharmacotherapy approach to the treatment-refractory patient?

Twenty-two randomized controlled trials (RCTs), more than 50 open trials, and several case reports were found concerning pharmacotherapy of PTSD. Placebo-controlled trials have been undertaken with the tricyclic antidepressants imipramine (1), amitriptyline (1), and desipramine (1), the monoamine oxidase inhibitor (MAOI) phenelzine (2), the reversible MAOI (RIMA) brofaromine (2), the SSRIs fluoxetine (5), paroxetine (3), and sertraline (3), the anticonvulsant lamotrigine (1), the antipsychotic olanzapine (1), the benzodiazepine alprazolam (1), and inositol (1). Imipramine has also been compared with phenelzine (Table 6.1).

Table 6.1 Randomized controlled trials for the short-term pharmacotherapy of posttraumatic stress disorder (PTSD)

Medication	Authors	Subjects on medication	Subjects on placebo	Duration	Outcome	Effect sizes[a]		Effect size[a] Medication > placebo
						Medication	Placebo	
RIMA								
Brofaromine	Baker *et al.* (1995)	56	58	10	CAPS total	1.67	1.56	−
	Katz *et al.* (1995)	22	23	14	CAPS total	1.71	1.56	+
MAOI								
Phenelzine	Kosten *et al.* (1991) Frank *et al.* (1988)[b]	19	18	8	IES total	1.03	0.12	+
	Shestatzky *et al.* (1988)	13	13	5	IES total	0.09	0.39	−
TCA								
Imipramine	Kosten *et al.* (1991) Frank *et al.* (1988)[b]	23	18	8	IES total	0.55	0.12	+
Desipramine	Reist *et al.* (1989)[c]	18	18	4	IES avoidance	0.04	0.01	−
					IES intrusion	0.13	0.04	−
Amitriptyline	Davidson *et al.* (1990) Davidson *et al.* (1993)[b]	25	21	8	IES total	0.68	0.48	+
SSRI								
Fluoxetine	Hertzberg *et al.* (2000)	6	6	12	SIP	0.12	0.09	−
	Connor *et al.* (1999a)	27	27	12	SIP	2.57	1.35	+
	Van de Kolk *et al.* (1994)[c]	33	33	5	–	*f*	*f*	+
	Nagy *et al.* (2000)[d]	22[e]		10	–	*f*	*f*	−
	Martenyi *et al.* (2002a)	226	75	12	TOP8	2.57	2.22	+
					CAPS	1.57	1.29	+
Paroxetine	Tucker *et al.* (2001)	151	156	12	CAPS total	*e*	*e*	+
	Marshall *et al.* (2001)	183*	186	12	CAPS total	2.46	1.59	+
		182**	186	12	CAPS total	2.43	1.59	+
	Stein *et al.* (2003)	160	162	12	CAPS2	*f*	*f*	+
					CGI-S	*f*	*f*	+
Sertraline	Davidson *et al.* (2001a)	100	108	12	CAPS total	2.04	1.63	+
	Brady *et al.* (2000)	94	98	12	CAPS total	1.46	1.00	+
					IES total	0.97	0.37	+
				10	CAPS2 CGI-S			

(cont.)

Table 6.1 (cont.)

Medication	Authors	Subjects on medication	Subjects on placebo	Duration	Outcome	Effect sizes[a]		Effect size[a] Medication > placebo
						Medication	Placebo	
	Zohar et al. (2002)	23	19			1.87	1.42	+
						1.38	0.88	+
Various								
Olanzapine	Butterfield et al. (2001)	10	5	10	SIP	2.23	2.25	–
					TOP8	1.26	1.88	–
					SPRINT	2.01	2.17	–
Lamotrigine	Hertzberg et al. (1999)	10	4	12	SIP	0.99	1.12	–
Inositol	Kaplan et al. (1996)[c]	13	13	4	IES	0.30	–0.3	–
Alprazolam	Braun et al. (1990)[c]	16	16	5	Observer-rated PTSD	0.54	0.13	–
					IES	0.49	0.03	–

RIMA, reversible monoamine oxidase inhibitor; MAOI, monoamine oxidase inhibitor; TCA, tricyclic antidepressant; SSRI, selective serotonin reuptake inhibitor.

[a] Effect size: Cohen's *d* was calculated by subtracting the posttest from the pretest score and dividing the difference by the pooled standard deviation.

[b] Excluded from this review: Frank et al. (1988): an extension of this database was subsequently published by Kosten et al. (1991); Davidson et al. (1993): this database had been published before by Davidson et al. (1990).

[c] Crossover design.

[d] Poster presentation.

[e] Impossible to calculate.

[f] Total PTSD subjects = 22.

* Paroxetine 20 mg; ** paroxetine 40 mg.

Caps (Clinician Administered Posttraumatic Stress (observer-rated)): Weathers et al. (2002). Clinician administered PTSD scale: a review of the first ten years of research. *Depression and Anxiety*, **13**, 132–56.

IES (Impact of Events Scale (self-rating)): Horowitz et al. (1979). Impact of event scale: a measure of subjective stress. *Psychosomatic Medicine*, **41**, 209–18.

CGI-S (Clinical Global Impression of Severity scale (observer-rated)): Guy, W. (1976). *ECDEU Assessment Manual for Psychopharmacology*. US Department of Health, Education, and Welfare publication (ADM) 76–338. Rockville, MD: National Institute of Mental Health, pp. 218–22.

SIP (Structured Interview for PTSD (observer-rated)): Davidson et al. (1997). Structured interview for PTSD (SIP): psychometric validation for DSM-IV criteria. *Depression and Anxiety*, **5**, 127–9.

TOP8 (the eight-item treatment outcome PTSD scale (observer-rated)): Davidson et al. (1997). The eight- item treatment outcome PTSD scale: a brief measure to assess outcome in posttraumatic stress disorder. *International Journal of Clinical Psychopharmacology*, **12**, 41–5.

SPRINT (Short PTSD Rating Interview (observer-rated)): Connor et al. (2001). SPRINT: a brief global assessment of post-traumatic stress disorder. *International Journal of Clinical Psychopharmacology*, **16**, 279–84.

Pharmacological treatment can be effective in reducing PTSD symptoms. All symptom clusters can be influenced, irrespective of comorbid anxiety and depressive episodes. Nevertheless, nine of the 22 controlled studies found no superiority of the active drug over placebo: 1 (out of 2) trial with phenelzine, 1 (out of 2) trial with brofaromine, 2 (out of 5) trials with fluoxetine, and the trials with desipramine, alprazolam, inositol, olanzapine, and lamotrigine (Table 6.1). A number of these pharmacological agents may not be effective for PTSD, but methodological weaknesses (including small subject numbers and short durations of treatment) may also have led to negative results.

What is the first-line pharmacotherapy of PTSD?

TCAs, MAOIs, and RIMAs

The earliest controlled medication trials in PTSD investigated tricyclic antidepressants (TCAs) and MAOIs in war veterans. Although these early studies had methodological problems (e.g., short duration, use of non-standardized rating scales), they nevertheless suggested that some of these medications are effective in the treatment of PTSD.

Three placebo-controlled trials on the efficacy of TCAs in combat-related PTSD have been published, with different results. Both amitriptyline and imipramine were found to be effective in war veterans with chronic PTSD (Kosten *et al.*, 1991; Davidson *et al.*, 1990). Desipramine was effective for depressive symptoms, but not for PTSD symptoms (Reist *et al.*, 1989). Two placebo-controlled trials of phenelzine have been published, again with varying results. In one trial phenelzine was not superior to placebo (Shestatzky *et al.*, 1988), but in another it was more effective than both imipramine and placebo, and was associated with lower dropout rates than imipramine (Kosten *et al.*, 1991).

The efficacy of the reversible inhibitor of MAO-A (RIMA) brofaromine has been investigated in two controlled trials. Brofaromine was more effective than placebo in patients suffering from PTSD after different traumatic experiences, but no difference in efficacy could be demonstrated in war veterans (Baker *et al.*, 1995; Katz *et al.*, 1995). Moclobemide, another RIMA, had a positive effect on reexperiencing, avoidance, numbing, and hyperarousal in an open trial (Neal *et al.*, 1997).

SSRIs

Several studies of the treatment of PTSD with SSRIs have been published. There are placebo-controlled trials with fluoxetine, paroxetine, and sertraline. Some of the studies report efficacy of SSRIs on the core symptoms of PTSD, as well as comorbid symptoms (depression, anxiety).

Two placebo-controlled trials (Van der Kolk *et al.*, 1994; Connor *et al.*, 1999a) have confirmed early open-label results (Burdon *et al.*, 1991; Davidson *et al.*, 1991; McDougle *et al.*, 1991; Shay, 1992; Nagy *et al.*, 1993) on the efficacy of fluoxetine in PTSD. Van der Kolk *et al.* found efficacy of fluoxetine with respect to numbing and hyperarousal. A subgroup analysis showed that symptom reduction was significant in civilians with PTSD (mostly women), but not in war veterans. Connor *et al.* confirmed efficacy of fluoxetine in a civilian population with PTSD in a placebo-controlled trial. Meltzer-Brody *et al.* concluded in a later publication that fluoxetine improved all symptom clusters of PTSD (Meltzer-Brody *et al.*, 2000). In contrast, in combat-related PTSD, there have been two small negative trials (Hertzberg *et al.*, 2000; Nagy *et al.*, 2000). However, a large multisite trial of fluoxetine that included many subjects with combat-related PTSD had sufficient power to show efficacy for this agent (Martenyi *et al.*, 2002a).

Paroxetine has been studied in three RCTs, all of which found that this medication is effective in the treatment of chronic PTSD in predominantly civilian subjects (Stein *et al.*, 2000a; Marshall *et al.*, 2001; Tucker *et al.*, 2001). An analysis of the pooled data set indicated that paroxetine improved all three symptom clusters of PTSD (Stein *et al.*, 2003). Therapy response was not dependent on gender, trauma type, time since trauma, severity of baseline PTSD, or comorbid diagnoses.

Sertraline has been studied in three placebo-controlled trials. Two RCTs in predominantly civilian samples found that sertraline was effective. The medication was effective for the range of symptom clusters (Brady *et al.*, 2000; Davidson *et al.*, 2001a). In a smaller sample of combat-related PTSD, significance was not reached (Zohar *et al.*, 2002). In an interesting open-label trial of subjects with both PTSD and alcohol dependence, both sets of symptoms appeared to respond to sertraline (Brady *et al.*, 1995).

While fluvoxamine and citalopram have not been studied in RCTs, there is open-label evidence to suggest that these agents are also effective in PTSD (De Boer *et al.*, 1992; Marmar *et al.*, 1996; Davidson *et al.*, 1998a; Seedat *et al.*, 2000; Tucker *et al.*, 2000; Khouzam *et al.*, 2001).

Other antidepressants

There are promising open-label data for venlafaxine (Smakjic *et al.*, 2001), mirtazapine (Connor *et al.*, 1999b), nefazodone (Davidson *et al.*, 1998b; Hertzberg *et al.*, 1998; Hidalgo *et al.*, 1999; Mellman *et al.*, 1999; Zisook *et al.*, 2000) and trazodone (Hertzberg *et al.*, 1996; Davis *et al.*, 2000; Warner *et al.*, 2001). Although these agents have not to date been found effective in published RCTs, they may offer advantages in terms of their side-effect profiles.

From the studies that have been published so far, it may be argued that SSRIs are the first choice in medication treatment of PTSD. First, there is good evidence of their efficacy in controlled trials; the largest studies demonstrating efficacy of medication in PTSD are those of the SSRIs (Table 6.1). Second, many PTSD patients have comorbid depression and anxiety, and depressive and anxiety symptoms in subjects with SSRIs respond to these agents. Third, the SSRIs are safer and better tolerated than older antidepressants; dropout rates in the sertraline, fluoxetine, and paroxetine trials are in the range of the dropout rates in their placebo control group, which is consistent with evidence that these agents are reasonably well-tolerated in patients with mood and anxiety disorders. Problems with the SSRIs include sexual dysfunction and weight changes. Certainly, a number of consensus guidelines have reached the conclusion that SSRIs are the first-line medication of choice in PTSD (Foa *et al.*, 1999, 2000; Ballenger *et al.*, 2000).

Other antidepressants, such as TCAs and MAOIs, which have proven effective in controlled trials can be considered in select patients. Nevertheless, the relatively poor tolerability of the TCAs and MAOIs are concerns. TCAs may be associated with daytime drowsiness, cardiac toxicity in overdose, impaired reaction times, and increased risk of road traffic accidents. Phenelzine requires strict adherence to a tyramine-free diet. The use of this medication is limited due to poor tolerance and concerns about the risk of administration (Foa *et al.*, 1999, 2000; Ballenger as above *et al.*, 2000). Some of the newer-generation antidepressants are less likely than the SSRIs to be associated with sexual dysfunction, and may also be effective in PTSD.

There are few fixed-dose studies of antidepressants in PTSD. It would seem reasonable to use similar dosages as are effective in depression, titrating upwards to maximum recommended doses if necessary. Many of the recent SSRI trials have been 12 weeks in length. Although response may be seen before endpoint, given that some subjects responded only late in the trial, it seems reasonable for an initial trial of medication to continue for this period of time. Indeed, there is some evidence that clinical response in PTSD can occur even after 12 weeks of treatment with an SSRI (see below).

How long should maintenance therapy be continued?

There have been few long-term controlled pharmacotherapy trials in PTSD (Davidson *et al.*, 2001b; Londborg *et al.*, 2001; Martenyi *et al.*, 2002b). Patients who responded during the acute treatment phase (12 weeks double-blind with fluoxetine or placebo) were rerandomized and continued in a 24-week relapse prevention phase with fluoxetine ($n = 69$) or placebo ($n = 62$). Patients in the fluoxetine/fluoxetine group were less likely to relapse than patients in the fluoxetine/placebo group. Participants in the fluoxetine/fluoxetine treatment group continued to experience statistically significant improvement in mean TOP8 (eight-item treatment outcome PTSD scale) score throughout the relapse prevention period and showed statistically significant better improvement at endpoint than did fluoxetine/placebo participants. Moreover they showed statistically significant improvement in illness severity (Clinical Global Impressions – severity of illness scale CGI-S scale) and in the CAPS avoidance subscore compared with fluoxetine/placebo-treated participants (Guy, 1976; Martenyi *et al.*, 2002b). Patients included in the sertraline treatment groups of the two large RCTs of this agent (Brady *et al.*, 2000; Davidson *et al.*, 2001a) were subsequently continued for 24 weeks of open-label sertraline (Londborg *et al.*, 2001). The majority of the patients who were responders after 12 weeks' treatment continued to be responders during this follow-up. Moreover, more than 50% of the patients who were non-responders after the initial 12 weeks became responders during continued treatment with sertraline in the following 24 weeks. Sixty-nine of the subjects were then randomized to sertraline and placebo for an additional 28 weeks. Sertraline was effective for maintaining the reduction in symptoms and preventing relapse (Davidson *et al.*, 2001b). These data provide support for consensus recommendations that treatment with an SSRI should be continued for at least a year.

The treatment-refractory patient

There are relatively few controlled trials addressing the optimal pharmacotherapy of patients who fail to respond to a first-line medication. Options include augmenting with a second agent, or switching to a different agent (either within the same class of medication or to a medication with a different mechanism of action). There is little information available on the rate of response to a second medication, but work in depression and anxiety disorders indicates that this can be a useful strategy. There have also been few controlled augmentation trials in PTSD, but there is now some evidence that augmentation of SSRIs with antipsychotic agents may be useful in treatment-refractory PTSD. Mood stabilizers have also been suggested as augmenting agents in PTSD, and we begin by briefly reviewing the data on these agents.

Mood stabilizers

A double-blind trial (12 weeks) among 15 patients with PTSD (war veterans and civilians) found that lamotrigine was more effective than placebo in reducing re-experiencing, avoidance, and numbing (Hertzberg *et al.*, 1999). There are also open-label data suggesting the value of lithium (Kitchner and Greenstein, 1987; Forster *et al.*, 1995; Stein *et al.*, 2000b), valproate (Fesler, 1991; Clark *et al.*, 1999; Szymanski and Olympia, 1991), carbamazepine (Lipper *et al.*, 1986; Wolf *et al.*, 1988), topiramate (Berlant, 2001), and vigabatrine (Macleod, 1996) in PTSD; in some of this work these medications have been added as augmenting agents

(Clark *et al.*, 1999; Macleod, 1996). It is possible that some of these mood stabilizers are particularly effective in decreasing impulsive and aggressive symptoms (Wolf *et al.*, 1988; Forster *et al.*, 1995).

Antipsychotics

Antipsychotic agents have long been reported effective in PTSD, but there have been few controlled trials (Ahearn *et al.*, 2003a; Dillard *et al.*, 1993; Hamner, 1996). Olanzapine was studied in a randomized placebo-controlled trial in 15 patients, mostly female rape victims. PTSD symptoms improved in both the olanzapine and the placebo group, without significant differences (Butterfield *et al.*, 2001). However, there is also evidence that new-generation antipsychotics can be useful as augmenting agents in treatment-refractory PTSD. There are several case reports and open-label studies suggesting improvement of treatment-resistant PTSD by adjunctive risperidone, olanzapine or quetiapine (Leyba and Wampler, 1998; Krashin and Oates, 1999; Monnelly and Ciraulo, 1999; Labatte and Douglas, 2000; Petty *et al.*, 2001; Prior, 2001; Sattar *et al.*, 2002; Ahearn *et al.*, 2003b; Filteau *et al.*, 2003; Hamner *et al.*, 2003a, b; Jakovljevic *et al.*, 2003; Monnelly *et al.*, 2003; States and St. Dennis, 2003; Sokolski *et al.*, 2003). There are three RCTs comparing adjunctive use of antipsychotics and placebo in treatment-resistant PTSD. Risperidone reduced irritability and intrusive thoughts (Monnelly *et al.*, 2003), and reduced psychotic symptoms (Hamner *et al.*, 2003a) in war-related PTSD. Olanzapine augmentation reduced PTSD, depressive, and sleep disorder symptoms (Stein *et al.*, 2002).

Various medications

Propranolol (Kolb *et al.*, 1984; Kinzie, 1989; Pitmann *et al.*, 2002; Vaiva *et al.*, 2003), clonidine (Kolb *et al.*, 1984; Kinzie, 1989), buspirone (Duffy and Malloy, 1994; Hamner *et al.*, 1997), naltrexone (Roth *et al.*, 1996), nalmefene (Glover, 1993), and cryptoheptadine (Gupta *et al.*, 1998; Brophy, 1991) have all been suggested helpful in PTSD. Nevertheless, controlled trials are needed before these agents can be routinely recommended. There is growing evidence that propranolol may be effective in the prophylaxis of PTSD symptoms after exposure to severe trauma (Pitmann *et al.*, 2002; Vaiva *et al.*, 2003).

The benzodiazepines do not seem effective in the treatment of PTSD. A placebo-controlled trial of alprazolam in 16 patients (10 completers) found no advantage of the medication over placebo in treating PTSD (Braun *et al.*, 1990). Also, a double-blind, crossover study showed that inositol (a second-messenger precursor that can affect the function of several neurotransmitters, including serotonin) was not effective in the treatment of PTSD (Kaplan *et al.*, 1996).

Conclusions

There is growing evidence that specific medications are effective in the treatment of PTSD. This is consistent with the modern understanding of PTSD as a medical disorder, characterized by specific psychobiological dysfunctions. In large controlled trials of antidepressants, these are effective in reducing the major symptom clusters of PTSD, comorbid depressive and anxiety symptoms, as well as associated disability. This evidence base represents a significant step forward in the management of PTSD.

Given the extent of the positive evidence for the efficacy and safety of SSRIs, these agents are currently the first-line pharmacotherapy for PTSD. A number of other antidepressants have, however, also been found useful in this disorder, and can be considered in individual patients who are suffering from side-effects associated with SSRIs or who are treatment-refractory. Antidepressant dose should be raised to maximal doses if necessary, and an initial trial of treatment should last up to 12 weeks.

In those who respond to pharmacotherapy, medication should be continued for at least a year. If response to an SSRI is insufficient, there is evidence that augmentation with an atypical antipsychotic may be effective in some patients. Other strategies include augmentation with mood stabilizers, or switching to a different SSRI or different class of medication. There is relatively little controlled work on the pharmacotherapy of treatment-refractory subjects, and additional work in this area is needed.

REFERENCES

Ahearn, E. P., Krohn, A., Connor, R. M., and Davidson, J. R. (2003a). Pharmacological treatment of post-traumatic stress disorder: a focus on antipsychotic use. *Annals of Clinical Psychiatry*, **15**, 193–200.

Ahearn, E. P., Winston, E., Mussey, M., and Howell, T. (2003b). Atypical antipsychotics, improved intrusive symptoms in patients with post-traumatic stress disorder. *Military Medicine*, **168**, x–xi.

American Psychiatric Association (1994). *Diagnostic and Statistical Manual of Mental Disorders*, 4th edn. Washington, DC: American Psychiatric Association.

Baker, D. G., Diamond, B. I., Gillette, G., *et al.* (1995). A double-blind, randomized, placebo-controlled, multi-center study of brofaromine in the treatment of posttraumatic stress disorder. *Psychopharmacology*, **122**, 386–9.

Ballenger, J. C., Davidson, J. R. T., Lecrubier, Y., *et al.* (2000). Consensus statement on posttraumatic stress disorder from the international consensus group on depression and anxiety. *Journal of Clinical Psychology*, **61** (suppl. 15), 60–6.

Berlant, J. L. (2001). Topiramate in posttraumatic stress disorder: preliminary clinical observations. *Journal of Clinical Psychiatry*, **62** (suppl. 17), 60–3.

Brady, K. T., Sonne, S. C., and Roberts, J. M. (1995). Sertraline treatment of comorbid posttraumatic stress disorder and alcohol dependance. *Journal of Clinical Psychiatry*, **56**, 502–5.

Brady, K. T., Pearlstein, T., Asnis, G. M., *et al.* (2000). Efficacy and safety of sertraline treatment of posttraumatic stress disorder, a randomized controlled trial. *Journal of the American Medical Association*, **283**, 1837–44.

Braun, P., Greenberg, D., Dasberg, H., *et al.* (1990). Core symptoms of posttraumatic stress disorder unimproved by alprazolam treatment. *Journal of Clinical Psychiatry*, **51**, 236–8.

Brophy, M. H. (1991). Cryptoheptadine for combat nightmares in posttraumatic stress disorder and dream anxiety disorder. *Military Medicine*, **156**, 100–1.

Brunello, N., Davidson, J. R. T., Deahl, M., *et al.* (2001). Posttraumatic stress disorder: diagnosis and epidemiology, comorbidity and social consequences, biology and treatment. *Neuropsychobiology*, **43**, 150–62.

Burdon, A. P., Sutjer, P. B., Foulks, E. F., *et al.* (1991). Pilot program of treatment for PTSD. *American Journal of Psychiatry*, **148**, 1269–70.

Butterfield, M. I., Becker, M. E., Connor, K. M., *et al.* (2001). Olanzapine in the treatment of post-traumatic stress disorder: a pilot study. *International Clinics in Psychopharmacology*, **16**, 197–203.

Clark, R. D., Canive, J. M., Calais, L. A., *et al.* (1999). Divalproex in post-traumatic stress disorder: an open label clinical trial. *Journal of Trauma and Stress*, **12**, 395–401.

Connor, K. M., Sutherland, S. M., Tupler, L. A., *et al.* (1999a). Fluoxetine in posttraumatic stress disorder. Randomized, double blind study. *British Journal of Psychiatry*, **175**, 17–22.

Connor, K. M., Davidson, J. R. T., Weisler, R. H., *et al.* (1999b). A pilot study of mirtazapine in posttraumatic stress disorder. *International Clinics in Psychopharmacology*, **14**, 29–31.

Davidson, J. R. T., Kudler, H., Smith, R., *et al.* (1990). Treatment of posttraumatic stress disorder with amitriptyline and placebo. *Archives of General Psychiatry*, **47**, 259–66.

Davidson, J. R. T., Roth, S., and Newman, E. (1991). Fluoxetine in posttraumatic stress disorder. *Journal of Trauma and Stress*, **4**, 419–23.

Davidson, J. R. T., Kudler, H., Erickson, W. B. *et al.* (1993). Predicting response to amitriptyline in posttraumatic stress disorder. *American Journal of Psychiatry*, **150**, 1024–9.

Davidson, J. R., Malik, M. A., and Travers, J. (1997). Structured interview for PTSD (SIP). *Depression and Anxiety*, **5**, 127–9.

Davidson, J. R. T., Weisler, R. H., Malik, M. L., *et al.* (1998a). Fluvoxamine in civilians with posttraumatic stress disorder. *Journal of Clinical Psychopharmacology*, **18**, 93–5.

Davidson, J. R. T., Weisler, R. H., Malik, M. L., and Connor, K. M. (1998b). Treatment of posttraumatic stress disorder with nefazodone. *International Clinics in Psychopharmacology*, **13**, 111–13.

Davidson, J. R. T., Pearlstein, T., and Londborg, P. (2001a). Efficacy of sertraline in preventing relapse of posttraumatic stress disorder: results of a 28-week double blind, placebo controlled study. *American Journal of Psychiatry*, **158**, 1974–81.

Davidson, J. R. T., Rothbaum, B. O., and Van der Kolk, B. A. (2001b). Multicenter, double-blind comparison of sertraline and placebo in the treatment of posttraumatic stress disorder. *Archives of General Psychiatry*, **58**, 485–92.

Davis, L. L., Nugent, A. L., Murray, J., *et al.* (2000). Trazodone treatment for chronic posttraumatic stress disorder: an open trial. *Journal of Clinical Psychopharmacology*, **20**, 159–63.

De Boer, M., Op den Velde, W., and Falger, P. J. (1992). Fluvoxamine treatment for chronic PTSD: a pilot study. *Psychotherapy and Psychosomatics*, **57**, 158–63.

Dillard, M. L., Bendfeldt, F., and Jernigan, P. (1993). Use of thioridazine in post-traumatic stress disorder. *Southern Medical Journal*, **86**, 1276–8.

Duffy, J. D. and Malloy, P. F. (1994). Efficacy of buspirone in the treatment of posttraumatic stress disorder. *Annals of Clinical Psychiatry*, **6**, 33–7.

Fesler, F. A. (1991). Valproate in combat-related posttraumatic stress disorder. *Journal of Clinical Psychiatry*, **52**, 361–4.

Filteau, M. J., Leblanc, J., and Bouchard, R. H. (2003). Quetiapine reduces flashbacks in chronic post-traumatic stress disorder. *Canadian Journal of Psychiatry*, **48**, 282–3.

Foa, E. B., Davidson, J. R. T., and Frances, A. (1999). The expert consensus guideline series: treatment of posttraumatic stress disorder. *Journal of Clinical Psychiatry*, **60** (suppl. 16), 18–23.

Foa, E. B., Keane, T. M., and Friedman, M. J. (2000). *Effective Treatments for PTSD: Practice Guidelines from the International Society for Traumatic Stress Studies*. New York, NY: Guildford Press.

Forster, P. L., Schoenfeld, F. B., and Marmar, C. R. (1995). Lithium for irritability in posttraumatic stress disorder. *Journal of Trauma and Stress*, **8**, 143–50.

Frank, J. B., Kosten, T. R., Giller, E. L., and Dan, E. (1988). A randomized clinical trial of phenelzine and imipramine for posttraumatic stress disorder. *American Journal of Psychiatry*, **145**, 1289–91.

Glover, H. (1993). A preliminary trial of nalmefene for the treatment of emotional numbing in combat veterans with posttraumatic stress disorder. *Israel Journal of Psychiatry and Related Science*, **30**, 255–63.

Gupta, S., Popli, A., Bathurst, E., *et al.* (1998). Efficacy of cryptoheptadine for nightmares associated with posttraumatic stress disorder. *Comprehensive Psychiatry*, **39**, 160–4.

Guy, W. (1976). *ECDEU Assessment Manual for Psychopharmacology*. US Department of Health, Education and Welfare publication (ADM) 76–338. Rockville, MD: National Institute of Mental Health, pp. 218–22.

Hamner, M. B. (1996). Clozapine treatment for a veteran with comorbid psychosis and PTSD. *American Journal of Psychiatry*, **153**, 841.

Hamner, M. B., Ulmer, H., and Horne, D. (1997). Buspirone potentiation of antidepressants in the treatment of PTSD. *Depression and Anxiety*, **5**, 137–9.

Hamner, M. B., Deitsch, S. E., Brodrick, P. S., Ulmer, H. G., and Loberbaum, J. P. (2003a). Quetiapine treatment in patients with post-traumatic stress disorder: an open trial of adjunctive therapy. *Journal of Clinical Psychopharmacology*, **23**, 15–20.

Hamner, M. B., Faldowski, R. A., Ulmer, H. G., *et al.* (2003b). Adjunctive risperidone treatment in post-traumatic stress disorder a preliminary controlled trial of effects on comorbid psychotic symptoms. *International Clinics in Psychopharmacology*, **18**, 1–8.

Hertzberg, M. A., Feldman, M. E., Beckham, J. C., and Davidson, J. R. T. (1996). Trial of trazodone for posttraumatic stress disorder using a multiple baseline group design. *Journal of Clinical Psychopharmacology*, **16**, 294–8.

Hertzberg, M. A., Feldman, M. E., Beckham, J. C., Moore, S. D., and Davidson, J. R. T. (1998). Open trial of nefazodone for combat-related posttraumatic stress disorder. *Journal of Clinical Psychiatry*, **59**, 460–4.

Hertzberg, M. A., Butterfield, M. I., Feldman, M. E., *et al.* (1999). A preliminary study of lamotrigine for the treatment of post-traumatic stress disorder. *Biological Psychiatry*, **45**, 1226–9.

Hertzberg, M. A., Feldman, M. E., Beckham, J. C., *et al.* (2000). Lack of efficacy for fluoxetine in PTSD: a placebo controlled trial in combat veterans. *Annals of Clinical Psychiatry*, **12**, 101–5.

Hidalgo, R., Hertzberg, M. A., Mellman, T., *et al.* (1999). Nefazodone in posttraumatic stress disorder: results from six open-label trials. *International Clinics in Psychopharmacology*, **14**, 61–8.

Jakovljevic, M., Sagud, M., and Mihaljevic-Peles, A. (2003). Olanzepine in the treatment resistant combat related post-traumatic stress disorder: a series of case reports. *Acta Psychiatrica Scandinavica*, **107**, 394–6.

Kaplan, Z., Amir, M., Schwartz, M., and Levine, J. (1996). Inositol treatment of posttraumatic stress disorder. *Anxiety*, **2**, 51–2.

Katz, R. J., Lott, M. H., Arbus, P., *et al.* (1995). Pharmacotherapy for posttraumatic stress disorder with a novel psychotropic. *Anxiety*, **1**, 169–74.

Kessler, R. C., Sonnega, A., Bromet, E., *et al.* (1995). Posttraumatic stress disorder in the national comorbidity survey. *Archives of General Psychiatry*, **52**, 1048–60.

Kessler, R. C. (2000). Posttraumatic stress disorder: the burden to the individual and to society. *Journal of Clinical Psychiatry*, **61** (suppl. 5), 4–12.

Khouzam, H. R., El Gabalauri, F., and Donnelly, N. J. (2001). The clinical experience of citalopram in the treatment of posttraumatic stress disorder: a report of two Persian Gulf War veterans. *Military Medicine*, **166**, 921–2.

Kinzie, J. D. (1989). Therapeutic approaches to traumatized Cambodian refugees. *Journal of Trauma and Stress*, **2**, 207–28.

Kitchner, I. and Greenstein, R. (1987). Low dose lithiumcarbonate in the treatment of posttraumatic stress disorder. *Military Medicine*, **150**, 378–81.

Kolb, L. C., Burris, B., and Griffith, S. (1984). Propranolol and clonidine in the treatment of the chronic posttraumatic stress of war. In: *Posttraumatic Stress Disorder: Psychological and Biological Sequelae*, ed. B. A. van der Kolk. Washington, DC: American Psychiatric Press, pp. 97–107.

Kosten, T. R., Frank, J. B., Dan, E., *et al.* (1991). Pharmacotherapy for posttraumatic stress disorder using phenelzine or imipramine. *Journal of Nervous and Mental Disease*, **179**, 366–70.

Krashin, D. and Oates, E. W. (1999). Risperidone as an adjunct therapy for posttraumatic stress disorder. *Military Medicine*, **164**, 605–6.

Labatte, L. A. and Douglas, S. (2000). Olanzepine for nightmares and sleep disturbance in post-traumatic stress disorder. *Canadian Journal of Psychiatry*, **45**, 667–8.

Leon, A. C., Olfson, M., Portera, L., *et al.* (1997). Assessing psychiatric impairment in primary care with the Sheehan disability scale. *International Journal of Psychiatry Medicine*, **27**, 93–105.

Leyba, C. M. and Wampler, T. P. (1998). Risperidone in PTSD. *Psychiatric Services*, **49**, 245–6.

Lipper, S., Davidson, J. R. T., Grady, T. A., *et al.* (1986). Preliminary study of carbamazepine in posttraumatic stress disorder. *Psychosomatics*, **27**, 849–54.

Londborg, P. D., Hegel, M. T., Goldstein, S., *et al.* (2001). Sertraline treatment of posttraumatic stress disorder: a result of 24 weeks of open label continuation treatment. *Journal of Clinical Psychiatry*, **62**, 325–31.

Macleod, A. D. (1996). Vigabatrin and posttraumatic stress disorder. *Journal of Clinical Psychopharmacology*, **16**, 190–1.

Marmar, C. R., Schoenfeld, F., Weiss, D. S., *et al.* (1996). Open trial of fluvoxamine treatment for combat related posttraumatic stress disorder. *Journal of Clinical Psychiatry*, **57** (suppl. 8), 66–72.

Marshall, R. D., Beebe, K. L., Oldham, M., *et al.* (2001). Efficacy and safety of paroxetine treatment for chronic PTSD: a fixed dose, placebo-controlled study. *American Journal of Psychiatry*, **158**, 1982–8.

Martenyi, F., Brown, E. B., Zhang, H., Koke, S. C., and Prakash, A. (2002a). Fluoxetine versus placebo in prevention of relapse in posttraumatic stress disorder. *British Journal of Psychiatry*, **181**, 315–20.

Martenyi, F., Brown, E. B., Zhang, H., Prakash, A., and Koke, S. C. (2002b). Fluoxetine versus placebo in PTSD. *Journal of Clinical Psychiatry*, **63**, 199–206.

McDougle, C. J., Southwick, S. M., Charney, D. S., *et al.* (1991). An open trial of fluoxetine in the treatment of posttraumatic stress disorder. *Journal of Clinical Psychopharmacology*, **11**, 325–7.

Mellman, T. A., David, D., and Barza, L. (1999). Nefazodone treatment and dream reports in chronic PTSD. *Depression and Anxiety*, **9**, 146–8.

Meltzer-Brody, S., Connor, K. M., Churchill, E., *et al.* (2000). Symptom specific side effects of fluoxetine in posttraumatic stress disorder. *International Clinics in Psychopharmacology*, **15**, 227–31.

Monnelly, E. P. and Ciraulo, D. A. (1999). Risperidone effects on irritable aggression in posttraumatic stress disorder. *Journal of Clinical Psychopharmacology*, **19**, 377–8.

Monnelly, E. P., Ciraulo, D. A., Knapp, C., and Keane, T. (2003). Low dose risperidone as adjunctive therapy for irritable aggression in post traumatic stress disorder. *Journal of Clinical Psychopharmacology*, **23**, 193–6.

Nagy, L. M., Morgan, C. A., Southwick, S. M., *et al.* (1993). Open prospective trial of fluoxetine for posttraumatic stress disorder. *Journal of Clinical Psychopharmacology*, **13**, 107–13.

Nagy, L. M., Southwick, S. M., and Charney, D. S. (2000). Placebo controlled trial of fluoxetine in PTSD. In: *Posttraumatic Stress Disorder: Diagnosis, Management and Treatment*, ed. D. Nutt. London: Martin Dunitz, 2000, p. 135.

Neal, L. A., Shapland, W., and Fox, C. (1997). An open trial of moclobemide in the treatment of posttraumatic stress disorder. *International Clinics in Psychopharmacology*, **12**, 231–7.

Petty, F., Brannan, S., Casada, J., *et al.* (2001). Olanzapine treatment for post-traumatic stress disorder: an open label study. *International Clinics in Psychopharmacology*, **16**, 331–7.

Pitmann, S. K., Sanders, R. M., Zusman, R. M., *et al.* (2002). Pilot study of secondary prevention of post-traumatic stress disorder with propanolol. *Biological Psychiatry*, **51**, 189–92.

Prior, T. I. (2001). Treament of post traumatic stress disorder with olanzapine. *Canadian Journal of Psychiatry*, **46**, 182.

Reist, C., Kaufmann, C. D., Haier, R. J., *et al.* (1989). A controlled trial of desipramine in 18 men with posttraumatic stress disorder. *American Journal of Psychiatry*, **146**, 513–16.

Roth, A. S., Ostroff, R. B., and Hoffman, R. E. (1996). Naltrexone as a treatment for repetitive self-injurious behaviour: an open label trial. *Journal of Clinical Psychiatry*, **57**, 233–7.

Sattar, S. P., Ucci, B., Grant, K., Bhatia, S. C., and Petty, F. (2002). Quetiapine therapy for post-traumatic stress disorder. *Annals of Pharmacotherapy*, **36**, 1875–8.

Seedat, S., Stein, D. J., and Emsley, R. A. (2000). Open trial of citalopram in adults with post-traumatic stress disorder. *International Journal of Neuropsychopharmacology*, **3**, 135–40.

Shay, J. (1992). Fluoxetine reduces explosiveness and elevates mood of Vietnam combat veterans with PTSD. *Journal of Trauma and Stress*, **5**, 97–101.

Shestatzky, M., Greenberg, D., and Lerer, B. (1988). A controlled trial of phenelzine in posttraumatic stress disorder. *Psychological Research*, **24**, 149–55.

Smajkic, A., Weine, S., Djuric-Bijedic, Z., *et al.* (2001). Sertraline, paroxetine, and venlafaxine in refugee posttraumatic stress disorder with depression symptoms. *Journal of Trauma and Stress*, **14**, 445–52.

Sokolski, K. N., Denson, T. F., Lee, R. T., and Reist, C. (2003). Quetiapine for treatment of refractory symptoms of combat related post-traumatic stress disorder. *Military Medicine*, **168**, 486–9.

Solomon, S. D. and Davidson, J. R. (1997). Trauma: prevalence, impairment, service use, and cost. *Journal of Clinical Psychiatry*, **58** (suppl. 9), 5–11.

Spitzer, R. L., Williams, J. B. W., Gibbon, M., *et al.* (1994). *Structured Clinical Interview for DSM-IV (SCID-IV)*. New York, NY: Biometric Research, New York State Psychiatric Institute.

States, J. H. and St. Dennis, C. D. (2003). Chronic sleep disruption and reexperiencing cluster of post-traumatic stress disorder symptoms are improved by olanzapine: brief review of the literature and a case based series. Primary Care Companion to the Journal of Clinical Psychiatry, **5**, 74–9.

Stein, D. J., Davidson, J. R. T., and Hewett, K. (2000a). Paroxetine in the pharmacotherapy of post-traumatic stress disorder. Cited in: Stein, D. J., Davidson, J., Seedat, S., and Beebe, K. (2003). Paroxetine in the treatment of post-traumatic stress disorder: pooled analysis of placebo-controlled studies. *Expert Opinion in Pharmacotherapy*, **4**, 1829–38.

Stein, D. J., Seedat, S., Van der Linden, G. J. H., and Zungu-Dirwayi, N. (2000b). Selective serotonin reuptake inhibitors in the treatment of post-traumatic stress disorder: a meta analysis of randomised controlled trials. *International Clinics in Psychopharmacology*, **15** (suppl. 2), S31–9.

Stein, D. J., Seedat, S., Van der Linden, G., and Kaminer, D. (2000c). Pharmacotherapy of post-traumatic stress disorder. In: *Post-Traumatic Stress Disorder, Diagnosis, Management and Treatment*. London: Martin Dunitz.

Stein, M. B., Kline, N. A., and Matloff, J. L. (2002). Adjunctive olanzepine for SSRI resistant combat related post-traumatic stress disorder: a double blind, placebo controlled study. *American Journal of Psychiatry*, **159**, 1777–9.

Stein, D. J., Davidson, J., Seedat, S., and Beebe, K. (2003). Paroxetine in the treatment of post-traumatic stress disorder: pooled analysis of placebo controlled studies. *Expert Opinion in Pharmacotherapy*, **4**, 1829–38.

Szymanski, H. V. and Olympia, J. (1991). Divalproex in posttraumatic stress disorder. *American Journal of Psychiatry*, **148**, 1086–7.

Tucker, P., Smith, K. L., Marx, B., *et al.* (2000). Fluvoxamine reduces physiologic reactivity to trauma scripts in posttraumatic stress disorder. *Journal of Clinical Psychopharmacology*, **20**, 367–72.

Tucker, P., Zaninelli, R., Yehuda, R., *et al.* (2001). Paroxetine in the treatment of chronic posttraumatic stress disorder: results of a placebo-controlled, flexible-dosage trial. *Journal of Clinical Psychiatry*, **62**, 860–8.

Vaiva, G., Ducrocq, F., Jezequel, K., *et al.* (2003). Immediate treatment with propanolol decreases post-traumatic stress disorder two months after trauma. *Biological Psychiatry*, **54**, 97–9.

Van der Kolk, B. A., Dreyfuss, D., Michaels, M., *et al.* (1994). Fluoxetine in posttraumatic stress disorder. *Journal of Clinical Psychopharmacology*, **55**, 517–22.

Vermetten, E., Vythillinga, M., Southwick, S. M., Charney, D. S., and Bremner, J. D. (2003). Long-term treatment with paroxetine increases verbal declarative memory and hippocampal volume in post-traumatic stress disorder. *Biological Psychiatry*, **54**, 693–702.

Warner, M. D., Dorn, M. R., and Peabody, C. A. (2001). Survey of the usefulness of trazodone in patients with PTSD with insomnia or nightmares. *Pharmacopsychiatry*, **34**, 128–31.

Wheaters, F. W., Keane, T. M., and Davidson, J. R. (2001). Clinician administered PTSD scale: a review of the first ten years of research. *Depression and Anxiety*, **13**, 132–56.

Wolf, M. E., Alavi, A., and Mosnaim, A. D. (1988). Posttraumatic stress disorder in Vietnam veterans, clinical and EEG findings; possible therapeutic effects of carbamazepine. *Biological Psychiatry*, **23**, 642–4.

Zisook, S., Chentsova-Dutton, Y. E., Smith-Vaniz, A., *et al.* (2000). Nefazodone in patients with treatment-refractory posttraumatic stress disorder. *Journal of Clinical Psychiatry*, **61**, 203–8.

Zohar, J., Miodownik, C., Kotler, M., *et al.* (2002). Double blind placebo-controlled study of sertraline in military veterans with post-traumatic stress disorder. *Journal of Clinical Psychopharmacology*, **22**, 190–5.

7

Evidence-based pharmacotherapy of social anxiety disorder

Carlos Blanco, Muhammad S. Raza, Franklin R. Schneier, and Michael R. Liebowitz

Columbia College of Physicians and Surgeons, New York, NY, USA

Social anxiety disorder is characterized by a fear of negative evaluation in social or performance situations and a strong tendency for sufferers to avoid feared social interactions or situations. While the Epidemiological Catchment Area (ECA) study of the early 1980s suggested that social anxiety disorder (as defined in *Diagnostic and Statistical Manual of Mental Disorders*, 3rd edition (DSM III), American Psychiatric Association (APA), 1980) affected 2–3% of women and 1–2% of men (Myers *et al.*, 1984), the more recent National Comorbidity Survey using broader DSM III-R criteria found lifetime prevalence of social anxiety disorder to be 13.3% in the USA (Kessler *et al.*, 1994). In this study, social anxiety disorder was the third most common mental disorder, following major depression and alcohol dependence. The 12-month prevalence of social anxiety disorder was also high (7.9%).

Social anxiety disorder begins early (characteristically in the mid-teens) and follows a chronic, unremitting course (Marks, 1970; Amies *et al.*, 1983; Öst, 1987). Impairments in vocational and social functioning are often substantial (Schneier *et al.*, 1992; Davidson *et al.*, 1993). The inability to work, attend school, socialize, or marry is common in clinical samples (Liebowitz *et al.*, 1985; Schneier *et al.*, 1994; Wittchen and Beloch, 1996).

The DSM-IV describes a generalized subtype. Individuals with generalized social anxiety disorder have distressing/disabling social fears in most social situations. It affects multiple aspects of life, including social, familial, and professional aspects. On the other hand, patients with non-generalized social anxiety disorder typically fear only a few social/performance situations, most commonly public speaking.

Given the prevalence and degree of impairment associated with social anxiety disorder, it is clear that the treatment of social anxiety disorder is of great public health importance. In this chapter, we first review the available evidence for the pharmacological management of social anxiety disorder, focusing on the published randomized clinical trials, which are summarized in Table 7.1. In considering the individual studies, it is important to realize that initial studies were conducted at

Table 7.1 Summary of placebo-controlled studies in the acute treatment of social anxiety disorder

Drug class	Drug	Author	Sample size	Duration	Dose (mg/day)	Response rates (%) Medication	Placebo
MAOIs	Phenelzine[a]	Liebowitz *et al.* (1992)	51	8 weeks	45–90	64	23
	Phenelzine[b]	Gelernter *et al.* (1991)	64	12 weeks	30–90	69	20
	Phenelzine[c]	Versiani *et al.* (1992)	52	8 weeks	15–90	81	27
	Phenelzine	Heimberg *et al.* (1998)	64	12 weeks	15–75	52	27
RIMAs	Moclobemide[b]	Versiani *et al.* (1992)	52	8 weeks	100–600	65	20
	Moclobemide	Katschnig *et al.* (1997)	578	12 weeks	300–600	44	32
	Moclobemide	Noyes *et al.* (1997)	506	12 weeks	75–900	35	33
	Moclobemide	Schneier *et al.* (1998)	75	8 weeks	100–400	18	14
	Moclobemide	Stein *et al.* (2002a)	390	12 weeks	450–750	43	30
	Brofaromine	van Vliet *et al.* (1992)	30	12 weeks	50–150	80	14
	Brofaromine	Fahlen *et al.* (1995)	77	12 weeks	150	78	23
	Brofaromine	Lott *et al.* (1997)	102	10 weeks	50–150	50	19
Benzodiazepines	Clonazepam	Davidson *et al.* (1993)	75	10 weeks	0.5–3	78	20
	Bromazepam	Versiani *et al.* (1997)	60	12 weeks	3–27	83	20
	Alprazolam[b]	Gelernter *et al.* (1991)	65	12 weeks	2.1–6.3	38	23
SSRIs	Fluvoxamine	van Vliet *et al.* (1994)	30	12 weeks	150	46	7
	Fluvoxamine	Stein *et al.* (1999)	86	12 weeks	202, mean dose	43	23
	Paroxetine	Stein *et al.* (1998)	182	12 weeks	10–50	55	22
	Paroxetine	Baldwin *et al.* (1999)	290	12 weeks	20–50	66	33
	Paroxetine	Allgulander (1999)		12 weeks	20–50	70	8
	Paroxetine	Liebowitz *et al.* (2002)	384	12 weeks	20–60	66	28
	Sertraline[d]	Katzelnick *et al.* (1995)	12	10 weeks	50–200	50	9
	Sertraline	van Ameringen *et al.* (2001)	204	20 weeks	50–200	53	29
	Sertraline	Liebowitz *et al.* (2003)	211	12 weeks	50–200	47	26
	Fluoxetine	Kobak *et al.* (2002)	60	8 weeks	20–60	40	30
Betablocker	Atenolol[a]	Liebowitz *et al.* (1992)	51	8 weeks	50–100	30	23
	Atenolol	Turner *et al.* (1994)	72	12 weeks	25–100	33	6
Other	Gabapentin	Pande *et al.* (1999)	69	14 week	900–3600	38	14
	Buspirone	van Vliet *et al.* (1997b)	30	12 weeks	15–30	27	13

MAOIs, monoamine oxidase inhibitors; RIMAs, reversible inhibitors of MAOIs; SSRIs, selective serotonin reuptake inhibitors.

[a] Study had three arms: phenelzine, atenolol, and placebo.

[b] Study had three arms: phenelzine, alprazolam, and placebo.

[c] Study had three arms: phenelzine, moclobemide, and placebo.

[d] Study had a crossover design.

academic centers using relatively small samples, whereas more recent studies have generally been sponsored by the pharmaceutical industry and have tended to have larger sample sizes. Because there are few head-to-head comparisons of medication treatments, we rely on meta-analytic reviews to estimate and compare the relative efficacy of different medications.

In order to provide some foundations for evidence-based pharmacological treatment of social anxiety disorder, we conducted a search using electronic databases (MEDLINE, PREMEDLINE, and PsychInfo) for the years 1980–2002 using a search strategy that combined the terms "social adj3 (anxiety or phobi$)" with "control$ or randomized or clinical trial or placebo$ or blind$." To complement the search strategy, we also consulted with other colleagues regarding published papers on trials involving medication for the treatment of social anxiety disorder. In this chapter we attempt to provide evidence-based answers to three main questions: (1) What should be the first-line pharmacological treatment of social anxiety disorder? (2) How long should this treatment last? and (3) What strategies can be used if first-line treatments fail? The overwhelming majority of the published work on the pharmacological treatment of social anxiety disorders is directed at answering the first question and our review of the literature reflects this fact. However, we also examine the limited available information regarding duration of pharmacological treatment, and suggest strategies for management of treatment-resistant cases. We conclude the review by outlining some future directions.

What is the first-line pharmacotherapy of social anxiety disorder?

Summary of published clinical trials

Monoamine oxidase inhibitors

Until recently, phenelzine was considered the best established treatment of social anxiety disorder. Direct evidence of the efficacy of phenelzine in social anxiety disorder has been provided by four double-blind placebo-controlled trials. In the first study (Liebowitz *et al.*, 1992), 85 patients meeting DSM-III criteria for social anxiety disorder were randomly assigned to phenelzine, atenolol, or placebo for 8 weeks. Patients were excluded from the study if they had current major depression or other major axis I disorders.

Patients were included in the statistical analysis ($n = 74$) if they had completed at least 4 weeks of medication with 2 weeks at therapeutic dose (atenolol 50 mg/day or phenelzine 45 mg/day). Mean doses of medication used per day were: phenelzine 75.7 mg/day (SD = 16; range 45–90) and atenolol 97.6 mg/day (SD = 10.9; range 50–100). Using a Clinical Global Impression (CGI) scale rating (Guy, 1976) score of 1–2 to define "responders," the response rate was as follows: phenelzine, 64%

(16 of 25), atenolol, 30% (7 of 23), and placebo, 23% (6 of 26). Phenelzine was significantly superior to both atenolol and placebo, but there were no significant differences between those two groups.

In a second study, Gelernter *et al.* (1991) randomized 60 patients meeting DSM-III criteria for social phobia to one of four groups for 12 weeks: phenelzine, alprazolam, placebo, or cognitive-behavioral group therapy. All patients assigned to medication (or placebo) received exposure instructions and were encouraged to engage in the feared situations. Medication dosages were increased until all social phobic symptoms had disappeared, until side-effects precluded further increases, or until the maximum medication dosage was reached. Mean doses at the end of the study were: phenelzine 55 mg/day (SD = 16) and alprazolam 4.2 mg/day (SD = 1.3). Phenelzine and alprazolam were superior to placebo on the Sheehan Disability Scale (SDS; Sheehan, 1983), which was only administered to patients in the medication groups, and phenelzine was better than all the other treatment groups on the State and Trait Anxiety Inventory (STAI) (Spielberger *et al.*, 1970). Response was defined as a final score on the social phobia subscale of the Fear Questionnaire (FQ) (Marks and Matthews, 1979) equal to or less than that established in the normative samples. Under that stringent criterion, 69% of patients on phenelzine were responders compared to 38% on alprazolam, 24% on cognitive-behavioral therapy (CBT), and 20% on placebo.

A third study, conducted by Versiani *et al.* (1992), compared phenelzine, moclobemide, and placebo in 78 patients with social anxiety disorder. The study comprised three phases, each lasting 8 weeks. Maximum allowed doses were 90 mg/day of phenelzine or 600 mg/day of moclobemide. Actual mean doses at the end of the study were: phenelzine 67.5 mg/day (SD = 15.0) and moclobemide 570.7 mg/day (SD = 55.6). At the end of the 8-week acute phase phenelzine was found to be more efficacious than placebo on all measures of social anxiety and more efficacious than moclobemide on the social avoidance subscale of the Liebowitz Social Anxiety Scale (LSAS; Liebowitz, 1987), although not on the other measures of efficacy. The LSAS, the most widely used scale for the assessment of social anxiety disorder severity in pharmacological trials, is a 24-item clinician-administered scale that rates the anxiety of individuals in a variety of social situations. Its value for total score is the sum of its two subscales ("Anxiety" and "Avoidance") and ranges from 0 to 144. The scale has been shown to have good psychometric properties (Heimberg *et al.*, 1999).

Most recently, Heimberg *et al.* (1998) randomized 133 patients to phenelzine, placebo, group CBT (CBGT) or an educational-supportive group. Efficacy was compared during a 12-week acute trial, a 6-month maintenance phase for responders to phenelzine and CBGT during the acute phase, and a 6-month treatment discontinuation phase (Liebowitz *et al.*, 1999). At the end of the 12-week acute phase, both

CBGT and phenelzine were significantly superior to the two control treatments in terms of rate of response and not different from each other (Heimberg *et al.*, 1998). On dimensional ratings, however, phenelzine appeared superior to CBGT.

Reversible inhibitors of monoamine oxidase A

Concerns regarding side-effects and safety of the standard nonreversible monoamine oxidase inhibitors (MAOIs) led to the development of the reversible MAOIs (RIMAs), for which clinical experience has shown that dietary restrictions are unnecessary.

Moclobemide

Five double-blind placebo-controlled studies of moclobemide have been published. The results of these studies indicate that, although RIMAs are considerably safer than non-reversible MAOIs, their efficacy appears inferior to that of phenelzine. As mentioned in the previous section, the first study by Versiani *et al.* (1992) compared moclobemide at a mean dose of 581 mg/day (sd = 56) with phenelzine and placebo. Moclobemide and phenelzine showed similar improvements on most measures. Phenelzine was superior on the social avoidance subscale of the LSAS, but had more severe side-effects.

The second study, a large multicenter trial (Katschnig *et al.*, 1997), randomized 578 patients to two doses of moclobemide (300 and 600 mg) or placebo in a 12-week fixed-dose study. Patients were encouraged to confront anxiety-provoking situations, although formal psychotherapy or any other concurrent treatment for social anxiety disorder was not allowed. The response rate was 47% in the 600 mg group, 41% in the 300 mg group, and 34% in the placebo group. The 600 mg dose was superior to placebo on all measures of social anxiety disorder, general anxiety, and disability. The 300 mg dose was superior to placebo on LSAS and Patient Impression of Change–Social Phobia scale. There were no differences in the side-effects of both groups of moclobemide.

In the third study (Noyes *et al.*, 1997) patients were randomized to one of five different doses of moclobemide (75, 150, 300, 600, and 900 mg) or placebo following a 12-week double-blind, fixed-dose, parallel-study design. None of the doses of moclobemide was superior to placebo.

In 1998, Schneier *et al.* conducted an 8-week flexible-dose study in 77 social phobic patients of moclobemide versus placebo. At week 8, only 7 out of 40 (17.5%) patients taking moclobemide and 5 out of 37 (13.5%) taking placebo were rated as "much" or "very much" improved in the CGI and considered responders, a nonsignificant difference.

In a recent study, Stein *et al.* (2002c) randomized 390 subjects with social anxiety disorder to moclobemide or placebo for 12 weeks. At week 12, 43% of patients in the moclobemide group and 31% in the placebo group were considered responders. Interestingly, exploratory analyses showed that the presence of a comorbid anxiety disorder was predictive of response. Subjects were offered the option of continuing for an additional 6 months of treatment. Moclobemide-treated patients continued to improve while some placebo-treated patients relapsed.

Brofaromine

Brofaromine differs from moclobemide in that, in addition to inhibiting MAO, it also inhibits the reuptake of serotonin. There are three published placebo-controlled studies of brofaromine for the treatment of social anxiety disorder. In the first study, conducted by van Vliet and colleagues (1992), 30 patients with social anxiety disorder were randomized to 12 weeks of fixed-dose (150 mg/day) brofaromine or matching placebo. Brofaromine was found to be superior to placebo on the LSAS.

Fahlen and colleagues (1995) also used a 12-week fixed-dose design to compare brofaromine 150 mg/day to placebo in 77 patients with social anxiety disorder. The brofaromine group experienced significantly greater improvement than the placebo group in both the CGI and LSAS. At endpoint 78% of the patients in the brofaromine group were much or very much improved, compared with 23% in the placebo group.

In the third published trial, Lott *et al.* (1997) compared brofaromine ($n = 52$) with placebo ($n = 50$) in a 10-week, flexible-dose design. Brofaromine was started at 50 mg and titrated up to 150 mg/day as clinically indicated. Brofaromine exceeded placebo in terms of response rates (50% versus 19%). Similarly, mean LSAS scores were significantly more improved with brofaromine (from 81.8 at baseline to 62.6 at endpoint) than with placebo (from 79.8 to 70.7). However, the endpoint LSAS score for the brofaromine group was 62.6, still in the clinical range, suggesting the need for additional treatment.

Selective serotonin reuptake inhibitors (SSRIs) and venlafaxine

The efficacy and tolerability of the SSRIs in the treatment of depression and other anxiety disorders encouraged researchers to study systematically the use of SSRIs in social anxiety disorder.

Paroxetine

Paroxetine is at present the most extensively studied and together with sertraline and venlafaxine, the only Food and Drug Administration (FDA)-approved medications for the treatment of social anxiety disorder. There are four published placebo-controlled studies of paroxetine. The first study compared paroxetine up to 50 mg/day versus placebo over 11 weeks after a 1-week single-blind placebo run-in (Stein *et al.*, 1998). On an intent-to-treat (ITT) basis with 183 patients, response rates were 55.0% for paroxetine versus 23.9% for placebo. Changes in total scores on the LSAS were 30.5 points for paroxetine versus 14.5 points for placebo, a highly significant difference.

A second multicenter flexible-dose study conducted in Europe and South Africa involved 290 randomized patients in a 12-week double-blind comparison of paroxetine 20–50 mg/day versus placebo, also after a 1-week placebo run-in period. The response rate for paroxetine was 65.7% versus 32.4% response rate for placebo (Baldwin *et al.*, 1999). Mean change on the total LSAS was 29.4 points for paroxetine versus 15.6 points for placebo. Paroxetine was statistically superior to placebo from week 4 onwards.

In a third study, conducted in Sweden by Allgulander (1999), 92 patients were randomized to paroxetine ($n = 44$) or placebo ($n = 48$) for 3 months. Patients were started at 20 mg/day of paroxetine or placebo, and the dose increased by 10 mg/day every week. Similar to the Baldwin *et al.* study, significant differences in efficacy between treatments were noted after 4 weeks, and increased through the trial. At the end of the study, 70% of the patients on paroxetine and 8% of the patients on placebo had a much or very much improved CGI and were considered responders.

In a fourth study (Liebowitz *et al.*, 2002), 384 patients meeting DSM-IV criteria for social anxiety disorder were randomly assigned to receive fixed-dose paroxetine, 20 ($n = 97$), 40 ($n = 95$), or 60 mg ($n = 97$), or placebo ($n = 95$) once daily in a 1:1:1:1 ratio for 12 weeks, after a 1-week, single-blind, placebo run-in. Patients treated with paroxetine 20 mg/day had significantly greater improvement on mean LSAS total scores compared with those receiving placebo ($P < 0.001$), while the incidence of responders, based on the CGI-I rating, was significantly greater with paroxetine, 40 mg/day, than with placebo ($P = 0.012$). Patients treated with paroxetine 20 and 60 mg also had significantly better responses on the social item of the SDS than did patients treated with placebo ($P < 0.019$).

Fluvoxamine

Two double-blind studies have investigated the efficacy of fluvoxamine in social anxiety disorder. van Vliet *et al.* (1994) randomized 30 patients to 12 weeks of fluvoxamine at 150 mg/day or placebo. Defining response as a reduction $\geq 50\%$ in LSAS, seven patients on fluvoxamine (46%) and one (7%) on placebo were classified as responders at the end of week 12. The fluvoxamine group also did better than the placebo group in a variety of other dimensions such as generalized anxiety, sensitivity rejection, and hostility.

Stein *et al.* (1999) conducted a larger, multicenter placebo-controlled study ($n = 92$) with a mean daily dose of 202 mg/day of fluvoxamine (SD = 86). The results showed that 43% on fluvoxamine responded compared with 23% on placebo, a significant difference. LSAS decreased by 22.0 points for fluvoxamine versus 7.8 points for placebo, a drug–placebo difference similar to the one found in the paroxetine trials. Fluvoxamine was also superior to placebo on the work functioning and family life/home functioning subscales but not the social life functioning subscale of the SDS.

Sertraline

The SSRI sertraline has been studied in four controlled trials. The first study consisted of a flexible-dose, crossover placebo-controlled trial that included 10 patients with generalized social anxiety disorder. Statistically significant changes were seen on the LSAS with sertraline at a mean dose of 134 mg/day (sd = 69) but not placebo (Katzelnick *et al.*, 1995). In a larger, controlled trial Van Ameringen *et al.* (2001) randomized 204 patients to sertraline or placebo for a period of 20 weeks. Sertraline was started at 50 mg/day and increased by 50 mg/day every 3 weeks after the fourth week of treatment. The maximum allowed dose was 200 mg/day. Mean dose of sertraline at the end of the study was 147 mg/day (sd = 57). Response was defined as a score of much improved or very much improved in the CGI. In the ITT sample, the response rate of sertraline (53%) was statistically superior to that of placebo (29%).

The third study (Blomhoff *et al.*, 2001) investigated the efficacy of sertraline, exposure therapy, or their combination administered alone or in combination in a general practice setting. Patients ($n = 387$) received sertraline 50–150 mg or placebo for 24 weeks. Patients were additionally randomized to exposure therapy or general medical care. Combined sertraline and exposure and sertraline were significantly superior to placebo. In contrast, no significant difference was observed between exposure- and non-exposure-treated patients.

In the most recent study, Liebowitz *et al.* (2003) randomly assigned 211 patients to sertraline or placebo using a flexible-dose design (maximum dose 200 mg/day). At week 12, sertraline produced a significantly greater reduction in the LSAS compared with placebo. Using a CGI-I score of 2 or less as a criterion for response, more patients in the sertraline group (47%) than in the placebo group (26%) were considered responders at the end of the study.

Fluoxetine

To date there is only one placebo-controlled study of fluoxetine for social anxiety disorder. Kobak *et al.* (2002) randomized 60 subjects to 14 weeks of double-blind fluoxetine or placebo. The dose was fixed at 20 mg for fluoxetine during the first 8 weeks of double-blind treatment; during the final 6 weeks, the dose could be increased every 2 weeks by 20 mg to a maximum of 60 mg/day. At the end of the study no significant differences were found between fluoxetine and placebo. In this study, there was a slightly higher than usual placebo response rate.

Venlafaxine

In a recent study (Liebowitz *et al.*, unpublished results), 279 adult outpatients with generalized social anxiety disorder were randomized to extended-release (ER) venlafaxine or placebo. The LSAS and the CGI were the primary outcome measures. Venlafaxine ER was superior to placebo on both measures. At week 12, the percentage of responders (defined as those patients who had a score of 1 or 2 on the CGI-improvement scale) and remitters (defined as individuals with an LSAS ≤ 30) was significantly greater in the venlafaxine ER group than in the placebo group (response: 44% versus 30%; remission: 20% versus 7%, respectively). Patients experienced no unexpected or serious adverse events.

There are at present other studies with SSRIs and venlafaxine that are at different stages in the prepublication process. Preliminary reports of those studies appear largely to confirm the findings presented here.

Benzodiazepines

Benzodiazepines have long been used for treatment of anxiety, although to date only clonazepam, alprazolam, and bromazepam have been studied for social anxiety disorder in the context of controlled clinical trials. Davidson *et al.* (1993) investigated the efficacy of clonazepam for the treatment of social anxiety disorder in a 10-week double-blind study with 75 patients. The mean dose of clonazepam at the end of the study was 2.4 mg/day. Seventy-eight percent of the patients on clonazepam and 20% of those on placebo had a much improved or very much improved CGI and were considered responders. The clonazepam group improved more than the placebo group in the LSAS and the work and social subscales of the SDS.

In the only published study of bromazepam for social anxiety disorder, Versiani and colleagues (1997) randomized 30 patients to bromazepam (up to 36 mg/day) or placebo for 12 weeks. Actual mean dose of bromazepam was 21 mg/day. At the end of the study, bromazepam was superior to placebo on the LSAS, CGI, SDS, and other secondary outcome measures. Main side-effects were sedation and some degree of cognitive disturbance.

There has been only one double-blind study of alprazolam, in which Gelernter *et al.* (1991) compared phenelzine, alprazolam, placebo, and CBT (see section on non-reversible MAOIs). Mean alprazolam dose was 4.2 mg/day (sd = 1.3). Only 38% of patients on alprazolam were considered responders at 12 weeks.

Other medications

Although most of the research on the pharmacological treatment of social anxiety disorder has investigated the efficacy of MAOIs, benzodiazepines, and SSRIs, there has also been some research on the efficacy of other medications. Pande *et al.* (1999) conducted a 14-week trial of gabapentin versus placebo in 69 patients with social anxiety disorder. Reductions in the LSAS were 27 points with gabapentin versus 12 points with placebo, a 15-point difference that was statistically significant. Using a rating of much or very much improved as the criterion for response, 32% of patients in the gabapentin group were classified as responders compared to 14% in the placebo group. Sixty-two percent of responders were on 3600 mg/day of gabapentin, the highest allowed dose in the study, suggesting that high doses of gabapentin may be needed to achieve response in social anxiety disorder.

Barnett *et al.* (2002) conducted an 8-week, double-blind, placebo-controlled evaluation of olanzapine. Patients ($n = 12$) were randomized to either olanzapine ($n = 7$) or placebo ($n = 5$). An initial dose of 5 mg/day was titrated to a maximum of 20 mg/day. Primary measures included the Brief Social Phobia Scale (BSPS; Davidson *et al.*, 1991) and Social Phobia Inventory (SPIN; Connor *et al.*, 2001). Seven subjects completed all 8 weeks of the study, four in the olanzapine group and three in the placebo group. In the ITT analysis, olanzapine yielded greater improvement than placebo on the primary measures: BSPS ($P = 0.02$) and SPIN ($P = 0.01$). Both treatments were well tolerated, although the olanzapine group had more drowsiness and dry mouth.

Beta-blockers are commonly used on an "as-needed" basis for non-generalized social phobia, based on anecdotal evidence and analog studies of anxious performers. While the results of controlled trials suggest that beta-blockers are not effective in the treatment of the generalized type, the subsamples of patients with non-generalized subtype have been too small to perform meaningful analysis. Beta-blockers have minimal side-effects but should be avoided in patients with asthma, diabetes, and certain heart diseases.

Finally, two studies with buspirone have failed to find differences from placebo for social anxiety disorder patients (Clark and Argas, 1991; van Vliet *et al.*, 1997b), although a small open trial suggests that it may have some value as an augmentation strategy (Van Ameringen *et al.*, 1996).

Use of the meta-analysis as a basis for evidence-based practice

Although clearly not a substitute for direct comparisons between medications within clinical trials, meta-analytic techniques can help resolve questions that individual studies may not be designed to answer. Meta-analysis is a statistical technique (or family of techniques) that allows the systematic combination and analysis of independent studies in order to obtain global estimates of the variable under investigation, such as medication efficacy. Meta-analytic techniques can provide more objective and precise (i.e., with smaller standard errors of the mean) estimates of group or subgroup treatment effects than narrative reviews of individual trials (Rosenthal, 1984). These techniques can assess the robustness of such estimates for each medication by testing for heterogeneity across studies and conducting sensitivity analyses (Greenhouse and Iyengar, 1994). They are more objective because they can eliminate the subjective differential weighting of studies that may occur in qualitative reviews. Meta-analytic techniques allow the comparison of individual studies and of a group of studies versus a single study, and take into account the number of patients and studies when generating confidence intervals (CIs) for such comparisons. Comparisons involving a smaller number of patients or studies tend to generate wider CIs, and are less likely to be statistically significant (Rosenthal, 1984; Wolff, 1986).

Meta-analysis of Gould and colleagues (1997)

The first meta-analysis to assess the efficacy of medication for social anxiety disorder was carried out by Gould and colleagues (1997). They conducted a comprehensive computer-based search using relevant key terms such as social phobia/social anxiety disorder, avoidant personality disorder, and others. The authors established *a priori* that only trials that employed a control group would be included in the meta-analysis. The authors' search included unpublished articles reported in the Dissertation Abstract database or presented in relevant conferences. In addition, they reviewed the reference sections of articles located using the prior references. The authors initially identified 41 articles, but only 24 finally met inclusion/exclusion criteria. Reasons for exclusion were lack of adequate comparison group and use of mixed samples (i.e., study patients with social anxiety disorder and patients with other anxiety disorders, such as agoraphobia or panic disorder). Of the 24 studies included, only 10 had a treatment arm that included medication, one of which was an interim report of a larger study.

One of the problems encountered by Gould *et al.* was the variety of measures used to assess treatment outcome in studies of social anxiety disorder. Those measures included behavioral avoidance tests, self-report questionnaires, blind and unblinded clinician-rated measures of change and physiological measures (e.g., heart rate or galvanic skin response). Following the recommendation of Rosenthal (1991), the authors decided to average across effect sizes when several dependent measures for the same construct were reported in a study. If a measure was mentioned in the Methods section but not presented in the Results section of a study, it was assumed to be non-significant and assigned a $P = 0.5$, and an effect size was

Table 7.2 Meta-analysis of Gould *et al.* (1997)

Drug group	Effect size	Dropout rate	Number of studies
MAOIs	0.64	13.8%	5
Benzodiazepines	0.72	12%	2
SSRIs	2.73	3%	2
Beta-blockers	−0.08	−22%	3
Buspirone	−0.5	22%	1

MAOIs, monoamine oxidase inhibitors; SSRIs, selective serotonin reuptake inhibitors.

subsequently derived using conventional methods. Effect sizes used Glass's delta procedure. Glass's delta is identical to the more frequently used Cohen's, except that in Glass's delta the denominator is the standard deviation of the control group, instead of the overall standard deviation of the treatment and control groups. In addition to calculation of effect sizes, the authors assessed the heterogeneity of effect sizes across studies using the chi-square test (Wolff, 1986).

Gould *et al.* found that the mean effect size for pharmacotherapy of social anxiety disorder was 0.62, with a 95% CI of 0.42–0.82. Because this CI did not include 0, it indicated that pharmacotherapy was superior to placebo. The overall dropout rate for all studies was 13.7%. The authors also reported effect sizes and dropout rates for groups of medications. The effect size of MAOIs (which included phenelzine and moclobemide) was 0.64, with a dropout rate of 13.8%. Benzodiazepines had an effect size of 0.72 and a dropout rate of 12%. The meta-analysis also included two studies conducted with SSRIs: the first study, conducted with fluvoxamine, had an effect size of 2.73 and a dropout rate of 3%, whereas the second one, a small crossover study, of sertraline had an effect size of 1.05, with zero dropout rate. In contrast, atenolol and buspirone were not different from placebo. The results of this meta-analysis are summarized in Table 7.2.

One interesting feature of this meta-analysis is that the authors assessed the effect of gender on effect size. Simple regression analysis found no difference between sex distribution and effectiveness of treatment. However, it is important to note that the studies did not report results separately for males and females and the meta-analysis assessed the pharmaco- and psychotherapy studies together, possibly introducing confounders in the analysis.

The authors also included a separate meta-analysis of long-term treatment outcome. Only one pharmacotherapy study reported data on long-term follow up. Although those data suggested a limited continued improvement, they have to be interpreted with great caution due to the obvious limitations. Gould *et al.* also conducted a comparison of pharmacotherapy versus CBT versus combined treatment.

They did not find any significant differences between the three conditions. However, given the differences in the control groups between pharmaco- and psychotherapy studies, and the limited statistical power of test of differences in effect sizes, these results are difficult to interpret.

Meta-analysis of Van der Linden and colleagues (2000)

A second meta-analysis was reported by Van der Linden and colleagues (Van der Linden *et al.*, 2000). In that paper, the authors first reviewed the efficacy of the SSRIs for social anxiety disorder using 25 reports of pharmacological clinical trials, eight of which were placebo-controlled. In the second part of the paper, they used the data of the randomized trials to conduct a formal meta-analysis. They estimated the effect size of the SSRIs and also presented data on the effect size of placebo-controlled trials of MAOIs, RIMAs, and clonazepam.

One innovative aspect of this meta-analysis is that it reported estimates using two measures of effect size, the odds ratio (OR) and Cohen's *d* (the mean difference between the treatments divided by the pretreatment standard deviation of the placebo and control groups combined), probably the two most commonly used measures in meta-analytic reviews. The OR was used to compare the percentage of responders in the drug and placebo drugs. Cohen's *d* was used to compare the improvement in LSAS scores between the active treatment and placebo groups.

Van der Linden and colleagues found a wide range in the estimates of effect size of the medications. However, with the exception of two moclobemide studies, all other studies showed superiority of drug over placebo. The results were consistent across the two measures of effect sizes used, increasing the credibility of their results. Although formal comparisons between drug classes were not performed, it appeared that SSRIs ($n = 8$) and clonazepam ($n = 1$) had the largest effect sizes.

One limitation of this study is that it did not report the search strategy, thus making it difficult to replicate. Similarly, inclusion and exclusion criteria were not clearly specified and may have been different from those used in the Gould study. However, the van der Linden study confirmed the initial finding of the Gould meta-analysis of large effect sizes of SSRIs and benzodiazepines.

Meta-analysis of Fedoroff and Taylor (2001)

A third meta-analysis, conducted by Fedoroff and Taylor (2001), included both psychological and pharmacological treatment of social phobia. The authors used computerized searches complemented by manual searches and consultation with social anxiety researchers and relevant drug companies. Criteria used to identify eligible trials included: participants had received a DSM-III, DSM-III-R, or DSM-IV diagnosis of generalized social anxiety disorder; four or more patients had been included in the study; sufficient information was provided to calculate effect sizes;

outcome measures were broad measures of social anxiety disorder with acceptable levels of reliability and validity. The authors examined drug classes (e.g., SSRIs) rather than specific medications (e.g., paroxetine or sertraline). However, they conducted tests of heterogeneity to determine whether there were any outlying effect sizes within these treatment conditions. Treatment conditions were only examined if there were four or more trials in that condition, as the authors considered this the minimal number of trials needed to make meaningful comparisons across conditions.

Effect size was calculated using Cohen's *d* and individual effect sizes were weighted by the sample size to obtain overall estimates of effect size for each condition. This procedure, not reported in previous meta-analyses of social anxiety disorder, allows for effect sizes of larger trials to make a greater contribution than effect sizes from small trials. Because ITT data were not available for many studies, the authors conducted their analyses based on completer data. In contrast to previous meta-analyses, which only included randomized trials, Fedoroff and Taylor also included uncontrolled trials.

One important innovation of this meta-analysis was the use of the random-effect model, which assumes that studies analyzed are a random sample of the studies that could have been conducted, allowing for a generalization of the results. In contrast, the fixed-effects model assumes that the studies included constitute the whole population of studies and thus does not allow for the generalization of the results beyond those studies (the random-effects model is generally preferred at present). In addition, Fedoroff and Taylor conducted the first comparison of effect sizes across drug classes by the use of 95% CIs. CIs that do not overlap are indicative of significant differences between the two groups compared, whereas overlapping intervals indicate that the differences are not significant.

Because there are reports suggesting that observer-rated measures tend to yield larger effect sizes than self-report measures, the authors performed separate meta-analyses for the two types of measure. Similar to the procedure used by Gould *et al.*, when several measures were reported in a trial, a composite measure was derived by averaging the effect sizes of the individual measures. Before constructing the combined effect sizes, the authors tested for within-study differences in effect sizes using different outcome measures and found those differences were not significant.

Federoff and Taylor found a remarkable homogeneity of effect sizes within each drug class, with only three studies generating heterogeneity according to the chi-square test for heterogeneity. In all three cases the effect sizes of the heterogeneous studies were greater than those of the other studies in their drug classes. The authors also found that the various drug treatments differed in terms of sex but not in terms of age. However, a one-way analysis of covariance (ANCOVA) using the (unweighted) effect size of the study as the outcome variable and the treatment condition and percentage of women in the study as covariates indicated that gender did not influence outcome.

Somewhat surprisingly, the authors also found that the CIs of double-blind and non-double-blind and controlled versus uncontrolled and group versus individual trials overlapped with one another, indicating no difference in effect size. Similarly, they also found that there were no differences in the rates of dropout by drug class. Consistent with the two previous meta-analyses, using self-report measures they found that the largest mean effect sizes for the acute treatment were for benzodiazepines and SSRIs, which were not significantly different from each other. However, when examining the 95% CI, there was no overlap between the CIs of benzodiazepines and the CI of MAOIs, cognitive therapy, or cognitive therapy with exposure, indicating a greater treatment efficacy for benzodiazepines. The CI of SSRIs, however, did overlap with these treatment conditions, indicating no difference between treatments. Results obtained using the observer-rated measures were in the same direction, but did not show any significant differences across treatment conditions.

Based on those results, Fedoroff and Taylor concluded that pharmacotherapies, particularly benzodiazepines and SSRIs, performed better than psychotherapies in the acute treatment of social anxiety disorder. There were not enough available data to evaluate the long-term course of treatment with pharmacotherapy.

Blanco and colleagues (in press)

We recently conducted a meta-analysis of the placebo-controlled studies of pharmacotherapy for social phobia using articles published between January 1980 and June 2001. In order to locate articles, we conducted computerized and manual searches of bibliographies in published manuscripts and consulted researchers in the treatment of social anxiety disorder. Following suggested guidelines, two authors extracted data independently. Relevance of examined papers was assessed using a hierarchical approach based on title, abstract, and the full manuscript. When the reviewers disagreed on assignment, the study was included in the next screening level, except at the last level, where decisions were made by consensus.

In order to improve the comparability of the results, it was decided *a priori* to use the LSAS (Liebowitz, 1987) as the primary outcome measure for the meta-analysis. The proportion of responders (defined as a score of 1 or 2 in the CGI) in each study was used as a secondary measure. Effect sizes for the LSAS were estimated using Hedges *g*, an unbiased measure of the difference between two means (Hedges and Olkin, 1985). Effect sizes for the proportion of responders were estimated using the OR (Fleiss, 1994).

For trials that included more than one dose of medication in their design (Katschnig *et al.*, 1997; Noyes *et al.*, 1997) a statistical adjustment was used to generate a unique effect size for each study (Glesser and Olkin, 1994). This adjustment compensates for the stochastic dependence of the effect sizes (one effect size per dose level) within each study to provide unbiased estimates of overall effect size within a study. Similar to Fedoroff and Taylor, we used a random-effects model for the estimation of effect sizes. The Q statistic was used to assess homogeneity across trials. Innovative features of this meta-analysis included the use of ITT data and the assessment of publication bias, i.e., testing whether studies with positive results were more likely to have been published than negative trials.

The authors also conducted a quality assessment of the clinical trials to evaluate whether standard procedures such as randomization of patients had been conducted, blind maintained throughout the trial, and appropriate statistical analyses performed. Finally, another innovative aspect of this meta-analysis was the performance of power analyses for the comparison between treatments.

Overall, the quality of clinical trials was very high. Our analysis found that clonazepam, based on a single study, had the largest mean effect size of all medications. The effect sizes of SSRIs and phenelzine were similar to each other and numerically (but not statistically) smaller than those of clonazepam. Because we found heterogeneity of effect sizes between moclobemide and brofaromine we estimated mean effect sizes for both medications separately. While the effect size of brofaromine was similar to that of SSRIs and MAOIs, the effect size of moclobemide was substantially lower. There were no significant differences across the three SSRIs that had been tested in placebo-controlled studies: paroxetine, sertraline, and fluvoxamine. Gabapentin, which had not been included in previous meta-analysis, had an effect size similar to that of the SSRIs, suggesting that further research on the efficacy of this medication for the treatment of social anxiety disorder might be warranted. The results were consistent across measures, i.e., LSAS and proportion of responders using the CGI. The effect sizes of the Blanco *et al.* meta-analysis are summarized in Table 7.3.

Surprisingly, there was no indication of publication bias, i.e., no evidence that papers reporting positive results had been published while those with negative results had been less likely to be published. Power was generally low, due mostly to relatively low number of studies in all categories, except the SSRIs (although power was also low to test individual SSRIs).

Choice of medication

The evidence from the reviewed clinical trials and meta-analyses suggests that a number of medications are efficacious in the treatment of social anxiety disorder. Moreover, based on the meta-analysis of Fedoroff and Taylor, they appear to be

Table 7.3 Effect sizes of meta-analysis of Blanco *et al.* (in press)

Drug	Number of studies	Effect size based on LSAS (95% CI)	Heterogeneity (LSAS)	Effect size based on the CGI (95% CI)	Heterogeneity based on the CGI
SSRIs	6	0.65 (0.50–0.81)	No	4.1 (2.01–8.41)	Yes
Benzodiazepines	2	1.54 (−0.03–3.32)	Yes	16.61 (10.18–27.39)	Yes
Phenelzine	3	1.02 (0.50–1.02)	Yes	5.53 (2.56–11.94)	Yes
Moclobemide	4	0.30 (0.00–0.6)	Yes	1.84 (0.89–3.82)	Yes
Brofaromine	3	0.66 (0.38–0.94)	No	6.96 (2.39–20.29)	No
Gabapentin[a]	1	0.78 (0.29–1.27)	Not applicable	3.78 (1.88–7.54)	Not applicable
Atenolol	2	0.10 (−0.44–0.64)	No	1.36 (0.87–2.12)	No
Buspirone[a,b]	1	0.02 (−0.70–0.73)	Not applicable	–	Not applicable

LSAS, Liebowitz Social Anxiety Scale; CI, confidence interval; CGI, Clinical Global Impression scale; SSRIs, selective serotonin reuptake inhibitors.

[a] At least two studies are necessary to test for heterogeneity.

[b] Study did not use the CGI.

superior to psychotherapy, at least in the acute phase of the treatment. Those data are consistent with recent findings of a randomized study of phenelzine versus cognitive-behavioral psychotherapy (Heimberg *et al.*, 1998), although more direct comparison would be highly desirable to confirm those findings.

Despite the use of slightly different approaches and inclusion criteria for the clinical trials, the meta-analyses also consistently indicate that benzodiazepines are the medication with the largest effect size for the treatment of social anxiety disorder independently of whether the analysis included only the placebo-controlled or also the open-label studies. Other medications with moderate to large side-effects included the SSRIs, phenelzine, brofaromine, and gabapentin. Based on those results, what should the practicing clinician do? We believe that choice of medication should be guided by three principles: (1) highest efficacy, based on the effect size of the medication (or medication group) and its reproducibility (determined by number of clinical trials published and overall number of patients in those clinical trials); (2) lowest potential for side-effects of the drug; and (3) ability to treat commonly comorbid conditions. In addition, special considerations pertaining to each individual patient, such as presence of specific comorbidity or contraindications, should always be taken into account.

Based on those considerations, we believe that at present SSRIs constitute the first-line medication treatment of social anxiety disorder. They have been more extensively tested in clinical trials than any other medication for social anxiety

disorder, have a moderate effect size, are generally well tolerated, and are efficacious for the treatment of other disorders that are frequently comorbid with social
anxiety disorders, including major depressive disorder and other anxiety disorders.
It is important to note, however, that although double-blind studies support the
efficacy of paroxetine, sertraline, and fluvoxamine, there are no published placebo-
controlled studies of citalopram, and a recent study found no significant differences
between fluoxetine and placebo (Kobak *et al.*, 2002). The serotonin-norepinephrine
(noradrenaline) reuptake inhibitor venlafaxine also appears to have efficacy based
on preliminary reports and FDA approval.

Benzodiazepines constitute a reasonable alternative to SSRIs as a first-line treatment for social anxiety disorder. Clonazepam and bromazepam, considered separately, have shown large effect sizes in the individual randomized trials. However,
as shown in our meta-analysis, the results of those two studies show heterogeneity
of effect sizes. When combined into a single category, the CI for the effect size of
clonazepam and bromazepam included 0, suggesting that the estimates of their
effect sizes are unstable. In addition, the only published study of alprazolam did
not show significant differences from placebo, raising further reservations to the
use of benzodiazepines as first-line treatment, although it is possible that there
may be intragroup differences in their efficacy for the treatment of social anxiety
disorder.

Part of the difficulty in assessing the effect size of benzodiazepines is that it is based
on only three controlled trials that included a relatively low number of patients.
Furthermore, benzodiazepines, in contrast to SSRIs, are not efficacious in the treatment of some of the psychiatric disorders, such as major depressive disorder, that are
frequently comorbid with social anxiety disorder. One additional consideration in
the use of benzodiazepines is that epidemiological and clinical studies have shown
high comorbidity of social anxiety disorder with alcohol abuse and dependence.
However, there is no evidence that use of prescribed benzodiazepines is associated
with abuse liability in individuals without a history of substance abuse disorders.
Overall, we think that these considerations make benzodiazepines a less preferred
initial option for most patients.

Another alternative would be the use of phenelzine (or another irreversible
MAOI, although those have been less systematically studied). Until relatively
recently, phenelzine was considered the gold standard in the treatment of social
anxiety disorder. However, results from the meta-analyses suggest that its efficacy is
not superior to that of the SSRIs or clonazepam, although it has never been directly
compared to those medications. Phenelzine is often well tolerated, and, as shown
by the Gould meta-analysis, does not seem to be associated with higher dropout
rates than other medications. The main barrier to treatment with phenelzine and

other irreversible MAOIs is the need for the patient to follow a low-tyramine diet, and the subsequent risk of hypertensive crisis if the diet is not followed. In addition, although clinical experience with MAOIs is extensive, relatively few patients with social anxiety disorder have been treated in clinical trials using phenelzine compared to SSRIs. Thus, there is less systematic evidence to support the use of MAOIs than the use of SSRIs as first-line treatment.

Gabapentin showed an effect size similar to those of the SSRIs in the only published trial and it is safe and generally well tolerated. Therefore, it is a promising alternative to the other agents. However, the gabapentin trial is somewhat unusual in that response rates to placebo and drug were substantially lower than in other clinical trials of social anxiety disorder. It is possible that the sample may have had some atypical characteristics that may account for this pattern of response. In any case, further studies to confirm the efficacy of gabapentin in social anxiety disorder appear warranted.

The RIMA brofaromine also appeared as a promising alternative. Unfortunately, its development was stopped by the manufacturer before marketing, for reasons unrelated to its safety or efficacy in social anxiety. The results of our analyses suggest that brofaromine may have found a therapeutic niche in the treatment of social phobia. In contrast, the clinical trials of moclobemide provide much less support for its use, although it is probably efficacious in some patients.

How long should pharmacotherapy of social anxiety disorder continue?

Although the research to date has provided answers to the most pressing questions regarding acute treatment of social anxiety disorder, a number of questions remain unanswered. Only recently have researchers started to conduct the studies that can provide evidence-based answers for those questions. One important question, frequently asked by patients, is how long to continue in treatment once they respond to medication. A number of studies have looked at that question.

Versiani *et al.* (1992) reported 50% loss of treatment gains in the 2 months following discontinuation of phenelzine responders under double-blind conditions after 16 weeks of treatment. Liebowitz *et al.* (1992) also reported relapse in one-third of patients over 2 months following discontinuation after 16 weeks of phenelzine treatment. In our initial collaborative study, responders to 12 weeks of acute treatment were maintained on phenelzine for an additional 6 months, during which there was a 23% relapse (Liebowitz *et al.*, 1999). Continued responders were then discontinued from medication and followed for an additional 6 months, during which time there was an additional 30% relapse. Supporting the concept that concomitant CBT may help maintain the gains following cessation of medication is the finding of Gerlernter *et al.* (1991), who reported no loss of phenelzine's effectiveness after 2 months of untreated follow-up. In this study, unlike those of Versiani *et al.* or Liebowitz *et al.*, cited above, phenelzine was combined with detailed self-exposure instructions during acute treatment.

In the first study of discontinuation using an SSRI, patients were treated with paroxetine in an 11-week open trial followed by 12 weeks of double-blind placebo-controlled discontinuation (Stein *et al.*, 1996). Relapse rates were 13% with continued paroxetine versus 63% with gradual switch to placebo. Given that the discontinuation of paroxetine was gradual, and placebo was substituted, the high relapse rate may indicate that 11 weeks is too brief a treatment period for most patients. In a more recent study, Stein *et al.* (2002a) treated 437 patients with social anxiety disorder with paroxetine for 12 weeks. Of those, 323 responded and agreed to continue treatment for an additional 24 weeks. Patients continuing treatment were randomized to paroxetine ($n = 162$) or placebo ($n = 161$). Two hundred and fifty-seven patients completed the study (136 paroxetine-treated and 121 placebo-treated patients). Significantly fewer patients relapsed in the paroxetine group than in the placebo group (14% versus 39%; OR 0.24; 95% CI 0.14–0.43; $P < 0.001$). Furthermore, at the end of the study, a significantly greater proportion of patients in the paroxetine group showed improvement as shown on the CGI global improvement rating compared with the placebo group (78% versus 51%; OR 3.66; 95% CI 2.22–6.04; $P < 0.001$).

In another study 203 patients were randomized to sertraline or placebo. Sertraline was superior to placebo with response rates of 53% versus 29% in the ITT sample at the end of 20 weeks (Van Ameringen *et al.*, 2001). Responders to sertraline were entered into a 24-week discontinuation trial, where they were randomized to continue on drug or switch abruptly to placebo (Walker *et al.*, 2000). Relapse rates were 4% for patients continued on sertraline versus 36% for those switched to placebo, a significant difference. An additional 20% of patients switched to placebo were prematurely discontinued due to adverse events versus 0% for those continued on sertraline. Total premature discontinuation by the end of the 24-week follow-up was 60% for patients switched to placebo versus only 12% for those continued on sertraline, a highly significant difference. Thus, these data again suggest that even after 5 months of SSRI treatment, relapse rates are high after discontinuation.

Although data are still limited, the available evidence suggests that discontinuation of medication after 12–20 weeks of treatment results in an increased risk for relapse compared to maintenance on medication after that time period. Whether longer treatment periods with medication or the addition of psychotherapy can protect against such relapse is unknown at present. At present it appears reasonable to maintain treatment for at least 3–6 months after the patient responds to treatment, with longer periods considered in individual cases, due to the lack of available systematic evidence.

What is the best pharmacotherapy approach to resistant social anxiety disorder?

The first question in the management of treatment-resistant cases is how to define them. Stein *et al.* (2002b) recently analyzed pooled data from three placebo-controlled studies of paroxetine, including a total of 829 patients, to determine predictors of response. Demographic, clinical, baseline disability, duration of treatment, and trial variables were included. After adjusting for the other covariates, only duration of treatment was a predictor of treatment response. The authors found that 46 (27.7%) of 166 non-responders to paroxetine at week 8 were responders at week 12. The authors concluded that an optimal trial of medication should continue beyond 8 weeks. At present there is no information on the probability of response of patients who have not responded by week 12. It appears reasonable to try a new medication if the patient has not shown any response at that time. If there has been a partial response, it may be preferable to try to augment the response using another efficacious medication, such as a benzodiazepine or neurontin, although no study has systematically tested any of those strategies.

Reasons for treatment resistance

As with any other medical condition, the next step is to identify the sources of non-response. Again, there is a paucity of information to guide this search. Probably an important source of therapeutic failure is non-adherence to treatment, which may have resulted in suboptimal medication doses or duration of treatment. If that is the case, the reasons for departures from recommended treatment should be explored and remedied.

A second potential source of treatment resistance is the presence of a comorbid psychiatric disorder. Clinical trials tend to exclude patients with comorbid disorders. Those that allow for comorbidity do not report treatment response stratified by presence or absence of comorbidity. Thus, there is a lack of systematic knowledge regarding the influence of comorbidity on treatment response. We recently completed an open-label study of citalopram in patients with primary social anxiety disorder and comorbid depression. Sixty-seven percent of patients completed the study, and the response rate was 67% for social anxiety disorder and 76% for major depressive disorder (Schneier *et al.*, 2003). Therefore, in that study response rates were similar to those found in clinical trials without comorbid depression. Whether the presence or absence of other comorbid disorders will result in similar (lack of) impact is unknown.

Other specific reasons for decreased efficacy may include comorbid medical conditions or individual pharmacokinetic characteristics (such as in rapid metabolizers or drug interactions).

Management strategies

Augmentation with medication

To the best of our knowledge, only two studies have partially addressed augmentation strategies. In the first study, conducted by Van Ameringen *et al.* (1996), 10 patients with generalized social phobia and who had obtained only partial response to an adequate trial of an SSRI were studied for 8 weeks. At endpoint the mean dose of buspirone was 45.0 mg/day (sD = 10.8) and the dose range was 30–60 mg/day. Seven (70%) patients were considered responders with a CGI of 1 or 2 and 3 (30%) patients were considered non-responders. However, the small sample size and the lack of control conditions limit the interpretability of this study.

Stein and colleagues (2001) reported a double-blind, placebo-controlled study about pindolol potentiation of paroxetine for social anxiety disorder. Patients on paroxetine were randomly assigned to receive either 5 mg of pindolol or placebo for 4 weeks. Responders were identified by a CGI rating of change as "very much improved" relative to the start of treatment. The results showed that pindolol was not superior to placebo for augmenting the actions of paroxetine. In this study pindolol was not used in treatment-resistant cases. However, the fact that it failed to increase response rates in non-resistant patients and that there are no clinical trials supporting the efficacy of beta-blockers in generalized social anxiety disorder suggests that it may not be a first-line agent for augmentation.

Pharmacological alternatives for augmentation include any combination of drugs with demonstrated efficacy for social anxiety disorder, provided their combined use is not contraindicated. Thus, an SSRI plus clonazepam or gabapentin, or clonazepam plus phenelzine, appear as reasonable options. In contrast, the combination of phenelzine and an SSRI is absolutely contraindicated. However, these recommendations are purely based on clinical experience. There are no systematic data to evaluate the efficacy of those combinations.

Psychotherapy

Although not the topic of this review, there is substantial evidence demonstrating the efficacy of CBT for social anxiety disorder. Therefore, it is intuitively appealing to combine, either simultaneously or sequentially, two treatments that are efficacious in their own right (medication and psychotherapy) and that probably have very different mechanisms of action. Very preliminary data from our group suggest that this may be a beneficial strategy. However, much more evidence is needed to confirm these initial findings.

The treatment of non-generalized social anxiety disorder

This review has focused on social anxiety disorder's generalized subtype, which is most impairing and is the most common form among treatment-seeking patients. The non-generalized subtype, most commonly characterized by phobia of public speaking or other performance situations, has been much less studied. Prominent sympathetic nervous system symptoms of racing heart, tremor, and sweating in anxious performers led early researchers to study the acute effects of beta-adrenergic blockers in these "analog" subjects, who were not formally assessed for social anxiety disorder. Nearly a dozen small single-dose placebo-controlled crossover studies in the 1970s and 1980s reported efficacy for propranolol and other beta-blockers for anxious musical performers, public speakers, and students taking a test (see Potts and Davidson, 1995, for review). On this basis, beta-blockers are currently widely used on an as-needed basis for persons with non-generalized social anxiety disorder, since as-needed medication is often preferred by patients who fear predictable and occasional performance situations.

Benzodiazepines have also seen clinical use in this population, and may have the benefit of decreasing the anticipatory anxiety, such as not being able to sleep the night before a performance. However, some patients find that the benzodiazepine effects of sedation or cognitive slowing may outweigh their anxiolytic benefits. Although SSRIs and MAOIs have not been studied in non-generalized subtype samples, clinical impressions suggest that, when used daily, they may also benefit performance anxiety.

Conclusions

Over the last few years the empirical basis for the pharmacological treatment of social anxiety disorder has expanded substantially and there are now a number of medications with substantial evidence of treatment efficacy. Future, cumulative meta-analyses should continue to update our base of knowledge about the relative efficacy of different medications in the treatment of social anxiety disorder. At the same time, as pointed out in the second section of this review, there are still important gaps in our knowledge. Those gaps constitute important second-generation questions for research in social anxiety disorder. Another area of future research should be the progressive linkage of biological findings and therapeutic strategies, so that treatment becomes not only evidence-based, but also theory-driven. Unfortunately, our understanding of the biology of social anxiety disorder is quite limited.

Finally, although social anxiety disorder often begins in childhood or adolescence, only one published randomized trial, recently completed by the Research Unit on Pediatric Psychopharmacology Anxiety Study Group (2001), has specifically addressed pharmacotherapy in these populations, and preliminary results from another study appear to confirm these findings (Wagner, 2003). Early treatment of social anxiety disorder in children holds theoretical promise for reduction of long-term morbidity and comorbidity. Carefully designed studies are needed to assess the risks and benefits of medication treatment in social anxiety disorder and to compare it to other alternatives such as age-adapted CBT.

Acknowledgment

This research was supported in part by grant DA-00482, a NARSAD Young Investigator Award, and a grant from the Alcohol Beverage Medical Research Foundation (Dr. Blanco).

REFERENCES

Allgulander, C. I. (1999). Paroxetine in social anxiety disorder: a randomized placebo-controlled study. *Acta Psychiatrica Scandinavica*, **100**, 196–8.

American Psychiatric Association (1980). *Diagnostic and Statistical Manual for Mental Disorders*, 3rd edn. Washington, DC: American Psychiatric Press.

Amies, P. L., Gelder, M. G., and Shaw, P. M. (1983). Social phobia: a comparative clinical study. *British Journal of Psychiatry*, **142**, 174–9.

Baldwin, D., Bobes, J., Stein, D. J., Scharwaechter, I., and Faure, M. (1999). Paroxetine in social phobia/social anxiety disorder: randomized, double-blind, placebo-controlled study. *British Journal of Psychiatry*, **175**, 120–6.

Barnett, S. D., Kramer, M. L., Casat, C. D., Connor, K. M., and Davidson, J. R. (2002). Efficacy of olanzapine in social anxiety disorder: a pilot study. *Journal of Psychopharmacology*, **16**, 365–8.

Blanco, C., Antia, S., and Liebowitz, M. R. (2002). Pharmacotherapy of social anxiety disorder. *Biological Psychiatry*, **51**, 109–20.

Blanco, C., Schneier, F. R., Schmidt, A. B., *et al.* (2003). Pharmacological treatment of social anxiety disorder: a meta-analysis. *Depression and Anxiety*, **18**, 29–40.

Blomhoff, S., Haug, T. T., Hellstrom, K., *et al.* (2001). Randomised controlled general practice trial of sertraline, exposure therapy and combined treatment in generalised social phobia. *British Journal of Psychiatry*, **179**, 23–30.

Clark, D. and Agras, W. S. (1991). The assessment and treatment of performance anxiety in musicians. *American Journal of Psychiatry*, **148**, 598–605.

Connor, K. M., Kobak, K. A., Churchill, L. E., Katzelnick, D., and Davidson, J. R. (2001). Mini-SPIN: a brief screening assessment for generalized social anxiety disorder. *Depression and Anxiety*, **14**, 137–40.

Davidson, J. R. T., Potts, N. L. S., Richichi, E. A., *et al.* (1991). The Brief Social Phobia Scale. *Journal of Clinical Psychiatry*, **52** (suppl. 11), 48–51.

Davidson, J. R. T., Potts, N., Richichi, E., *et al.* (1993). Treatment of social phobia with clonazepam and placebo. *Journal of Clinical Psychopharmacology*, **13**, 423–8.

Fahlen, T., Nilsson, H. L., Bog, K., Humble, H., and Pauli, U. (1995). Social phobia: the clinical efficacy and tolerability of the monoamine oxidase-A and serotonin uptake inhibitor brofaromine. *Acta Psychiatrica Scandinavica*, **92**, 351–8.

Fedoroff, I. C. and Taylor, S. (2001). Psychological and pharmacological treatments of social phobia; a meta-analysis. *Journal of Clinical Psychopharmacology*, **21**, 311–23.

Fleiss, J. L. (1994). Measures of effect size for categorical data. In: *The Handbook of Research Synthesis*, ed. H. Cooper and L. Hedges. New York, NY: Russell Sage Foundation, pp. 245–60.

Gelernter, C. S., Uhde, T. W., Cimbolic, P., *et al.* (1991). Cognitive-behavioral and pharmacological treatments of social phobia: a controlled study. *Archives of General Psychiatry*, **48**, 938–45.

Glesser, L. J. and Olkin, I. (1994). Stochastically dependent effect sizes. In: *The Handbook of Research Synthesis*, ed. H. Cooper and L. Hedges. New York, NY: Russell Sage Foundation, pp. 339–56.

Gould, R. A., Buckminister, S., Pollack, M. H., Otto, M. W., and Yap, L. (1997). Cognitive-behavioral and pharmacological treatments of social phobia: a meta-analysis. *Clinical Psychology: Science and Practice*, **4**, 291–306.

Greenhouse, J. B. and Iyengar, S. (1994). Sensitivity analysis and diagnostics. In: *The Handbook of Research Synthesis*, ed. H. Cooper and L. Hedges. New York, NY: Russell Sage Foundation, pp. 383–98.

Guy, W. (1976). *ECDEU Assessment Manual for Psychopharmacology*. US Department of Health, Education and Welfare publication ADM 76-338. Rockville, MD: National Institute of Mental Health, pp. 217–22.

Hedges, L. V. and Olkin, I. (1985). *Statistical Methods for Meta-Analysis*. Orlando, FL: Academic Press.

Heimberg, R. G., Liebowitz, M. R., Hope, D. A., *et al.* (1998). Cognitive-behavioral group therapy vs phenelzine therapy for social phobia. *Archives of General Psychiatry*, **55**, 1133–41.

Heimberg, R. G., Horner, K. J., Juster, H. R., *et al.* (1999). Psychometric properties of the Liebowitz Social Anxiety Scale. *Psychological Medicine*, **29**, 199–212.

Katschnig, H., Stein, M. B., and Buller, R. (1997). Moclobemide in social phobia. A double-blind, placebo-controlled clinical study. *European Archive of Psychiatry and Clinical Neuroscience*, **247**, 71–80.

Katzelnick, D. J., Kobak K. A., Greist, J. H., *et al.* (1995). Sertraline for social phobia: a double-blind, placebo-controlled cross over study. *American Journal of Psychiatry*, **152**, 1368–71.

Kessler, R. C., McGonagle, K. A., Zhao, S., *et al.* (1994). Lifetime and 12 month prevalence of DSM III-R psychiatric disorders in the United States. *Archives of General Psychiatry*, **51**, 8–19.

Kobak, K. A., Griest, J. H., Jefferson, J. W., and Katzelnick, D. J. (2002). Fluoxetine in social phobia: a double-blind placebo controlled pilot study. *Journal of Clinical Psychopharmacology*, **22**, 257–62.

Liebowitz, M. R. (1987). Social phobia. *Modern Problems in Pharmacopsychiatry*, **22**, 141–73.

Liebowitz, M. R., Gorman, J. M., Fyer, A. J., and Klein, D. F. (1985). Social phobia: review of a neglected anxiety disorder. *Archives of General Psychiatry*, **42**, 729–36.

Liebowitz, M. R., Schneier, F. R., Campeas, R., *et al.* (1992). Phenelzine vs. atenolol in social phobia: a placebo-controlled comparison. *Archives of General Psychiatry*, **49**, 290–300.

Liebowitz, M. R., Heimberg, R. G., Schneier, F. R., *et al.* (1999). Cognitive-behavioral group therapy versus phenelzine in social phobia: long-term outcome. *Depression and Anxiety*, **10**, 89–98.

Liebowitz, M. R., Stein, M. B., Tancer, M., *et al.* (2002). A randomized, double-blind, fixed-dose comparison of paroxetine and placebo in the treatment of generalized social anxiety disorder. *Journal of Clinical Psychiatry*, **63**, 66–74.

Liebowitz, M. R., DeMartinis, N. A., Weihs, K., *et al.* (2003). Efficacy of sertraline in severe generalized social anxiety disorder: results of a double-blind, placebo-controlled study. *Journal of Clinical Psychiatry*, **64**, 785–92.

Lott, M., Greist, J., Jefferson, J. W., *et al.* (1997). Brofaromine for social phobia: a multicenter, placebo-controlled, double-blind study. *Journal of Clinical Psychopharmacology*, **17**, 255–60.

Marks, I. M. (1970). The classification of phobic disorders. *British Journal of Psychiatry*, **116**, 377–86.

Marks, I. M. and Matthews, A. M. (1979). Brief standard self-rating for phobic patients. *Behavior Research and Therapy*, **17**, 263–7.

Myers, J. K., Weissman, M. M., Tischler, G. I., *et al.* (1984). Six-month prevalence of psychiatric disorders in three communities. *Archives of General Psychiatry*, **41**, 959–67.

Noyes, R., Moroz, G., Davidson, J., *et al.* (1997). Moclobemide in social phobia: a controlled dose–response. *Journal of Clinical Psychopharmacology*, **17**, 247–54.

Öst, L. G. (1987). Age of onset in different phobias. *Journal of Abnormal Psychology*, **96**, 223–9.

Pande, A. C., Davidson, R. T., Jefferson, J. W., *et al.* (1999). Treatment of social phobia with gabapentine: a placebo controlled study. *Journal of Clinical Psychopharmacology*, **19**, 341–8.

Potts, N. L. S. and Davidson, J. R. T. (1995). Pharmacological treatments: literature review. In: *Social Phobia: Diagnosis, Assessment and Treatment*, ed. R. G. Heimberg, M. R. Liebowitz, D. A. Hope, and F. R. Schneier. New York: Guilford, pp. 334–65.

Research Unit on Pediatric Psychopharmacology Anxiety Study Group (2001). Fluvoxamine for the treatment of anxiety disorders in children and adolescents. *New England Journal of Medicine*, **344**, 1279–85.

Rosenthal, R. (1984). *Meta-Analytic Procedures for Social Research*. Beverly Hills, CA: Sage.
  (1991). Meta-Analysis: a review. *Psychosomatic Medicine*, **53**, 247–71.

Schneier, F. R., Johnson, J., Hornig, C. D., Liebowitz, M. R., and Weissman, M. M. (1992). Social phobia: comorbidity and morbidity in an epidemiological sample. *Archives of General Psychiatry*, **49**, 282–8.

Schneier, F. R., Liebowitz, M. R., Garfinkel, R., *et al.* (1994). Disability in work and social functioning and social phobia. *Journal of Clinical Psychiatry*, **55**, 322–31.

Schneier, F. R., Goetz, D., Campeas, R., *et al.* (1998). A placebo-controlled trial of moclobemide in social phobia. *British Journal of Psychiatry*, **172**, 70–7.

Schneier, F. R., Blanco, C., Campeas, R., *et al.* (2003). Citalopram treatment of social anxiety disorder and comorbid major depression. *Depression and Anxiety*, **17**, 191–6.

Sheehan, D. V. (1983). *The Anxiety Disease*. New York: Charles Scribner's Sons.

Spielberger, C. D., Gorsuch, R. L., and Lushene, R. E. (1970). *STAI, Manual for the State-Trait Anxiety Inventory*. Palo Alto, CA: Consulting Psychologists Press.

Stein, M. B., Chartier, M. J., Hazen, A. L., *et al.* (1996). Paroxetine in the treatment of generalized social phobia: open-label treatment and double-blind placebo-controlled discontinuation. *Journal of Clinical Psychopharmacology*, **16**, 218–22.

Stein, M. B., Liebowitz, M. R., Lydiard, R. B., *et al.* (1998). Paroxetine treatment of generalized social phobia (social anxiety disorder): a randomized, double-blind, placebo-controlled study. *Journal of the American Medical Association*, **280**, 708–13.

Stein, M. B., Fyer, A. J., Davidson, J. R. T., Pollack, M. H., and Wiita, B. (1999). Fluvoxamine treatment of social phobia (social anxiety disorder): a double-blind placebo-controlled study. *American Journal of Psychiatry*, **156**, 756–60.

Stein, M. B., Sareen, J., Hami, S., and Chao, J. (2001). Pindolol potentiation of paroxetine for generalized social phobia. A double-blind, placebo-controlled, cross-over study. *American Journal of Psychiatry*, **158**, 1725–7.

Stein, D. J., Cameron, A., Amrein, R., *et al.* (2002a). Moclobemide is effective and well tolerated in the long-term pharmacotherapy of social anxiety disorder with or without comorbid anxiety disorder. *International Clinics in Psychopharmacology*, **17**, 161–70.

Stein, D. J., Stein, M. B., Pitts, C. D., Kumar, R., and Hunter, B. (2002b). Predictors of response to pharmacotherapy in social anxiety disorder, an analysis of three placebo-controlled paroxetine trials. *Journal of Clinical Psychiatry*, **63**, 152–5.

Stein, D. J., Versiani, M., Hair, T., and Kumar, R. (2002c). Efficacy of paroxetine for relapse prevention in social anxiety disorder: a 24-week study. *Archives of General Psychiatry*, **59**, 1111–18.

Turner, S. M., Beidel, D. C., and Jacob, R. G. (1994). Social phobia: a comparison of behavior therapy and atenolol. *Journal of Consulting and Clinical Psychology*, **62**, 350–8.

Van Ameringen, M., Mancini, C., and Wilson, C. (1996). Buspirone augmentation of selective serotonin reuptake inhibitors (SSRIs) in social phobia. *Journal of Affective Disorders*, **39**, 115–21.

Van Ameringen, M. A., Lane, R. M., Walker, J. R., *et al.* (2001). Sertraline treatment of generalized social phobia: a 20-week double-blind, placebo-controlled study. *American Journal of Psychiatry*, **158**, 275–81.

Van der Linden, G. J. H., Stein, D. J., and Van Balkom., A. (2000). The efficacy of the selective serotonin reuptake inhibitors for social anxiety disorder: a meta-analysis of randomized controlled trials. *International Clinics in Psychopharmacology*, **15** (suppl. 2), S15–23.

van Vliet, I. M., den Boer, J. A., and Westenberg, H. G. M. (1992). Psychopharmacological treatment of social phobia: clinical and biochemical effects of brofaromine, a selective MAO-A inhibitor. *European Neuropsychopharmacology*, **2**, 21–9.

van Vliet, I. M., den Boer, J. A., and Westenberg, H. G. M. (1994). Psychopharmacological treatment of social phobia: a double blind controlled study with fluvoxamine. *Psychopharmacology*, **115**, 128–34.

van Vliet, I. M., den Boer, J. A., Westenberg, G. A., and Ho Pian, K. L. (1997a). Clinical effects of buspirone in social phobia. A double-blind, placebo-controlled study. *Journal of Clinical Psychiatry*, **58**, 164–8.

van Vliet, I. M., Den Boer, J. A., Westenberg, G. A., and Ho Pian, K. L. (1997b). Clinical effects of buspirone in social phobia. A double-blind placebo controlled study. *Journal of Clinical Psychiatry*, **58**, 164–8.

Versiani, M., Nardi, A. E., Mundim, F. D., *et al.* (1992). Pharmacotherapy of social phobia: a controlled study with moclobemide and phenelzine. *British Journal of Psychiatry*, **161**, 353–60.

Versiani, M., Nardia, A. E., Figueira, I., Mendlowicz, M., and Marques, C. (1997). Double-blind placebo controlled trials with bromazepam. *Jornal Brasileiro de Psiquiatria*, **46**, 167–71.

Wagner, K. D. (2003). Paroxetine treatment of mood and anxiety disorders in children and adolescents. *Psychopharmacology Bulletin*, **37** (suppl. 1), 167–75.

Walker, J. R., Van Ameringen, M. A., Swinson, R., *et al.* (2000). Prevention of relapse in generalized social phobia: results of a 24-week study in responders to 20 weeks of sertraline treatment. *Journal of Clinical Psychopharmacology*, **20**, 636–44.

Wittchen, H. U. and Beloch, E. (1996). The impact of social phobia on quality of life. *International Clinics in Psychopharmacology*, **11** (suppl. 3), 15–23.

Wolff, F. M. (1986). *Meta-analysis: Quantitative Methods for Research Synthesis*. Beverly Hills, CA: Sage.

8

Evidence-based pharmacotherapy of obsessive-compulsive disorder

Naomi A. Fineberg[1] and Tim M. Gale[2]

[1] Queen Elizabeth II Hospital, Welwyn Garden City, and
[2] Department of Psychology, University of Hertfordshire, Hatfield, UK

Obsessive-compulsive disorder (OCD) is now recognized to be a common, treatable illness with a distinctive pathophysiology and pharmacology. Wide-ranging epidemiological surveys have repeatedly demonstrated high lifetime prevalence, amounting to 2–3% of the population worldwide under *Diagnostic and Statistical Manual*, 3rd edition (DSM-III) and DSM-IIIR criteria (Robins *et al.*, 1984; Weissman *et al.*, 1994). However only a fraction of sufferers present for treatment and the diagnosis is often missed. OCD is somewhat more common in women than men (ratio 1.5:1) and the mean age of onset is reported as 20 years, with bimodal peaks at 12–14, and 20–22 years (Rasmussen and Eisen, 1990). There is a high childhood incidence and, if untreated, OCD runs a fluctuating, unremitting course with greatest prevalence in early–middle adult life. A substantial lifetime comorbidity with several DSM-IV axis I and II disorders has been identified (Hollander *et al.*, 1998), including depression, which supervenes in approximately two-thirds of cases, simple phobia (22%), social phobia (18%), eating disorder (17%), alcohol dependence (14%), panic disorder (12%), and Tourette's syndrome (7%; Piggott *et al.*, 1994), and increased rates of suicidal behavior. The costs of OCD to society, in terms of individual suffering, diminished human potential, and lost revenue, are high (Hollander and Wong, 1998).

The systematic investigation of OCD has depended, to a large extent, on the introduction of universally accepted diagnostic criteria and the development of comprehensive and sensitive rating scales that measure small changes in symptoms, such as the six- and eight-item CPRS-OC scales (Montgomery and Montgomery, 1980; Thoren *et al.*, 1980, respectively) derived from the Comprehensive Psychopathological Rating Scale (CPRS; Asberg *et al.*, 1978) and the Yale-Brown Obsessive Compulsive Scale (Y-BOCS; Goodman *et al.*, 1984). However, in spite of such advances, OCD remains poorly recognized and undertreated. Although surveys suggest the time lag between symptom onset and correct diagnosis is shortening, patients still wait an average of 17 years before appropriate treatment is initiated (Hollander and Wong, 1998). It is often only when depression supervenes that OCD sufferers present for treatment. At this point it is vital to the success of clinical intervention that the OCD is not overlooked.

This review considers the evidence base for the pharmacological management of OCD based upon, wherever possible, randomized controlled trials (RCTs). Three fundamental clinical issues are addressed: (1) what are the first-line treatments? (2) how long should treatment continue? and (3) what is the preferred treatment for those who do not respond to first-line agents? Uncontrolled studies are cited where systematic data are lacking and meta-analyses are cited where adequate head-to-head comparator studies do not exist. Expert consensus guidelines are considered and practical recommendations made for the clinical setting. A systematic search of electronic databases (Embase (1974–date), MEDLINE (1966–date), PsychInfo (1987–date)) was run using combinations of the terms "obsessive compulsive, randomised or control$ or clinical trial$ or placebo$ or blind$" and "systematic or review$ or meta-analysis," as well as individual drug names. This was complemented by consulting with colleagues in the field and reviewing recent data presented at international peer-reviewed symposia. Most published studies have investigated acute treatment of OCD, with a shortage of long-term and relapse prevention data. The results from a growing number of studies on children suggest they respond similarly to adults. There is a regrettable shortage of data on pharmacotherapy of OCD in the elderly.

The weight of evidence shows that OCD responds preferentially to drugs which powerfully inhibit the synaptic reuptake of serotonin, i.e., clomipramine and selective serotonin reuptake inhibitors (SSRIs). Drugs lacking potent SRI actions have not been effective in controlled studies. This selective pharmacological response has generated hypotheses about the role of serotonin in the etiology of OCD but, so far, no unifying theory has emerged and the mechanisms by which SSRIs exert anti-obsessional benefits remain poorly understood (Fineberg et al., 1997). It is widely believed that OCD encompasses a heterogeneous group of illnesses, and that other neurotransmitters are involved in its pathophysiology.

What is the first-line pharmacotherapy of OCD?

Clomipramine

The first uncontrolled case series showing successful treatment with clomipramine appeared in the 1960s (Fernandez and Lopez-Ibor, 1967; Reynghe de Voxrie, 1968) and, by 1990, a collection of double-blind, placebo-controlled trials demonstrated conclusively that clomipramine is efficacious in OCD, both in the presence (Marks et al., 1980; Thoren et al., 1980; Insel et al., 1983; Flament et al., 1985; Mavissakalian *et al.*, 1985; Jenike *et al.*, 1989) and absence of comorbid depression (Marks *et al.*, 1988; De Veaugh-Geiss *et al.*, 1989; Katz *et al.*, 1990).

Clomipramine in OCD without depression

Early reports suggested that clomipramine may exert benefit on obsessional symptoms within depression, and it was unclear if this was an antidepressant effect or a more specific effect on OCD. The first study of "pure" OCD patients (Montgomery, 1980) employed a crossover design with randomized allocation to 4 weeks' treatment, and a low fixed daily dose (75 mg) to protect blinding. Early onset of action was detected on the six-item, CPRS-OC scale, with significant advantages over placebo at 1, 3, and 4 weeks in the group comparison, and 2, 3, and 4 weeks in the crossover analysis, despite only 14 patients taking part. This finding was replicated by Marks *et al.* (1988), who reported efficacy over concurrent exposure therapy *and* placebo, and by Greist *et al.* (1990), who demonstrated clear efficacy using only 32 cases. Two multicenter studies of clomipramine, comprising 238 and 263 cases respectively, and where concomitant depression was excluded, have been published (De Veaugh-Geiss *et al.*, 1989; Clomipramine Collaborative Study Group, 1991). Placebo response did not exceed 5% reduction in Y-BOCS total over 10 weeks, with significant differences emerging for clomipramine groups at weeks 1–2. The benefits of clomipramine, given in flexible doses up to 300 mg/day, increased slowly and gradually after 1 week of treatment up to the 10-week endpoint. The resulting 38% and 44% (respective) improvements in baseline OC ratings represented substantial improvement in emotional and social well-being. Another 10-week study by Katz *et al.* (1990) stratified patients by Hamilton Depression Scale (Hamilton, 1960) scores. In the non-depressed subgroup, 134 patients improved significantly on the National Institute of Mental Health (NIMH) global OC scale (Insel *et al.*, 1983), approaching a 40% reduction of baseline score (cf. 129 on placebo who remained essentially unchanged).

Clomipramine in OCD with depression

Eight placebo-controlled studies have investigated clomipramine in OCD with comorbid depression. A 5-week study by Thoren *et al.* (1980) comparing clomipramine to nortriptyline and placebo showed significant improvement on the CPRS-OC for clomipramine over nortriptyline and placebo. In Insel *et al.*'s (1983) crossover study ($n = 12$), clomipramine was superior to clorgyline and placebo at 4 and 6 weeks. Moreover, Marks *et al.* (1980) showed significance at 4 weeks for clomipramine in 40 ritualizers, although these findings relied on self-rated instruments. Further small studies by Mavissakalian *et al.* (1985) and Jenike *et al.* (1989) also showed significance for clomipramine (100–300 mg) over placebo.

The controlled study by Flament *et al.* (1985) was the first to demonstrate efficacy of a pharmacological treatment in childhood OCD. Nineteen children with primary OCD aged 6–18 years entered the 5-week crossover study. A significant improvement in obsessional scores was seen for clomipramine (mean dose 141 mg/day), and this was irrespective of baseline depression. Significant post-baseline improvements were also observed in the placebo group, suggesting that children may be susceptible to non-specific treatment effects. However, a positive study by De Veaugh-Geiss *et al.* (1992) on children and adolescents reported only an 8% improvement in the placebo group ($n = 29$) at the 8-week endpoint, compared with 37% on clomipramine ($n = 31$), with significant differences evident from 3 weeks.

Most of the above studies are small by today's standards but the pattern of results is highly consistent. Such consistency is rare in psychopharmacological research and, together, the results offer unequivocal support for the efficacy of clomipramine in OCD. They also reflect the special qualities of patients under investigation at that time. Most had long histories of stable, severe, untreated illness with few treatment-refractory cases. The studies' power also depended on low placebo response rates and these distinguish OCD from depression and other anxiety disorders, where placebo response rates are higher.

SRIs compared with other antidepressants lacking strong serotonergic activity

Clomipramine is distinguished from other tricyclics by its more powerful SRI activity, though its effects are not exclusively serotonergic. In the first crossover study comparing clomipramine with the noradrenergic tricyclic desipramine (Insel *et al.*, 1985), the response to desipramine was indistinguishable from placebo, whereas clomipramine was superior. Failure of desipramine relative to clomipramine was seen more clearly in two crossover studies in children (Leonard *et al.*, 1988, 1991), and in later comparisons with SSRIs such as fluvoxamine (Goodman *et al.*, 1990) and sertraline (Hoehn-Saric *et al.*, 2000). Likewise, in studies comparing clomipramine with imipramine, the former was superior at 6 and 12 weeks (Volavka *et al.*, 1985). Antidepressant responses were reported in imipramine-treated patients (Foa *et al.*, 1987), but while clomipramine exerted antiobsessional benefits, imipramine did not. In a small, three-way study by Thoren *et al.* (1980), clomipramine was superior to placebo but nortriptyline was not; and in a small study by Ananth *et al.* (1981) there was a significant advantage for clomipramine but not amitriptyline. The small placebo-controlled crossover study by Insel *et al.* (1983) found clomipramine to be superior to clorgyline in 13 patients. And although the study by Vallejo *et al.* (1992) was probably too small to discriminate between phenelzine and clomipramine, Jenike *et al.* (1997) demonstrated a significant advantage for fluoxetine over phenelzine, the latter being indistinguishable from placebo. No study to date has demonstrated a convincing advantage for a monoamine oxidase inhibitor (MAOI) over placebo in OCD.

In some studies, comparator agents may have shown some antiobsessional benefit, but the effect is consistently weaker than that of SRIs. Demonstrating a significant difference between active treatments usually requires a large sample size, so the fact that several small studies show superiority for SRIs strongly suggests that non-SRIs have little, if any, efficacy in OCD.

SSRIs

Although clomipramine is a powerful SRI, it has an active metabolite with strong noradrenergic properties. That the more highly selective SSRIs are also beneficial, showing a similar slow, incremental effect, suggests their antiobsessional actions are related to this pharmacological property. Early promising reports suggesting efficacy for zimelidine were curtailed by the withdrawal of the drug for safety reasons.

Placebo-controlled studies of fluvoxamine

Perse *et al.* (1987) reported a double-blind crossover study of fluvoxamine in 20 patients. Efficacy was evident after 8 weeks, based on 16 completers. Fluvoxamine also showed superiority over placebo in the 8- and 24-week analysis by Cottraux *et al.* (1990), in spite of concurrent exposure therapy in the placebo group, thereby emphasizing the strength of the drug effect relative to psychotherapy. The study has been criticized for not including an intent-to-treat analysis and for relying on behavioral ratings for the OCD. Goodman *et al.* (1989) demonstrated similar response profiles in depressed and non-depressed OCD patients with significant placebo-referenced improvement on the Y-BOCS from week 2 onwards. Similar results were reported by Jenike *et al.* (1990a), although significant differences only appeared at week 10. The multicenter study by Goodman *et al.* (1996), looking at two groups of 78 patients receiving either 10 weeks of fluvoxamine (100–300 mg) or placebo, confirmed superiority for fluvoxamine on all outcome measures from week 4 onwards. Obsessions and compulsions both improved, with a possible earlier benefit for obsessions. Only 10 cases discontinued because of side-effects.

Another multicenter study by Hollander *et al.* (2003a) compared 127 patients on flexible, once-daily doses of controlled-release (CR) fluvoxamine (100–300 mg) with 126 on placebo. Fluvoxamine CR was superior in decreasing Y-BOCS scores from as early as week 2. By the 12-week endpoint fluvoxamine CR-treated individuals showed a 32% improvement, compared to 21% on placebo, with significantly greater improvements on CGI(S), CGI-I and responder analyses. Remission was defined as either a Y-BOCS total <16, or subscore <8, and remission rates for fluvoxamine CR were 44% and 18% respectively. In the fluvoxamine-treated group, 19% (cf. 6% placebo) withdrew early through adverse effects (mainly nausea, insomnia, somnolence, dizziness, and diarrhea).

Riddle et al. (2001) reported the first RCT of fluvoxamine (50–200 mg) in 120 children aged 8–17 years. Improvement on the C-Y-BOCS was superior to placebo from weeks 1 to 6 and at the 10-week endpoint. Only 3 patients on fluvoxamine and 1 on placebo withdrew through adverse effects. This finding supports the rapid efficacy and tolerability of fluvoxamine in childhood OCD.

Placebo-controlled studies of sertraline

Jenike et al. (1990b) found no group differences in a study comparing sertraline ($n = 10$) and placebo ($n = 9$), although this study was arguably underpowered. Chouinard et al. (1990) demonstrated superiority for flexible doses of sertraline (50–200 mg) on the Y-BOCS and NIMH Global OC scale, but not on the Maudsley Obsessive-Compulsive Inventory (Hodgson and Rachman, 1977), suggesting that the latter may lack sensitivity for monitoring clinical change. Kronig et al. (1999) replicated this work in a larger sample, demonstrating superiority for sertraline (50–200 mg; $n = 86$) over placebo ($n = 81$) as early as 3 weeks. Ten percent of the sertraline group and 5% of the placebo group discontinued because of side-effects. The subsequent fixed-dose study by Greist et al. (1995a), which was hampered by a strong placebo response, showed efficacy on the Y-BOCS for pooled sertraline (50–200 mg; $n = 240$) at week 2 onwards compared to placebo ($n = 84$). However, at the 12-week endpoint almost as many in the placebo group (30%) were much or very much improved compared with those on sertraline (39%). March et al. (1998) evaluated the efficacy of sertraline, titrated up to 200 mg, in a cohort of 107 children and 80 adolescents, finding a significant advantage on the C-Y-BOCS over placebo as early as 3 weeks. Insomnia, nausea, agitation, and tremor were overrepresented in the drug-treated condition and 13% of sertraline patients discontinued early because of adverse effects (cf. 3% placebo). Cardiovascular parameters were systematically monitored and showed no clinically meaningful abnormalities, suggesting that sertraline is safe up to doses of 200 mg in children (Wilens et al., 1999).

Placebo-controlled studies of fluoxetine

Fluoxetine has also been extensively investigated in OCD. Two multicenter studies benefited from a design that allowed comparison of different fixed doses. In the 8-week study by Montgomery et al. (1993), the 20 mg dose ($n = 52$) fared no better than placebo ($n = 56$), while the 40 mg dose ($n = 52$) was superior on the responder analysis and the 60 mg dose ($n = 54$) was superior on both reduction of Y-BOCS scores and responder rate. Side-effects were low and <6% withdrew early because of them. In the larger, longer study by Tollefson *et al.* (1994), all fixed doses of fluoxetine emerged as superior to placebo by the 13-week endpoint, but there was a trend toward superiority for the 60 mg dose on the Y-BOCS analysis. Side-effects of fluoxetine included nausea, dry mouth, tremor, and sexual problems. A meta-analysis of separate study data showed no association between fluoxetine and suicidality in OCD (Beasley *et al.*, 1992). The placebo-controlled study by Jenike *et al.* (1997) investigated doses of fluoxetine up to 80 mg, and included a comparison with the MAOI phenelzine. Fluoxetine ($n = 23$) was superior to placebo ($n = 21$) and phenelzine ($n = 20$), which did not differentiate from placebo.

Three studies have looked at fluoxetine in childhood OCD, all showing some level of superiority over placebo. Riddle *et al.*'s (1992) crossover study on 14 children used fixed doses of 20 mg. A significant advantage was observed on the CGI but not C-Y-BOCS, which showed a 44% improvement after 8 weeks' treatment, compared with 27% on placebo. Behavioral activation occurred as an adverse effect in a few children, and one left the study early because of suicidal ideation. The authors considered these side-effects to be dose-related, advocating initiating treatment at lower doses. Geller *et al.* (2001) took a larger cohort, titrating doses upwards from 10 to 60 mg over 13 weeks, according to clinical response. Fluoxetine was superior to placebo on the C-Y-BOCS from week 6 and was well-tolerated across all doses, with similar dropout rates from adverse events on drug (8.5%) and placebo. Leibowitz *et al.* (2002) extended the dose range to 80 mg after the first 6 weeks in a trial spanning 7 years. After 8 weeks, responders could continue double-blind treatment for a further 8 weeks. Fluoxetine's effects were slow to develop, and superiority over placebo did not emerge until after 8 weeks. No patient withdrew as a result of adverse effects.

Placebo-controlled studies of paroxetine

Positive results from a fixed-dose study reported in poster form by Wheadon *et al.* (1993) were confirmed in a multinational study by Zohar and Judge (1996), which included clomipramine as a comparator agent. Paroxetine, given in doses up to 60 mg ($n = 201$), was significantly more effective than placebo ($n = 99$) on all *a priori* efficacy measures, and of comparable efficacy to clomipramine (50–250 mg; $n = 99$). Only 9% of paroxetine-treated patients withdrew because of side-effects (mainly asthenia, headache, dry mouth, and nausea) compared to 6% given placebo. In a large trial of 348 OCD patients, Hollander *et al.* (2003b) tested paroxetine in fixed doses (20, 40, and 60 mg) with placebo. Respective Y-BOCS score reductions were 16%, 25%, 29%, and 13% in the acute phase of the study. Both higher doses were significantly different from placebo by week 6 and from the 20 mg dose by week 3. Paroxetine was well tolerated at all doses.

Placebo-controlled studies of citalopram

The multinational placebo-controlled study by Montgomery *et al.* (2001) showed efficacy for fixed doses of 20 mg ($n = 102$), 40 mg ($n = 98$) and 60 mg citalopram ($n = 100$), compared with placebo ($n = 101$). A significant reduction in baseline Y-BOCS score was seen from week 3 for the 60 mg group, and from weeks 7 to 12 for other doses. Citalopram was well tolerated (4% withdrew through adverse effects, mainly nausea, headache, fatigue, insomnia) and improved psychosocial disability on the Sheehan Disability Scale (Sheehan *et al.*, 1996). To date, there are no studies relating to the active S-isomer, escitalopram in OCD.

Changes in study populations have affected treatment studies

The data on SSRIs provides conclusive evidence of efficacy in OCD. The success of clomipramine and SSRIs has led to their rapid acceptance as first-line treatments, and it is increasingly difficult for specialist research centers to recruit patients who are not already receiving one of these pharmacotherapies. This has compromised the recruitment of treatment-naive patients in more recent studies of SSRIs, where greater numbers of treatment-refractory individuals have been included. Moreover, exclusion of comorbid depression has reduced the numbers of severely ill individuals at baseline. Accordingly, the magnitude of the observed treatment effect has diminished from 40–50% average reduction in baseline scores in the clomipramine studies to around 30% in the later SSRI studies. Between 32% and 65% of the SSRI-treated study participants showed a clinically meaningful improvement using the various recognized criteria for clinical response. Table 8.1 summarizes the rates of clinical response in those studies that report them. Furthermore, increased placebo response rates, in some cases exceeding 20% improvement in baseline scores, have also been observed in more recent studies, probably resulting from inclusion of milder, atypical cases, some of whom undergo spontaneous remission. The rise in the placebo response rate cautions against drawing conclusions about efficacy from open, naturalistic reporting, and emphasizes the importance of controlled investigation. Finally, the application of increasingly stringent inclusion criteria in recent studies, often driven by requirements of regulatory authorities, may well contribute to the changing pattern of response rates, since treatment groups are less heterogeneous. By contrast, response rates in general psychiatry clinics are probably closer to the original clomipramine results. The net effect of these changes has been to reduce the statistical power of the studies, so that larger numbers are now needed to test the efficacy of new treatments. Meta-analyses of existing studies can, to some extent, compensate by pooling data, but if they fail to take these changes into account they may be misleading.

Table 8.1 Rates of clinical response in placebo-controlled studies of selective serotonin reuptake inhibitors for patients with obsessive-compulsive disorder

Study	Definition of clinical response				
	Much or very much improved on CGI-I (criterion A)	>25% improved on baseline Y-BOCS (criterion B)	>35% improved on baseline Y-BOCS	Criteria A and B	Drug (duration in weeks)
Goodman et al. (1989)	9/21				Fluvoxamine (8)
Goodman et al. (1996)	33.3%				Fluvoxamine (10)
Hollander et al. (2003a)	34% from graph	63%	45%		Fluvoxamine CR (12)
Riddle et al. (2001)		42% (CY-BOCS)			Fluvoxamine (10)
Kronig et al. (1999)	41%				Sertraline (12)
Greist et al. (1995a)	38.9%				Sertraline (12)
March et al. (1998)	42%				Sertraline (12)
Montgomery et al. (1993)				36%	Fluoxetine 20 mg (8)
				48%	Fluoxetine 40 mg (8)
				47%	Fluoxetine 60 mg (8)
Tollefson et al. (1994)					Fluoxetine 20 mg (13)
		32%	34%		Fluoxetine 40 mg (13)
		35%			Fluoxetine 60 mg (13)
Geller et al. (2001)	55%				Fluoxetine (13)
Leibowitz et al. (2002)	57%				Fluoxetine (16)
Zohar and Judge (1996)	55.1%				Paroxetine (12)
	55.3%				Clomipramine (12)
Montgomery et al. (2001)	57.4%				Citalopram 20 mg (12)
	52%				Citalopram 40 mg (12)
	65%				Citalopram 60 mg (12)

CGI-I, Clinical Global Impression I; Y-BOCS, Yale-Brown Obsessive Compulsive Scale.

Meta-analyses of SRIs in OCD

Meta-analyses combine data from separate studies using specific rules and provide more objective and quantifiable measures of treatment effect size than narrative reviews. However, problems may arise in controlling for between-study differences such as dose, duration, blindness, method of assessment, and population differences, so results must be viewed cautiously (Pigott and Seay, 1999). In short, meta-analyses cannot substitute for high-quality head-to-head comparator trials.

Meta-analyses of existing OCD studies all suggest superior efficacy for clomipramine over SSRIs. An analysis by Jenike et al. (1990a) of their work on SSRIs showed that efficacy correlated negatively with serotonin-selectivity. Stein et al. (1995) examined effect sizes for studies that employed validated rating scales and were of at least 6 weeks duration. However, although the effect size for clomipramine was larger than that of comparators, several methodological and statistical shortcomings were acknowledged, which limit the conclusions drawn. Piccinelli *et al.*'s (1995) meta-analysis related exclusively to double-blind RCTs of clomipramine and SSRIs, using Y-BOCS or NIMH-OC scales. All treatments were significantly superior to placebo, but clomipramine was associated with significantly greater mean Y-BOCS reduction (61%) compared with fluoxetine (28.5%), fluvoxamine (28%), and sertraline (22%), with no significant difference between individual SSRIs. The authors concluded that large-scale controlled comparator studies are needed to draw firmer conclusions about relative efficacy. Greist and colleagues (1995c) reported on data from four multicenter, placebo-controlled studies of clomipramine, fluoxetine, fluvoxamine, and sertraline. Clomipramine was significantly more effective than SSRIs, which did not differ in calculated effect size using the Y-BOCS. Whereas dropout rates associated with adverse effects were similar across all groups (8%, 12%, 15%, and 10% respectively), withdrawal from all causes was significantly lower in the clomipramine group.

Abramowitz (1997) investigated effect sizes of SRIs and psychological interventions in RCT data. Using clinician ratings, clomipramine was again superior to fluvoxamine, fluoxetine, and sertraline (in decreasing order), and side-effect contrast was significantly correlated to effect size. Abramowitz suggested the apparent supremacy of clomipramine may, in part, be caused by unblinding because it has more noticeable side-effects. Kobak *et al.* (1998) extended the procedure to look at all available studies relating to SRIs and exposure therapy, regardless of publication mode and methodology. Data were analyzed before and after attempts to control for methodological variables, such as year of publication and experimental design. The results were consistent with previous meta-analyses, in as much as clomipramine had the largest effect size compared to all the SSRIs, apart from fluoxetine. However, after attempts to control for methodological variables, clomipramine was not significantly more effective than fluoxetine or fluvoxamine, but was still superior to other SSRIs. In their analysis of head-to-head comparisons, however, there was no significant difference between SRIs. The authors remarked on the consistency with which meta-analyses had favored clomipramine over more selective SRIs. In spite of its less favorable side-effect profile, the dropout rate for clomipramine was no different from the other SRIs. As predicted, year of publication was negatively correlated with treatment effect size. These authors also postulated several additional biases in favour of clomipramine: for example, patients may have been more willing to continue on clomipramine, in spite of side-effects, because they inferred they were receiving the active drug, particularly when no other known alternatives were available. The unblinding effect may also have biased patients' and clinicians' assessment of improvement. This article also acknowledged that its findings were not supported by the evidence from head-to-head trials.

Ackerman and Greenland's (2002) meta-analysis attempted to quantify characteristics of published trials that might account for differences in effect size. Although they used different techniques, their findings broadly agreed with previous analyses. The considerable heterogeneity across studies appeared to be associated with factors such as year of publication, length of single-blind prerandomisation period, length of trial and severity of OCD, and confirmed the recent rise in placebo response rates. They concluded that superiority of clomipramine in placebo-controlled trials persisted after controlling for these factors, but that there was no difference in studies comparing clomipramine directly with SSRIs.

Geller *et al.* (2003a) performed the first meta-analysis on pharmacotherapy for childhood OCD. Twelve trials were considered and the results were consistent with the adult literature, showing modest but significant advantages for all SRIs over placebo, and superiority for clomipramine over SSRIs. SSRIs were more or less comparable and the findings were not dependent on publication date or placebo response rate. The authors noted an absence of head-to-head studies and recommended that clomipramine should not generally be used first-line in children because of its side-effect profile.

Direct comparison of SRIs in OCD

So far, only two controlled studies have compared the relative efficacy of different SSRIs, and the results are inconclusive. The single-blind study by Mundo *et al.* (1997a) that failed to detect differences between fluvoxamine, paroxetine, and citalopram was undoubtedly underpowered with only 10 patients per group. Bergeron *et al.* (2001) compared 77 patients on sertraline with 73 on fluoxetine, under double-blind conditions. At the 24-week endpoint, no significant difference was seen on primary efficacy measures, but there was a non-significant trend toward an earlier effect in the sertraline group, and a higher number of sertraline patients reached remission, defined as a CGI-I ≤ 2 and Y-BOCS score ≤ 11. In conjunction with meta-analysis data, these results do not support the superior efficacy of any one SSRI. The selection of a particular compound should therefore take account of other factors, such as possible interactions with other drugs being prescribed. In this respect, fluoxetine, paroxetine, and, to a much lesser extent, sertraline, inhibit the P450 isoenzyme CYP 2D6 which metabolizes tricyclic antidepressants, antipsychotics, antiarrythmics, and beta-blockers, whereas fluvoxamine inhibits both CYP 1A2 and CYP 3A4, which eliminate warfarin, tricyclics, benzodiazepines, and some antiarrhythmics. Citalopram is relatively free from hepatic interactions. Fluoxetine has a long half-life, and has fewer discontinuation effects, which can be advantageous for patients who forget to take their tablets.

Whereas meta-analyses consistently report a smaller effect size for SSRIs relative to clomipramine, many head-to-head studies demonstrate equivalent efficacy (Table 8.2). While many of these were underpowered (Montgomery *et al.*, 1990), the trial by Bisserbe *et al.* (1997) was large enough to detect a significant advantage for sertraline. However the advantage, apparent for certain measures in the intent-to-treat analysis, was not clear-cut. Another smaller study found an advantage for clomipramine over fluoxetine (40 mg) on secondary outcome measures (Lopez-Ibor *et al.*, 1996). The larger study first presented by Rouillon (1998; see also Mundo *et al.*, 2001) showed equivalent efficacy for clomipramine and SSRI on all visits and measures. In the comparator study by Zohar and Judge (1996), paroxetine and clomipramine showed similar placebo-referenced efficacy at weeks 6, 8, and 12. Paroxetine was superior to placebo on depression ratings whereas clomipramine was not. Response was defined as 25% or more improvement in baseline Y-BOCS scores and, at endpoint, 55% of both paroxetine- and clomipramine-treated patients met this criterion, compared with 35% in the placebo group.

Improved tolerability favors SSRIs

Altogether, the evidence does not appear strong enough to support superior efficacy of clomipramine over SSRIs. In the face of equivalence, choice of SRI depends greatly on the side-effect profile of the compound. An important advantage of the SSRIs, compared with clomipramine, lies in their improved acceptability and tolerability (Table 8.2). In the comparator study of Zohar and Judge (1996), the dropout rate from adverse effects on clomipramine (approximately 17%) was consistently higher than for paroxetine (9%), and Rouillon (1998) reported that clomipramine was associated with significantly more early withdrawals associated with side-effects than fluvoxamine. Moreover, in Bisserbe *et al.*'s (1997) intent-to-treat analysis, it was concluded that superior tolerability of sertraline over clomipramine explained its greater benefit.

The risk of dangerous side-effects such as convulsions (occurring in up to 2% on clomipramine, compared with 0.1–0.5% on high-dose SSRIs), cardiotoxicity, and cognitive impairment is substantially lower with SSRIs. Clomipramine shares anticholinergic side-effects associated with tricyclics including dry mouth, constipation, and blurred vision, and is lethal in overdose. All SRIs are associated with impaired sexual performance but clomipramine (up to 80% of cases, Monteiro *et al.*, 1987) appears more problematic than SSRIs (up to 30% cases). SSRIs are responsible for more asthenia, insomnia, and nausea. Maina *et al.* (2003a) reported clinically relevant weight gain in approximately 14.5% of cases (mainly females)

Table 8.2 Controlled studies comparing selective serotonin reuptake inhibitors with clomipramine (CMI)

Drug and study	*n*	Design	Outcome Efficacy	Tolerability
Fluoxetine (FLX)				
Pigott *et al.* (1990)	11	CMI (50–250 mg) versus FLX (20–80 mg)	CMI = FLX	FLX > CMI
Lopez-Ibor *et al.* (1996)	30 vs. 24	CMI 150 mg versus FLX 40 mg	CMI = FLX on primary criterion CMI > FLX on other criteria	FLX = CMI
Fluvoxamine (FLV)				
Smeraldi *et al.* (1992)	10	CMI 200 mg versus FLV 200 mg	CMI = FLV	FLV = CMI
Freeman *et al.* (1994)	30 vs. 34	CMI (150–250 mg) versus FLV (150–250 mg)	CMI = FLV	FLV > CMI (on severe effects)
Koran *et al.* (1996)	42 vs. 37	CMI (100–250 mg) versus FLV (100–250 mg)	CMI = FLV	FLV = CMI
Milanfranchi *et al.* (1997)	13 vs.13	CMI (50–300 mg) versus FLV (50–300 mg)	CMI = FLV	FLV = CMI
Rouillon (1998)	105 vs. 112	CMI (150–300 mg) versus FLV (150–300 mg)	CMI = FLV	FLV > CMI
Paroxetine (PAR)				
Zohar and Judge (1996)	99 vs. 201 vs. 99	CMI (50–250 mg) versus PAR (20–60 mg) versus Placebo	CMI > Placebo PAR > Placebo	PAR > CMI
Sertraline (SER)				
Bisserbe *et al.* (1997)	82 versus 86	CMI (50–200 mg) versus SER (50–200 mg)	SER = CMI	SER > CMI
Citalopram (CIT)				
Pidrman and Tuma (1998)	24	CIT versus CMI	CIT = CMI	CIT = CMI

Y-BOCS, Yale-Brown Obsessive Compulsive Scale.

over 30 months of open SRI monotherapy, with clomipramine producing more weight gain than sertraline and fluoxetine.

The concept of a "gold-standard" drug for OCD is, perhaps, misleading. According to Y-BOCS analyses, SSRIs appear equally effective at relieving obsessional thoughts and compulsive rituals. Their improved safety and tolerability offer considerable benefits for the long-term treatment of OCD, and indicate that the SSRIs should usually be considered the treatments of choice, with clomipramine reserved for those who cannot tolerate or who have failed to respond to them.

Expert consensus guidelines for OCD

Expert consensus has a role in complementing and supplementing empirical evidence. By synthesizing combined views on best practice, a broader range of pertinent clinical questions can be addressed. Moreover, such opinions reflect experience with a range of cases and not just the highly selected groups that meet study criteria. The Expert Consensus Panel for OCD (March *et al.*, 1997) comprised 65–100 worldwide experts and the guidelines present specific judgments on a comprehensive range of issues relating to pharmacological and psychological treatments. The guidelines recommended initial treatment either with cognitive-behavioral therapy (CBT) alone or in conjunction with an SRI. Although the guidelines did not distinguish between clomipramine and SSRIs, improved tolerability of SSRIs was acknowledged. Combined CBT and medication was preferred by experts in terms of speed, efficacy, durability, tolerability, and acceptability, and was thought the best approach for most patients. Inclusion of medication should depend on illness severity and age. More recently, a smaller group of members of the World Council on Anxiety met to agree recommendations for long-term treatment (Greist *et al.*, 2003).

What is the most effective dose?

Traditionally, OCD has been thought to require higher doses of medication than depression and anxiety. Head-to-head studies comparing different fixed doses of active drug with placebo are needed to examine this issue. Clomipramine has not been tested in this way. Whereas the single-dose studies showed efficacy for relatively low fixed daily doses (75 and 125 mg) compared with placebo, most studies used flexible doses titrated toward the upper end of the range (200–300 mg/day). Similarly, fluvoxamine was found to be effective in doses ranging from 150 to 300 mg/day.

Available evidence suggests that exposure therapy is associated with similar rates of improvement as pharmacotherapy, and that combining the two forms of treatment is beneficial, although properly controlled head-to-head studies have not been performed. A review of behavior therapy is beyond the scope of this article.

Table 8.3 Placebo-controlled comparator studies of fixed-doses of selective serotonin reuptake inhibitors

Drug and studies	Fixed dose	n	Duration	Positive dose–response relationship?
Fluoxetine				
Montgomery *et al.* (1993)	20/40/60 mg	214	8 weeks	Yes[a]
Tollefson *et al.* (1994)	20/40/60 mg	355	13 weeks	No
Sertraline				
Greist *et al.* (1995b)	50/100/200 mg	324	12 weeks	No
Paroxetine				
Wheadon *et al.* (1993)	20/40/60 mg	348	12 weeks	Yes
Hollander *et al.* (2003b)	20/40/60 mg	348	12 weeks	Yes
Citalopram				
Montgomery *et al.* (2001)	20/40/60 mg	352	12 weeks	No

[a] Marginally significant benefit for medium and higher doses on primary analysis (total Yale-Brown Obsessive Compulsive Scale; $P = 0.059$); significant on responder analysis ($P < 0.05$).

Fluoxetine, paroxetine, and sertraline have each been investigated in a series of multiple fixed doses (Table 8.3). In the case of paroxetine, a positive dose–response relationship was clearly demonstrated; in two studies a 40 and 60 mg dose showed efficacy while a 20 mg dose did not (Hollander *et al.*, 2003b; Wheadon *et al.*, 1993). Similar results are seen for fluoxetine: whereas all three fixed doses (20, 40, and 60 mg/day) were effective, the greatest benefit was seen in patients receiving the highest dose, although this did not reach statistical significance. Adverse effects appear to be dose-related, with no differences between 20 mg and placebo groups, compared to 18.5% early withdrawal in the 60 mg group (Tollefson *et al.*, 1994). A meta-analysis of the contemporaneous grouped data showed that the 60 mg dose was significantly more effective than 20 mg (Wood *et al.*, 1993). A smaller fixed dose comparison of 20, 40, and 60 mg of fluoxetine produced clearer findings. In this study the 40 and 60 mg doses were effective, but the 20 mg dose was not (Montgomery *et al.*, 1993). The existence of a dose–response relationship is less clear-cut in the case of sertraline and citalopram. In a multiple fixed-dose study of sertraline (Greist *et al.*, 1995b), the 50 and 200 mg doses were superior to placebo, whereas the 100 mg dose was not, possibly because of increased withdrawal rates in the 100 mg group. A smaller study (Ushijima *et al.*, 1997) suggested that a dose–response relationship exists for sertraline as well. In the fixed-dose study of citalopram (Montgomery *et al.*, 2001), a numerical advantage was seen for higher dose levels, and a significant reduction in baseline Y-BOCS score was seen from week 3 in the 60 mg group, compared to weeks 7–12 in the other two groups. However, these differences did not reach statistical significance.

These mixed results suggest that higher doses (e.g., 60 mg paroxetine, fluoxetine, citalopram, 200 mg sertraline) produce better antiobsessional efficacy. Controlled studies demonstrate efficacy and tolerability for doses as high as 80 mg fluoxetine (Jenike et al., 1997; Leibowitz et al., 2002) and 300 mg clomipramine (de Veaugh-Geiss et al., 1989). The expert guidelines advocate treatment at moderate dose levels in most cases, only titrating upwards to the maximum after a period of assessment.

Strategies for dose titration in OCD

Acute studies of SRIs show a slow, gradual treatment effect and, unlike panic disorder, exacerbation of anxiety is rare in the first days of treatment. Improvements can take several weeks to become established, irrespective of dose, and patients should be warned about this from the outset. Individuals with OCD are notoriously poor at recognizing their own improvements, and it is useful to enlist the help of informants to report early signs of improvement. Observer-rated scales may also detect small improvements in a clinical setting, though in some cases observable benefits may not appear for several months. These cases can be extremely challenging, with pressure on the clinician to change treatments or escalate doses prematurely. Given the dose–response data, there are clear grounds for titrating doses upwards, but the clinician needs to strike a delicate balance between speed of increase and tolerability. Fast upwards titration may produce earlier responses, but the long-term benefits of this approach are unclear. A single-blind study compared rapid dose escalation with sertraline to 150 mg over 5 days, with slower dose escalation over 15 days, and found a significant difference in favor of the rapid titration group at weeks 4 and 6, but this advantage disappeared thereafter (Bogetto et al., 2002). The study was too small to discern differences in tolerability. In another study, pulse loading with intravenous clomipramine produced a large and rapid decrease in obsessive symptoms, but oral pulse loading did not, and the early advantages were not sustained over treatment (Koran et al., 1997). The arguments for slower dose increases may be more persuasive, particularly in children and the elderly. Early SSRI-related adverse effects such as nausea and agitation can be ameliorated by slowly titrating upwards over weeks and months. Longer-term side-effects such as sleep disturbance and headache are also dose-related, and need to be monitored. Sexual dysfunction is a common cause of drug discontinuation, and, if necessary, strategies such as dose reduction, short drug holidays, or use of drugs with restorative potency (e.g., nefazodone, Viagra, mianserin (Aizenberg et al., 1999)) can be considered in stable cases.

The Expert Guidelines recommend continuing treatment at average dose levels for 4–8 weeks. If there are no signs of improvement at that point, they suggest proceeding to the maximum licenced dose. In the case of partial improvement, the guidelines suggest waiting longer for the effect to increase (5–9 weeks) before titrating the dose upwards. When at the highest dose it is best to continue for at least 3 months (in some cases longer periods are required) to allow the treatment effect time to develop.

SRIs are the treatment of choice in comorbid depression

Moderate levels of depression do not interfere with the antiobsessional response (Zohar and Judge, 1996). However, comorbid depression has received relatively little attention because most studies have excluded depressed individuals. Clomipramine, fluvoxamine, and sertraline have been compared with desipramine in groups where comorbid depression was included. In the study by Hoehn-Saric *et al.* (2000), patients were specifically selected for the presence of significant depression. In general, comorbid depression responded in parallel with OCD, and shared its characteristic selectivity for the serotonergic drug. It is unusual for an antidepressant like desipramine to show such a poor response. These results suggest that the depression is either integral or secondary to OCD, and imply that depressed patients with OCD should be treated with an SRI. OCD frequently co-occurs with bipolar disorder, with lifetime comorbidity as high as 30% (Kruger *et al.*, 1995). This presents a challenge since SRIs can be associated with a switch to mania. SSRIs are less risky than clomipramine in this respect, and judicious administration of mood-stabilizing medication together with caution in dose escalation are advisable (Kaplan and Hollander, 2003). Unlike drugs, studies of behavior therapy suggest that moderately high levels of baseline depression adversely affect the treatment outcome (Kejsers *et al.*, 1994). This disadvantage may be neutralized by augmenting psychotherapy with an SSRI (Hohagen *et al.*, 1998), though studies investigating this have been unable to disentangle the antiobsessional effects of medication from those of behavioral interventions. These findings suggest that the first-line treatment for depressed patients with OCD should be an SSRI.

Other treatments

Preliminary reports hinting at benefits for a variety of agents acting on serotonin, such as mianserin and mirtazapine (Koran *et al.*, 2001a), and the serotonin precursor L-tryptophan (Montgomery *et al.*, 1992), are of theoretical value. There has been particular interest in the role of venlafaxine in OCD which, in low doses, acts mainly as an SSRI, but in doses exceeding 225 mg combines this activity with norepinephrine (noradrenaline) reuptake inhibition. A small, placebo-controlled trial ($n = 30$) failed to separate venlafaxine from placebo (Yaryura-Tobias and Neziroglu, 1996). Venlafaxine was also compared to paroxetine in a non-placebo double-blind study of non-depressed OCD cases (Denys *et al.*, 2003a) where 75 individuals

Table 8.4 Placebo-controlled studies of long-term treatments for patients with obsessive-compulsive disorder (OCD)

Study	Active treatment	n	Duration (weeks)	Outcome
Cottraux *et al.* (1990)	Fluvoxamine + exposure[a]	50 44 37	8 24 48	Fluvoxamine superior to placebo in follow-up phase, but only for depression
Katz *et al.* (1990)	Clomipramine[b]	124	(10 +) 52	Superiority of clomipramine sustained in follow-up phase
Tollefson *et al.* (1994)	Fluoxetine[b]	76	(13 +) 24	Improvement on all doses, 60 mg significant above others
Greist *et al.* (1995a)	Sertraline[b]	118	(12 +) 40	Significant additional improvements in OCD symptoms for sertraline

[a] Extended double-blind study.
[b] Double-blind continuation in acute-phase ($\times$ weeks) responders.

received paroxetine (60 mg) and 75 venlafaxine (300 mg). Both treatments appeared equally effective at reducing Y-BOCS scores. An evaluation of quality-of-life measures from the study also showed equivalent improvements (Tenney *et al.*, 2003). A smaller single-blind study comparing venlafaxine with clomipramine also failed to reach significance, though 42.6% (20/47) of the clomipramine group were responders compared to 34.6% (9/26) on venlafaxine on the intent-to-treat analysis (Albert *et al.*, 2002). Further evaluation of the relative efficacy and tolerability of venlafaxine is warranted.

How long should pharmacotherapy of OCD continue?

OCD is a long-term illness and we need to know if acute treatments maintain efficacy in the longer term. In comparison to the evidence base for acute treatment of OCD, long-term outcome is less clear. Evidence for long-term efficacy can be derived from a variety of sources. Some investigators have followed treatment-responders from acute-phase studies on uncontrolled SRIs for up to 2 years, without tolerance developing. The study by Wagner *et al.* (1999) reported ongoing efficacy for open-label sertraline up to 1 year in a large cohort of children and adolescents. Evidence from controlled studies is more convincing (Table 8.4). Cottraux *et al.* (1990) reported a significant benefit for fluvoxamine over placebo, but only for depressive symptoms. Katz *et al.* (1990) randomized patients to either clomipramine (100–300 mg) or placebo for 10 weeks, after which they entered 124 responders into a 52-week double-blind extension period. Clomipramine's superiority over placebo was sustained over the extension phase, to the extent that OCD was no longer compromising the lives of half the clomipramine group. However, a high incidence of adverse effects in the clomipramine group resulted in 23% withdrawing early.

Tollefson *et al.* (1994) followed up 76 responders from the 13-week multiple fixed-dose, placebo-controlled fluoxetine study on their ascribed treatment up to 24 weeks. Patients on all doses of fluoxetine (20, 40, and 60 mg) continued to improve, with further significant improvements evident for the 60 mg group only. Only 6% of fluoxetine-treated individuals discontinued due to side-effects. In the large extension study by Greist *et al.* (1995a), 118 patients who had responded to 12 weeks' treatment with sertraline or placebo continued under double-blind conditions for 40 weeks. The patients maintained their improvements as long as they remained on sertraline. Compliance was good: only 13% of patients dropped out of treatment prematurely during the extension phase. Of these, one-third blamed side-effects and two-thirds blamed unsatisfactory clinical response. Side-effects improved over time, and there were no statistically significant differences between sertraline and placebo in vital signs or laboratory abnormalities. Fifty-nine completers were followed up for a further year on open-label sertraline, and showed significant additional improvements in OCD symptoms over the course of the second year, with a reduced incidence of side-effects compared with the earlier study (Rasmussen *et al.*, 1997).

How long should treatment continue?

One way of tackling this question is to explore whether continuation of pharmacotherapy provides ongoing protection against deterioration. A promising technique involves taking patients who have responded to active drug and comparing their "relapse" rates following randomization to either continuous drug treatment or drug discontinuation. Planning and interpretation of drug discontinuation studies are not always straightforward. There is still debate about the definition of a meaningful clinical response and the concept of "relapse" has been even more difficult to apply to an illness that runs a chronic course and shows partial response to long-term treatment. Indeed, the lack of agreed definitions for "relapse" makes interstudy comparison difficult. Criteria such as $\geq$50% worsening of postbaseline Y-BOCS improvement, five-point worsening of Y-BOCS, Y-BOCS total score of $\geq$19, and clinical global impression of improvement scores of "much" or "very much worse" have been proposed. Some studies have erred toward imposing too stringent qualifications, requiring more than two criteria to be present at any one time (Romano *et al.*, 2001), or requiring criteria to persist over several visits (Koran *et al.*, 2002). This has compromised the sensitivity to detect outcome differences. In addition, studies need to differentiate between early "withdrawal effects" occurring soon after drug termination, and a more gradual reemergence of OCD. Withdrawal effects are related to the pharmacological properties of the compound, and are believed to complicate clomipramine and paroxetine more than fluoxetine (Rosenbaum *et al.*, 1998).

A series of controlled studies has shown that discontinuation of treatment is positively associated with symptomatic relapse, irrespective of treatment duration (up to 2 years) (Table 8.5). For most agents, symptoms reemerged within only a few weeks of stopping medication. The earlier clomipramine studies showed relatively high early relapse rates, possibly related to stronger withdrawal symptoms. For example, in the discontinuation study by Pato *et al.* (1988), 16/18 patients exhibiting sustained improvements on clomipramine showed substantial worsening of symptoms within 4 weeks of crossing over to placebo. The reemergence of symptoms was gradual and progressive and unrelated to duration of clomipramine pretreatment, which exceeded 2 years in some cases. In this study, reinstatement of clomipramine resulted in improvement to a level close to pre-discontinuation, though other authors have reported less favorable results. Similarly, in the study by Leonard *et al.* (1988), 89% of patients relapsed within 2 months of switching to placebo.

In the relapse prevention study by Romano *et al.* (2001), responders to 20 weeks' fixed-dose fluoxetine were randomized to continuation or placebo and followed up for a year. Relapses were stringently defined, and 38% relapsed over 12 months following double-blind discontinuation. Patients remaining on the highest dose (60 mg) showed significantly lower relapse rates (17.5%), but the study still did not discriminate between continuation and switching. In spite of its larger size and longer duration, the study by Koran *et al.* (2002) was also unable to demonstrate a significant advantage for sertraline on the *a priori* criterion for preventing relapse, in this case almost certainly because the criterion for relapse was too strictly defined. However, those remaining on sertraline showed significantly fewer "dropouts due to relapse or insufficient clinical response" (9% versus 24% on placebo) and "acute exacerbation of symptoms" (12% versus 25% on placebo), and ongoing sertraline was associated with continued improvement in Y-BOCS, NIMH-OC, and CGI scores and quality-of-life measures.

A discontinuation study investigating adults who had responded to 6 months' paroxetine (Dunbar *et al.*, 1995) was presented at an international meeting but has not been published. Results showed that those who continued on paroxetine suffered significantly fewer relapses during the next 36 weeks than those who switched to placebo. Roughly 10% of paroxetine-treated patients had a full relapse, compared with 18% on placebo. The intent-to-treat analysis showed a significantly shorter time-to-relapse on placebo. Y-BOCS scores were maintained or slightly improved under paroxetine, but deteriorated under placebo. A more recent large-scale study of paroxetine by Hollander *et al.* (2003b) looked at 105 responders to 6-month

Table 8.5 Double-blind discontinuation studies of relapse prevention in obsessive-compulsive disorder (OCD)

Study	Drug	Duration of prior drug treatment	n in discontinuation phase	Follow-up after discontinuation (weeks)	Outcome
Yaryura-Tobias et al. (1976)	Clomipramine	4 or 6 weeks	13	1	Worsening of OCD on placebo
Flament et al. (1985)[a]	Clomipramine	5 weeks	19	5	Worsening of OCD on placebo
Pato et al. (1988)	Clomipramine	5–27 months	18	7	94.4% relapsed on placebo
Leonard et al. (1988)[b]	Clomipramine	17 months	21	5	89% relapsed on placebo
Dunbar et al. (1995)[c]	Paroxetine	9 months	104	36	Relapse rate on placebo > paroxetine
Romano et al. (2001)[c]	Fluoxetine	20 weeks	71	52	Relapse rate on placebo = pooled fluoxetine. Relapse rate on placebo > fluoxetine 60 mg
Koran et al. (2002)[c]	Sertraline	52 weeks	223	28	Relapse rate on placebo = sertraline. Acute OCD exacerbation on placebo > sertraline. Dropouts due to relapse on placebo > sertraline
Geller et al. (2003b)[b]	Paroxetine	16 weeks	193	16	Relapse rate on placebo = paroxetine
Hollander et al. (2003b)[c]	Paroxetine	12 weeks	105	36	Relapse rate on placebo > paroxetine

[a] In children.
[b] In children and adolescents survival analysis performed.
[c] Survival analysis performed.

treatment and demonstrated a significantly better outcome for those remaining on the active drug over the 6-month double-blind discontinuation phase: 59% of patients randomized to placebo relapsed, compared to 38% on paroxetine (20–60 mg), with paroxetine being well tolerated across the dose range. Geller *et al.* (2003b) investigated paroxetine in children and adolescents, of whom more than half had at least one comorbid illness, using a relapse prevention design. After 16 weeks' open-label paroxetine, 193 responders were randomized to a further 16 weeks' double-blind treatment on paroxetine or placebo. The overall relapse rate was not significantly higher in the placebo than paroxetine group (43.9% versus 34.7%), possibly because the duration of follow-up was too short. Post-hoc analyses showed a significantly greater relapse rate for patients with comorbid disorders than those with uncomplicated OCD randomized to placebo, but this did not apply under paroxetine. The authors argued that patients with comorbidity are at increased risk of relapse following discontinuation and that studies which too rigorously exclude comorbid disorders may underestimate relapse rates in clinical samples of OCD.

It is difficult to draw strong conclusions from these mixed findings. We may surmise that medication probably confers protection against relapse, as long as it is continued. The Expert Consensus Guidelines (March *et al.*, 1997) recommended pharmacotherapy maintenance for a minimum of 3–6 months after acute treatment, reserving long-term treatment for subsequent relapses. However, it was also noted that much longer periods, exceeding 2 years, were usually needed, and that lifelong treatment was warranted after 2–4 relapses. More recent guidelines (Greist *et al.*, 2003) have more strongly emphasized the importance of long-term treatment from the outset and recommended continuation of pharmacotherapy for a minimum of 1–2 years in treatment-responsive individuals. Discontinuation, if necessary, should be gradual to minimize discontinuation effects, and patients should be warned to look out for early signs of relapse, whereupon reinstatement of pharmacotherapy may achieve the same level of improvement as before, although this cannot be guaranteed (Ravizza *et al.*, 1998). Until clear predictors relating to relapse are available, lifelong medication may be the best option for most cases.

What is the best dose for long-term treatment?

There is little evidence supporting dose reduction in long-term treatment, apart from one small study where lowering the dose of clomipramine and fluvoxamine did not affect relapse rates (Mundo *et al.*, 1997b). Results from Romano *et al.*'s (2001) study, in which a 60 mg dose of fluoxetine appeared the most effective over the 24-week extension phase, support continuation of treatment at higher dose levels. On the basis of the limited data available, most experts recommend continuing treatment at the effective dose, and the adage "the dose that gets you well, keeps you well" probably applies.

What is the best pharmacotherapy approach to resistant OCD?

Predictors of treatment response

Although most patients experience substantial improvements, for many the treatment response is not complete. In about 30% of cases residual symptoms remain in spite of prolonged treatment with SRIs. The problem of partial responders is an area that has received inadequate controlled investigation and which is bedeviled by the lack of universally accepted definitions. Pallanti *et al.* (2002a) advocated the use of standardized operational criteria across treatment trials. Specifically, they proposed that an improvement of ≥35% in baseline Y-BOCS score, or "much" or "very much improved" on the CGI-I, represented a meaningful clinical response, while "remission" required a total Y-BOCS score of less than 16. Those showing between 25 and 35% improvement in Y-BOCS scores were considered partial responders. Relapse was defined as a 25% worsening in Y-BOCS (or a CGI score of 6), after a period of remission, and the term "treatment-refractory" was reserved for those who do not respond to "all available treatments." Levels of non-response, according to the numbers of failed treatments, were also defined.

Few studies provide information on response status, and the literature on pharmacological response predictors is sparse and inconsistent. Mataix-Cols *et al.*'s (1999) factor analysis suggests that adults with compulsive rituals, early-onset age, longer duration, chronic course, comorbid tics, and personality disorders (especially schizotypal), respond poorly to clomipramine and SSRIs. Additional analyses of large databases for clomipramine and fluoxetine reported better responses for previously SRI-naive patients, and poorer responses for those with subclinical depression. Patients with an earlier age of onset responded poorly to clomipramine, but not to fluoxetine (Ackerman and Greenland, 2002). The more recent analysis of data from a large trial of citalopram also reported that patients with a longer duration of illness or previous SSRI treatment, as well as greater illness severity, were less likely to respond well to the active drug (Stein *et al.*, 2001). One small study has identified better responses in females (Mundo *et al.*, 1999) and children with comorbid attention-deficit hyperactivity disorder, tic disorder, and oppositional defiant disorder showed a less favorable response (Geller *et al.*, 2003a).

Switching SRI, increasing dose, or changing mode of drug delivery

Given the limitations of data supporting alternative strategies, and the acceptability of switching from one SSRI to another, this remains the preferred option for many clinicians. Sometimes, however, it may be appropriate to persist for longer with a particular SRI even in patients who show little sign of improvement, since a delayed response may occur after 6 months or more. March et al. (1997) recommended changing the SRI after 8–12 weeks on the maximal dose if the clinical effect was incomplete. They proposed a 40% chance of responding to a second SRI, and a lesser response to a third, and suggested switching to clomipramine after 2–3 failed trials on SSRIs. An unpublished report by Ravizza et al. (2001) looked at patients who had failed to respond to at least two trials of SSRIs other than citalopram. Patients were randomized to clomipramine, venlafaxine, or citalopram for 12 weeks and 14% responded to citalopram, 37.5% to clomipramine, and 42% to venlafaxine. A single-blind study in 29 cases of SRI-resistant OCD showed encouraging results for venlafaxine (37.5–375 mg) as a monotherapy (Hollander et al., 2003c). These results hint that patients who have failed to respond to two SSRIs may benefit from switching to an agent with a different mode of action.

Results from uncontrolled case studies suggest that, for some patients, increasing SSRI doses above formulary limits can procure a better effect (Byerly et al., 1996; Bejerot and Bodlund, 1998). Although doses of clomipramine up to 300 mg have been systematically investigated and found to be acceptable, the risk of seizures and cardiotoxicity associated with this drug suggests that doses exceeding this should be generally avoided. Altering the mode of administration may be considered, though this is not practical in many cases. Intravenous clomipramine has been shown to be more effective than placebo in a single double-blind study investigating refractory OCD, with 6/29 randomized to clomipramine classed as responders after 14 daily infusions, compared to none for placebo (Fallon et al., 1998). A positive open study of 21 days' intravenous citalopram has also been reported (Pallanti et al., 2002b).

Combining SRIs and drugs exerting antidepressant or anxiolytic properties

If a patient fails to respond to successive SRI trials, augmented with CBT, the Expert Consensus Guideline recommends adding another agent to the SRI. The evidence is acknowledged to be limited, based on the results of small studies and open case series (Table 8.6). Combining clomipramine with an SSRI has been proposed for adults or children unresponsive to, or intolerant of, SRI monotherapy. This strategy should be approached with caution since the pharmacokinetic interactions on the hepatic cytochrome P 450 isoenzymes may lead to a build-up of clomipramine that could be dangerous, and electrocardiogram and plasma-level monitoring are advisable. Positive results have been reported from small, uncontrolled case series (Szegedi et al., 1996), although a fluoxetine–clomipramine combination resulted in electrocardiogram changes in some cases. Pallanti et al. (1999) compared 9 treatment-refractory patients given citalopram plus clomipramine with 7 given citalopram alone, in a randomized open-label trial. They reported a significantly larger improvement in Y-BOCS ratings for those given the combination, all of whom

Table 8.6 Treatment-refractory obsessive-compulsive disorder (OCD)

Double-blind, placebo-controlled pharmacotherapy studies

May be effective

- Intravenous clomipramine[a]
- Adding haloperidol[b]
- Adding risperidone
- Adding quetiapine
- Adding clonazepam[c]

Apparently ineffective

- Adding lithium
- Adding buspirone
- Adding triiodothyronine (liothyronine)
- Adding desipramine
- Adding inositol

Promising treatments warranting controlled study

- Higher-dose SSRI monotherapy
- Combined SSRI–clomipramine treatment
- Extended SSRI therapy
- Adding olanzapine
- Adding amisulpride
- Intravenous citalopram
- Triptans that enter the CNS, e.g., zolmitriptan
- Immunoglobulins and plasmapharesis
- Deep-brain stimulation
- Neurosurgery (gamma knife surgery)

[a] Remains investigational in many countries.
[b] Primarily in tic-related OCD.
[c] Small numbers and improvement not evident on all OCD rating scales.
SSRI, selective serotonin reuptake inhibitors; CNS, central nervous system.

experienced decreases $\geq 35\%$ from baseline. This combination is advantageous in not altering the metabolism of clomipramine, and was well tolerated. No controlled studies of the co-administration of different SSRIs have been published.

Controlled studies have confirmed the lack of efficacy of lithium augmentation in OCD (McDougle *et al.*, 1991; Pigott *et al.*, 1991). Similarly, three double-blind placebo controlled studies have demonstrated that combining buspirone with an SRI is not helpful (Pigott *et al.*, 1992a; Grady *et al.*, 1993; McDougle *et al.*, 1993). Clonazepam is a benzodiazepine with putative effects on serotonin neurotransmission. As a monotherapy it fails to impact on the core symptoms of OCD (Hollander *et al.*, 2003d), though it may help with associated anxiety.

Pigott *et al.* (1992b) reported limited efficacy for clonazepam given together with fluoxetine or clomipramine in a placebo-controlled study. Pindolol is a beta-blocker which also acts as an antagonist at presynaptic 5HT1A autoreceptors. Dannon *et al.* (2000) demonstrated efficacy for pindolol when combined with paroxetine in a double-blind, placebo-controlled study of 14 treatment-resistant cases, but another study combining it with fluvoxamine did not (Mundo *et al.*, 1998). Blier and Bergeron (1996) found a beneficial effect for pindolol only when L-tryptophan was openly added to the combination. The limitations of adding drugs acting on serotonin led investigators to reexamine the role of noradrenergic agents in resistant OCD. Barr *et al.* (1997) investigated the addition of desipramine to 20 patients who had failed SSRI monotherapy, in a double-blind, placebo-controlled study, and found no added benefit.

Combining SRIs and drugs with antipsychotic properties

No positive studies of antipsychotic monotherapy in OCD meet today's standards, and OCD is not recognized to respond to these drugs individually. McDougle *et al.* (1990) reported a benefit from adding open-label pimozide (6.5 mg) in 17 patients unresponsive to fluvoxamine. Patients with comorbid chronic tics or schizotypal disorder were most responsive. A subsequent double-blind placebo-controlled study by the same author demonstrated a significant Y-BOCS improvement for low-dose haloperidol (6.2 mg) added to fluvoxamine. Eleven of 17 patients receiving the active drug achieved responder status by as early as 4 weeks, compared to none on placebo. Again, a preferential response was seen in patients with comorbid tics (McDougle *et al.*, 1994). Antipsychotics such as haloperidol and sulpiride are first-line treatments for the Tourette syndrome, so this finding supports a theoretical link between these disorders. This combination increases the side-effect burden, including extrapyramidal effects. It is therefore wise to start treatment with very low doses, and increase cautiously subject to tolerability (e.g., 0.25–0.5 mg haloperidol, titrated slowly to 2–4 mg: McDougle and Walsh, 2001).

Newer second-generation antipsychotics, that modulate serotonin and dopamine neurotransmission, also offer promise and have lower side-effect risks. Positive reports from open case series were confirmed by McDougle *et al.* (2000) in the first reported double-blind placebo-controlled study showing efficacy for risperidone augmentation in 36 patients unresponsive to 12 weeks on an SRI. Risperidone (2.2 mg) was superior to placebo in reducing Y-BOCS scores as well as anxiety and depression, was well-tolerated, and there was no difference between those with and without comorbid tics or schizotypy. A smaller double-blind study by Hollander *et al.* (2003e) examined patients failing to respond to at least two trials of SRIs. Four of 16 patients randomized to risperidone (0.5–3 mg) turned out to be responders, defined as a CGI-I score of 1 or 2 and Y-BOCS decrease of >25% at the 8-week endpoint, compared with none of the 6 patients randomized to placebo.

Quetiapine has also been the subject of recent controlled investigation. There have been contradictory results from open (Sevincok and Topuz, 2003) and single-blind studies (Atmaca *et al.*, 2002). However, the recent double-blind placebo-controlled study by Denys *et al.* (2003b), published in abstract form, showed clear evidence of efficacy for 8 weeks' quetiapine (<300 mg) augmentation in 20 SRI-refractory patients, showing a mean decrease of 30% on baseline Y-BOCS, compared to 20 controls who showed only 6% improvement. Encouraging results from a small number of open-label studies of olanzapine (D'Amico *et al.*, 2003) and an open-label study of amisulpride (Metin *et al.*, 2003) suggest these drugs may also be helpful, and further investigation is underway. The results for clozapine have been less encouraging (McDougle *et al.*, 1995). Some authors report emergent obsessions during treatment with atypical antipsychotics, which may be related to their mixed receptor antagonist properties. Altogether, these results favor the use of second-generation antipsychotics as the first-line strategy for augmentation in resistant OCD. It remains uncertain as to how long patients need to remain on augmented treatment. A small retrospective study by Maina *et al.* (2003b) showed that the vast majority of patients who had responded to the addition of an antipsychotic to their SRI subsequently relapsed when the antipsychotic was withdrawn.

Other strategies for refractory OCD

Inositol (18 g/day) is an experimental compound that acts through intracellular messenger systems. It was thought to have mild antiobsessional efficacy but results from a placebo-controlled augmentation study by Fux *et al.* (1999) refute this. Sumatriptan is a 5HT1D agonist used to treat migraine. A small open case series suggested improvement over 4 weeks' treatment but, in a double-blind placebo-controlled study of 10 patients, 5-day treatment was associated with a worsening of OCD (Koran *et al.*, 2001b). Drugs that alter the immune system response may have a role in refractory OCD. For example, syndromes of sudden-onset OCD following childhood streptococcal infections are recognized, and these may respond to plasmapharesis and intravenous immunoglobulin (Perlmutter *et al.*, 1999). Preliminary reports that repetitive transcranial magnetic stimulation may reduce compulsions (Greenberg *et al.*, 1997) have not been substantiated in treatment studies. Neither is electroconvulsive therapy considered effective, although it may help relieve severe comorbid depression. Stereotactic neurosurgery should be viewed as a last option. Techniques such as cingulotomy and capsulotomy have produced improvements in some intransigent cases, but the absence of controlled trial data, including long-term follow-up on adverse effects, is discouraging. Deep-brain stimulation involves less intracerebral neuronal damage and holds promise for future investigation.

Conclusions

An extensive evidence base now exists for the pharmacological management of OCD. First-line treatment with an SSRI is uncontroversial, with improvements being sustained over time, although response is often incomplete, with many individuals failing to respond adequately. Treatment-resistant OCD is now receiving systematic evaluation: augmentation with second-generation antipsychotic agents appears a promising strategy and other techniques for resistant cases are under evaluation. Important questions requiring further investigation include identification of clinically relevant predictors relating to treatment response and relapse, the clarification of optimal duration of treatment, and the evaluation of antiobsessional treatment in comorbid disorders such as schizophrenia with OCD. Agreed definitions for response, relapse, resistance, and refractoriness will improve research in this area.

Acknowledgments

The authors wish to thank: Joan Lomas and Jill Jones, from the QEII Hospital Library, and Richard Jenkins, from the Royal College of Psychiatrists Research Unit, for help in obtaining manuscripts; and Kerry Foley and Penny Davy for assistance with reference formatting. Finally we are grateful to Professor B. Lerer and three anonymous reviewers for their insightful comments on an earlier draft.

Statement of interest

Naomi Fineberg has participated in several trials in OCD sponsored by the pharmaceutical industry, and has received honoraria for lectures and remuneration for consultation work, and sponsorship to attend scientific congresses. Companies include: Lundbeck (consultation, sponsorship for trials, lectures, and congresses), Astra-Zeneca (sponsorship for trials and attendance at congresses), Solvay (support for attendance at congresses), Lilley (sponsorship for trials and attendance at meetings), Novartis (sponsorship for attendance at congresses), Roche (trial sponsorship), Pfizer (sponsorship for lectures and attendance at conferences), Janssen (sponsorship for attendance at congresses). Tim Gale is participating in a trial sponsored by Lundbeck.

REFERENCES

Abramowitz, J. S. (1997). Effectiveness of psychological and pharmacological treatments for obsessive compulsive disorder: a quantitative review. *Journal of Consulting and Clinical Psychology*, **65**, 44–52.

Ackerman, D. L. and Greenland, S. (2002). Multivariate meta-analysis of controlled drug studies for obsessive compulsive disorder. *Journal of Clinical Psychopharmacology*, **22**, 309–17.

Aizenberg, D., Naor, S., Zemishlany, Z., and Weizman, A. (1999). The serotonin antagonist mianserin for treatment of serotonin-reuptake inhibitor-induced sexual dysfunction: an open-label study. *Clinical Neuropharmacology*, **22**, 347–50.

Albert, U., Aguglia, E., Maina, G., and Bogetto, F. (2002). Venlafaxine versus clomipramine in the treatment of obsessive compulsive disorder: a preliminary, single-blind 12-week controlled study. *Journal of Clinical Psychiatry*, **63**, 1004–9.

Ananth, J., Pecknold, J. C., Van Den Steen, N., and Engelsmann, F. (1981). Double-blind comparative study of clomipramine and amitriptyline in obsessional neurosis. *Progress in Neuro-Psychopharmacology*, **5**, 257–62.

Asberg, M., Montgomery, S. A., Perris, C., Schalling, D., and Sedvall, G. (1978). A comprehensive psychopathological rating scale. *Acta Psychiatrica Scandinavica*, **271** (suppl.), 5–27.

Atmaca, M., Kuloglu, M., Tezcan, E., and Gecici, O. (2002). Quetiapine augmentation in patients with treatment-resistant obsessive compulsive disorder. A single blind, placebo-controlled study. *International Clinical Psychopharmacology*, **17**, 115–19.

Barr, L. C., Goodman, W. K., Anand, A., McDougle, C. J., and Price, L. H. (1997). Addition of desipramine to serotonin reuptake inhibitors in treatment-resistant obsessive-compulsive disorder. *American Journal of Psychiatry*, **154**, 1293–5.

Beasley, C. M., Potvin, J. H., Masica, D. N., *et al.* (1992). Fluoxetine: no association with suicidality in obsessive-compulsive disorder. *Journal of Affective Disorders*, **24**, 1–10.

Bejerot, S. and Bodlund, O. (1998). Response to high doses of citalopram in treatment-resistant obsessive compulsive disorder. *Acta Psychopharmacologica Scandinavica*, **98**, 423–4.

Bergeron, R., Ravindran, A. V., Chaput, Y., *et al.* (2001). Sertraline and fluoxetine treatment of obsessive compulsive disorder: results of a double-blind, 6-month treatment study. *Journal of Clinical Psychopharmacology*, **22**, 148–54.

Bisserbe, J. C., Lane, R. M., and Flament, M. F. (1997). A double-blind comparison of sertraline and clomipramine in outpatients with obsessive-compulsive disorder. *European Psychiatry*, **12**, 82–93.

Blier, P. and Bergeron, R. (1996). Sequential administration of augmentation strategies in treatment resistant obsessive compulsive disorder: preliminary findings. *International Clinical Psychopharmacology*, **11**, 37–44.

Bogetto, F., Albert, U., and Maina, G. (2002). Sertraline treatment of obsessive-compulsive disorder: efficacy and tolerability of a rapid titration regimen. *European Neuropsychopharmacology*, **12**, 181–6.

Byerly, M. J., Goodman, W. K., and Christenen, R. (1996). High doses of sertraline for treatment-resistant obsessive compulsive disorder. *American Journal of Psychiatry*, **153**, 1232–3.

Chouinard, G., Goodman, W., Greist, J., *et al.* (1990). Results of a double-blind placebo-controlled trial of a new serotonin reuptake inhibitor, sertraline, in the treatment of obsessive-compulsive disorder. *Psychopharmacology Bulletin*, **26**, 279–84.

Clomipramine Collaborative Study Group (1991). Clomipramine in the treatment of patients with obsessive compulsive disorder. *Archives of General Psychiatry*, **48**, 730–8.

Cottraux, J., Mollard, E., Bouvard, M., *et al.* (1990). A controlled study of fluvoxamine and exposure in obsessive-compulsive disorder. *International Clinical Psychopharmacology*, **5**, 17–30.

D'Amico, G., Cedro, C., Muscatello, M. R., *et al.* (2003). Olanzapine augmentation of paroxetine-refractory obsessive-compulsive disorder. *Progress in Neuro-psychopharmacology and Biological Psychiatry*, **27**, 619–23.

Dannon, P. N., Sasson, Y., Hirschmann, S., *et al.* (2000). Pindolol augmentation in treatment-resistant obsessive compulsive disorder. A double-blind placebo-controlled trial. *European Neuropsychopharmacology*, **10**, 165–9.

Denys, D., van der Wee, N., van Megen, H. J., and Westenberg, H. G. (2003a). A double blind comparison of venlafaxine and paroxetine in obsessive-compulsive disorder. *Journal of Clinical Psychopharmacology*, **23**, 568–75.

Denys, D., De Geus, F., Van Megen, H. J., Salzman, C., and Westenberg, H. G. (2003b). A double-blind placebo-controlled trial of quetiapine augmentation in patients with obsessive compulsive disorder resistant to serotonin reuptake inhibitors. *European Neuropsychopharmacology*, **13** (suppl.), s361.

De Veaugh-Geiss, J., Landau, P., and Katz, R. (1989). Treatment of obsessive compulsive disorder with clomipramine. *Psychiatric Annals*, **19**, 97–101.

De Veaugh-Geiss, J., Moroz, G., Biederman, J., *et al.* (1992). Clomipramine hydrochloride in childhood and adolescent obsessive compulsive disorder: a multicenter trial. *Journal of the American Academy of Child and Adolescent Psychiatry*, **31**, 45–9.

Dunbar, G., Steiner, M., Bushnell, W. D., Gergel, I., and Wheadon, D. E. (1995). Long-term treatment and prevention of relapse of obsessive compulsive disorder with paroxetine. *European Neuropsychopharmacology*, **5**, 372 (P-D-11).

Fallon, B. A., Liebowitz, M. R., Campeas, R., *et al.* (1998). Intravenous clomipramine for obsessive-compulsive disorder refractory to oral clomipramine: a placebo-controlled study. *Archives of General Psychiatry*, **55**, 918–24.

Fernandez, C. E. and Lopez-Ibor, J. J. (1967). Monochlorimipramine in the treatment of psychiatric patients resistant to other therapies. *Actas Luso-Españolas de Neurología Psiquiatríay Ciencias Afines*, **26**, 119–47.

Fineberg, N. A., Roberts, A., Montgomery, S. A., and Cowen, P. H. (1997). Brain 5-HT function in obsessive-compulsive disorder: prolactin responses to *d*-fenfluramine. *British Journal of Psychiatry*, **171**, 280–2.

Flament, M. F., Rapoport, J. L., Berg, C. J., *et al.* (1985). Clomipramine treatment of childhood obsessive-compulsive disorder. A double-blind controlled study. *Archives of General Psychiatry*, **42**, 977–83.

Foa, E. B., Steketee, G., Kozak, M. J., and Dugger, D. (1987). Imipramine and placebo in the treatment of obsessive-compulsives: their effect on depression and obsessional symptoms. *Psychopharmacology Bulletin*, **23**, 8–11.

Freeman, C. P. L., Trimble, M. R., Deakin, J. F. W., Stokes, T. M., and Ashford, J. J. (1994). Fluvoxamine versus clomipramine in the treatment of obsessive compulsive disorder: a multicentre randomized double-blind parallel group comparison. *Journal of Clinical Psychiatry*, **55**, 301–5.

Fux, M., Benjamin, J., and Belmaker, R. H. (1999). Inositol versus placebo augmentation of serotonin reuptake inhibitors in the treatment of obsessive-compulsive disorder: a double-blind cross-over study. *International Journal of Neuropsychopharmacology*, **2**, 193–5.

Geller, D. A., Hoog, S. L., Heiligenstein, J. H., *et al.* (2001). Fluoxetine treatment for obsessive-compulsive disorder in children and adolescents: a placebo-controlled clinical trial. *Journal of the American Academy of Child and Adolescent Psychiatry*, **40**, 773–9.

Geller, D. A., Biederman, J., Stewart, S. E., *et al.* (2003a). Which SSRI? A meta-analysis of pharmacotherapy trials in paediatric obsessive-compulsive disorder. *American Journal of Psychiatry*, **160**, 1919–28.

Geller, D. A., Biederman, J., Stewart, S. E., *et al.* (2003b). Impact of comorbidity on treatment response to paroxetine in paediatric obsessive compulsive disorder: is the use of exclusion criteria empirically supported in randomised controlled trials? *Journal of Child and Adolescent Psychopharmacology*, **13** (suppl.), S19–29.

Goodman, W. K., Price, L. H., Rasmussen, S. A., *et al.* (1984). The Yale-Brown Obsessive Compulsive Scale: development, use and reliability. *Archives of General Psychiatry*, **46**, 1006–11.

Goodman, W. K., Price, L. H., Rasmussen, S. A., *et al.* (1989). Efficacy of fluvoxamine in obsessive-compulsive disorder. A double-blind comparison with placebo. *Archives of General Psychiatry*, **46**, 36–44.

Goodman, W. K., Price, L. H., Delgado, P. L., *et al.* (1990). Specificity of serotonin reuptake inhibitors in the treatment of obsessive-compulsive disorder: comparison of fluvoxamine and desipramine. *Archives of General Psychiatry*, **47**, 577–85.

Goodman, W. K., Kozak, M. J., Liebowitz, M., and White, K. L. (1996). Treatment of obsessive-compulsive disorder with Fluvoxamine: a multicentre, double-blind, placebo-controlled trial. *International Clinical Psychopharmacology*, **11**, 21–9.

Grady, T. A., Pigott, T. A., L'Heureux, F., *et al.* (1993). Double-blind study of adjuvant buspirone for fluoxetine-treated patients with obsessive-compulsive disorder. *American Journal of Psychiatry*, **150**, 819–21.

Greenberg, B. D., George, M. S., Martin, D. J., *et al.* (1997). Effect of prefrontal repetitive transcranial magnetic stimulation in obsessive-compulsive disorder: a preliminary study. *American Journal of Psychiatry*, **154**, 867–9.

Greist, J. H., Jefferson, J. W., Rosenfeld, R., *et al.* (1990). Clomipramine and obsessive compulsive disorder: a placebo-controlled double-blind study of 32 patients. *Journal of Clinical Psychiatry*, **51**, 292–7.

Greist, J. H., Jefferson, J. W., Kobak, K. A., *et al.* (1995a). A one year double-blind placebo-controlled fixed dose study of sertraline in the treatment of obsessive-compulsive disorder. *International Clinical Psychopharmacology*, **10**, 57–65.

Greist, J., Chouinard, G., DuBoff, E., *et al.* (1995b). Double-blind parallel comparison of three dosages of sertraline and placebo in outpatients with obsessive-compulsive disorder. *Archives of General Psychiatry*, **52**, 289–95.

Greist, J. H., Jefferson, J. W., Kobak, K. A., Katzelnick, D. J., and Serlin, R. C. (1995c). Efficacy and tolerability of serotonin transport inhibitors in obsessive-compulsive disorder: a metaanalysis. *Archives of General Psychiatry*, **52**, 53–60.

Greist, J. H., Bandelow, B., Hollander, E., *et al.* (2003). Long-term treatment of obsessive-compulsive disorder in adults. *CNS Spectrums*, **8**, 7–16.

Hamilton, M. (1960). A rating scale for depression. *Journal of Neurology, Neurosurgery and Psychiatry*, **23**, 56–62.

Hodgson, R. J. and Rachman, S. (1977). Obsessional-compulsive complaints. *Behavior Research and Therapy*, **15**, 389–95.

Hoehn-Saric, R., Ninan, P., Black, D. W., *et al.* (2000). Multicentre double-blind comparison of sertraline and desipramine for concurrent obsessive-compulsive and major depressive disorders. *Archives of General Psychiatry*, **57**, 76–82.

Hohagen, F., Winkelmann, G., Rasche-Ruchle, H., *et al.* (1998). Combination of behaviour therapy with fluvoxamine in comparison with behaviour therapy and placebo: results of a multicentre study. *British Journal of Psychiatry*, **173**, 71–8.

Hollander, E. and Wong, C. (1998). Psychosocial function and economic costs of obsessive compulsive disorder. *CNS Spectrums*, **3** (suppl. 1), 48–58.

Hollander, E., Greenwald, S., and Neville, D. (1998). Uncomplicated and comorbid obsessive-compulsive disorder in an epidemiological sample. *CNS Spectrums*, **3**, 10–18.

Hollander, E., Koran, L. M., Goodman, W. K., *et al.* (2003a). A double-blind placebo-controlled study of the efficacy and safety of controlled release fluvoxamine in patients with obsessive-compulsive disorder. *Journal of Clinical Psychiatry*, **64**, 640–7.

Hollander, E., Allen, A., Steiner, M., *et al.* (2003b). Acute and long-term treatment and prevention of relapse of obsessive-compulsive disorder with paroxetine. *Journal of Clinical Psychiatry*, **64**, 1113–21.

Hollander, E., Friedberg, J., Wasserman, S., *et al.* (2003c). Venlafaxine in treatment-resistant obsessive-compulsive disorder. *Journal of Clinical Psychiatry*, **64**, 546–50.

Hollander, E., Kaplan, A., and Stahl, S. M. (2003d). A double-blind placebo-controlled trial of clonazepam in obsessive-compulsive disorder. *World Journal of Biological Psychiatry*, **4**, 30–4.

Hollander, E., Rossi, N. B., Sood, E., and Pallanti, S. (2003e). Risperidone augmentation in treatment-resistant obsessive compulsive disorder: a double-blind, placebo controlled study. *International Journal of Neuropsychopharmacology*, **6**, 397–401.

Insel, T. R., Murphy, D. L., Cohen, R. M., *et al.* (1983). Obsessive-compulsive disorder – a double-blind trial of clomipramine and clorgyline. *Archives of General Pychiatry*, **40**, 605–12.

Insel, T. R., Mueller, E. A., Alterman, I., Linnoila, M., and Murphy, D. L. (1985). Obsessive-compulsive disorder and serotonin: is there a connection? *Biological Psychiatry*, **20**, 1174–88.

Jenike, M. A., Baer, L., Summergrad, P., *et al.* (1989). Obsessive-compulsive disorder: a double-blind, placebo-controlled trial of clomipramine in 27 patients. *American Journal of Psychiatry*, **146**, 1328–30.

Jenike, M. A., Hyman, S., Baer, L., *et al.* (1990a). A controlled trial of fluvoxamine in obsessive-compulsive disorder; implications for a serotonergic theory. *American Journal of Psychiatry*, **147**, 1209–15.

Jenike, M. A., Baer, L., Summergrad, P., *et al.* (1990b). Sertraline in obsessive-compulsive disorder: a double-blind comparison with placebo. *American Journal of Psychiatry*, **147**, 923–8.

Jenike, M. A., Baer, L., Minichiello, W. E., Raunch, S. L., and Buttolph, M. L. (1997). Placebo-controlled trial of fluoxetine and phenelzine for obsessive-compulsive disorder. *American Journal of Psychiatry*, **154**, 1261–4.

Kaplan, A. and Hollander, E. (2003). A review of pharmacologic treatments for obsessive-compulsive disorder. *Psychiatric Services*, **54**, 1111–18.

Katz, R. J., DeVeaugh-Geiss, J., and Landau, P. (1990). Clomipramine in obsessive-compulsive disorder. *Biological Psychiatry*, **28**, 401–4.

Kejsers, G., Hoogdiun, C., and Schaap, C. P. (1994). Predictors of treatment outcome in the behavioural treatment of obsessive-compulsive disorder. *British Journal of Psychiatry*, **165**, 781–6.

Kobak, K. A., Greist, J. H., Jefferson, J. W., Katzelnick, D. J., and Henk, H. J. (1998). Behavioural versus pharmacological treatments of obsessive compulsive disorder: a metaanalysis. *Psychopharmacology*, **136**, 205–16.

Koran, L. M., McElroy, S. L., Davidson, J. R., *et al.* (1996). Fluvoxamine versus clomipramine for obsessive compulsive disorder: a double-blind comparison. *Journal of Clinical Psychopharmacology*, **16**, 121–9.

Koran, L. M., Sallee, F. R., and Pallanti, S. (1997). Rapid benefit of intravenous pulse-loading of clomipramine in obsessive compulsive disorder. *American Journal of Psychiatry*, **154**, 396–401.

Koran, L. M., Quirk, T., Lorberbaum, J. P., and Elliott, M. (2001a). Mirtazepine treatment of obsessive-compulsive disorder. *Journal of Clinical Psychopharmacology*, **21**, 537–9.

Koran, L. M., Pallanti, S., and Querciolil, L. (2001b). Sumatriptan, 5-HT(1D) receptors and obsessive compulsive disorder. *European Neuropsychopharmacology*, **11**, 169–72.

Koran, L. M., Hackett, E., Rubin, A., Wolkow, R., and Robinson, D. (2002). Efficacy of sertraline in the long-term treatment of obsessive-compulsive disorder. *American Journal of Psychiatry*, **159**, 89–95.

Kronig, M. H., Apter, J., Asnis, G., *et al.* (1999). Placebo-controlled, multicenter study of sertraline treatment for obsessive-compulsive disorder. *Journal of Clinical Psychopharmacology*, **19**, 172–6.

Kruger, S., Cooke, R. G., Hasey, G. M., Jorna, T., and Persad, E. (1995). Comorbidity of obsessive compulsive disorder in bipolar disorder. *Journal of Affective Disorders*, **34**, 117–20.

Leibowitz, M. R., Turner, S. M., Piacentini, J., *et al.* (2002). Fluoxetine in children and adolescents with OCD: a placebo-controlled trial. *Journal of the American Academy of Child and Adolescent Psychiatry*, **41**, 1431–8.

Leonard, H. L., Swedo, S., Rapoport, J. L., Coffey, M., and Cheslow, D. (1988). Treatment of childhood obsessive compulsive disorder with clomipramine and desmethylimipramine: a double-blind crossover comparison. *Psychopharmacology Bulletin*, **24**, 93–5.

Leonard, H. L., Swedo, S. E., Lenane, M. C., *et al.* (1991). A double-blind desipramine substitution during long-term clomipramine treatment in children and adolescents with obsessive-compulsive disorder. *Archives of General Psychiatry*, **48**, 922–7.

Lopez-Ibor, J., Jr., Saiz, J., Cottraux, J., *et al.* (1996). Double-blind comparison of fluoxetine versus clomipramine in the treatment of obsessive compulsive disorder. *European Neuropsychopharmacology*, **6**, 111–18.

Maina, G., Salvi, V., and Bogetto, F. (2003a). Weight-gain during long-term drug treatment of obsessive compulsive disorder. *European Neuopsychopharmacology*, **13** (suppl.), s357.

Maina, G., Albert, U., Ziero, S., and Bogetto, F. (2003b). Antipsychotic augmentation for treatment-resistant obsessive compulsive disorder: what if antipsychotic is discontinued? *International Clinical Psychopharmacology*, **18**, 23–8.

March, J. S., Frances, A., Kahn, D. A., and Carpenter, D. (1997). The Expert Consensus Guideline series. Treatment of obsessive-compulsive disorder. *Journal of Clinical Psychiatry*, **58** (suppl.), 1–72.

March, J. S., Biederman, J., Wolkow, R., *et al.* (1998). Sertraline in children and adolescents with obsessive compulsive disorder: a multicentre randomised controlled trial. *Journal of the American Medical Association*, **28**, 1752–6.

Marks, I. M., Stern, R. S., Mawson, D., Cobb, J., and McDonald, R. (1980). Clomipramine and exposure for obsessive-compulsive rituals. *British Journal of Psychiatry*, **136**, 1–25.

Marks, I. M., Lelliott, P., Basoglu, M., *et al.* (1988). Clomipramine, self-exposure and therapist-aided exposure for obsessive-compulsive rituals. *British Journal of Psychiatry*, **152**, 522–34.

Mataix-Cols, D., Rauch, S. L., Manzo, P. A., Jenike, M. A., and Baer, L. (1999). Use of factor-analysed symptom dimensions to predict outcome with serotonin reuptake inhibitors and placebo in the treatment of obsessive-compulsive disorder. *American Journal of Psychiatry*, **156**, 1409–16.

Mavissakalian, M., Turner, S. M., Michelson, L., and Jacob, R. (1985). Tricyclic antidepressants in obsessive-compulsive disorder: antiobsessional or antidepressant agents? *American Journal of Psychiatry*, **142**, 572–6.

McDougle, C. J. and Walsh, K. H. (2001). Treatment of refractory OCD. In: *Obsessive Compulsive Disorder: A Practical Guide*, ed. N. A. Fineberg, D. Marazitti, and D. Stein. London, UK: Martin Dunitz, pp. 135–52.

McDougle, C. J., Goodman, W. K., Price, L. H., *et al.* (1990). Neuroleptic addition in fluvoxamine-refractory obsessive compulsive disorder. *American Journal of Psychiatry*, **147**, 652–4.

McDougle, C. J., Price, L. H., Goodman, W. K., Charney, D. S., and Heninger, G. R. (1991). A controlled trial of lithium augmentation in fluvoxamine-refractory obsessive compulsive disorder: lack of efficacy. *Journal of Clinical Psychopharmacology*, **11**, 175–84.

McDougle, C. J., Goodman, W. K., Leckman, J. F., *et al.* (1993). Limited therapeutic effect of addition of buspirone in fluvoxamine-refractory obsessive compulsive disorder. *American Journal of Psychiatry*, **150**, 647–9.

McDougle, C. J., Goodman, W. K., Leckman, J. F., *et al.* (1994). Haloperidol addition in fluvoxamine refractory obsessive-compulsive disorder: a double-blind placebo-controlled study in patients with and without tics. *Archives of General Psychiatry*, **51**, 302–8.

McDougle, C. J., Barr, L. C., Goodman, W. K., *et al.* (1995). Lack of efficacy of clozapine monotherapy in refractory obsessive-compulsive disorder. *American Journal of Psychiatry*, **152**, 423–9.

McDougle, C. J., Epperson, C. N., Pelton, G. H., Wasylink, S., and Price, L. H. (2000). A double-blind, placebo-controlled study of risperidone addition in serotonin re-uptake inhibitor-refractory obsessive-compulsive disorder. *Archives of General Psychiatry*, **57**, 794–801.

Metin, O., Yaziki, K., Tot, S., and Yazici, A. E. (2003). Amisulpride augmentation in treatment-resistant obsessive compulsive disorder: an open trial. *Human Psychopharmacology*, **18**, 463–7.

Milanfranchi, A., Ravagli, S., Lensi, P., Marazitti, D., and Cassano, G. B. (1997). A double-blind study of fluvoxamine and clomipramine in the treatment of obsessive compulsive disorder. *International Clinical Psychopharmacology*, **12**, 31–6.

Monteiro, W. O., Noshirvani, H. F., Marks, I. M., and Lelliott, P. T. (1987). Anorgasmia from clomipramine in obsessive-compulsive disorder: a controlled trial. *British Journal of Psychiatry*, **151**, 107–12.

Montgomery, S. A. (1980). Clomipramine in obsessional neurosis: a placebo-controlled trial. *Pharmacological Medicine*, **1**, 189–92.

Montgomery, S. A. and Montgomery, D. B. (1980). Measurement of change in psychiatric illness: new obsessional, schizophrenia and depression scales. *Postgraduate Medical Journal* (suppl.), 50–2.

Montgomery, S. A., Fineberg, N., and Montgomery, D. B. (1990). The efficacy of serotonergic drugs in OCD: power calculations compared with placebo. In: *Current Approaches in Obsessive Compulsive Disorder*, ed. S. A. Montgomery, W. K. Goodman, and N. Goeting. Southampton, UK: Ashford Colour Press for Duphar Medical Relations, pp. 54–63.

Montgomery, S. A., Fineberg, N. A., Montgomery, D. B. *et al.* (1992). L-tryptophan in obsessive compulsive disorder: a placebo-controlled study. *European Neuropsychopharmacology*, **2** (suppl. 2), 384.

Montgomery, S. A., McIntyre, A., Osterheider, M., *et al.* (1993). A double-blind placebo-controlled study of fluoxetine in patients with DSM-IIIR obsessive compulsive disorder. *European Neuropsychopharmacology*, **3**, 143–52.

Montgomery, S. A., Kasper, S., Stein, D. J., Bang Hedegaard, K., and Lemming, O. M. (2001). Citalopram 20 mg, 40 mg, and 60 mg are all effective and well tolerated compared with placebo in obsessive-compulsive disorder. *International Clinical Psychopharmacology*, **16**, 75–86.

Mundo, E., Bianchi, L., and Bellodi, L. (1997a). Efficacy of fluvoxamine, paroxetine, and citalopram in the treatment of obsessive-compulsive disorder; a single-blind study. *Journal of Clinical Psychopharmacology*, **17**, 267–71.

Mundo, E., Bareggi, S. R., Pirola, R., Bellodi, L., and Smeraldi, E. (1997b). Long-term pharmacotherapy of obsessive-compulsive disorder; a double-blind controlled study. *Journal of Clinical Psychopharmacology*, **17**, 4–10.

Mundo, E., Guglielmo, E., and Bellodi, L. (1998). Effect of adjuvant pindolol on the anti-obsessional response to fluvoxamine; a double-blind, placebo-controlled study. *International Clinical Psychopharmacology*, **13**, 219–24.

Mundo, E., Bareggi, S. R., Pirola, R., and Bellodi, L. (1999). Effect of acute intravenous clomipramine and antiobsessional response to proserotonergic drugs: is gender a predictive variable? *Biological Psychiatry*, **45**, 290–4.

Mundo, E., Rouillon, F., Figuera, M. L., and Stigler, M. (2001). Fluvoxamine in obsessive-compulsive disorder: similar efficacy but superior tolerability in comparison with clomipramine. *Human Psychopharmacology*, **16**, 461–8.

Pallanti, S., Quercioli, L., Paiva, R. S., and Koran, L. M. (1999). Citalopram for treatment-resistant obsessive-compulsive disorder. *European Psychiatry*, **14**, 101–6.

Pallanti, S., Hollander, E., Bienstock, C., *et al.* (2002a). Treatment-non-response in OCD: methodological issues and operational definitions. *International Journal of Neuropsychopharmacology*, **5**, 181–91.

Pallanti, S., Quercioli, L., and Koran, L. M. (2002b). Citalopram infusions in resistant obsessive compulsive disorder: an open trial. *Journal of Clinical Psychiatry*, **63**, 796–801.

Pato, M. T., Zohar-Kadouch, R., and Zohar, J. (1988). Return of symptoms after discontinuation of clomipramine in patients with obsessive compulsive disorder. *American Journal of Psychiatry*, **145**, 211–14.

Perlmutter, S. J., Leitman, S. F., Garvey, M. H., *et al.* (1999). Therapeutic plasma exchange and intravenous immunoglobulin for obsessive compulsive disorder and tic disorders in children. *Lancet*, **354**, 1153–8.

Perse, T., Greist, J. H., Jefferson, J. W., Rosenfeld, R., and Dar, R. (1987). Fluvoxamine treatment of obsessive compulsive disorder. *American Journal of Psychiatry*, **144**, 1543–8.

Piccinelli, M., Pini, S., Bellantuono, C., and Wilkinson, G. (1995). Efficacy of drug treatment in obsessive compulsive disorder. *British Journal of Psychiatry*, **166**, 424–43.

Pidrman, V. and Tuma, I. (1998). Citalopram versus clomipramine in double-blind therapy of obsessive compulsive disorder. *Abstracts of the 11th Congress of the European College of Neuropsychopharmacology*, Oct 31–Nov 4, Paris.

Pigott, T. A. and Seay, S. M. (1999). A review of the efficacy of selective serotonin re-uptake inhibitors in obsessive compulsive disorder. *Journal of Clinical Psychiatry*, **60**, 101–6.

Pigott, T. A., Pato, M. T., Bernstein, S. E., *et al.* (1990). Controlled comparisons of clomipramine and fluoxetine in the treatment of obsessive compulsive disorder. Behavioral and biological results. *Archives of General Psychiatry*, **47**, 926–32.

Pigott, T. A., Pato, M. T., L'Heureux, F., *et al.* (1991). A controlled comparison of adjuvant lithium carbonate or thyroid hormone in clomipramine-treated patients with obsessive compulsive disorder. *Journal of Clinical Psychopharmacology*, **11**, 242–8.

Pigott, T. A., L'Heureux, F., Hill, J. L., *et al.* (1992a). A double-blind study of adjuvant buspirone hydrochloride in clomipramine-treated patients with obsessive compulsive disorder. *Journal of Clinical Psychopharmacology*, **12**, 11–18.

Pigott, T. A., L'Heureux, F., Rubinstein, C. F., Hill, J. L., and Murphy, D. L. (1992b). A controlled trial of clonazepam augmentation in OCD patients treated with clomipramine or fluoxetine. New Research Abstracts NR 144. Presented at the *145th Annual Meeting of the American Psychiatric Association*. Washington, DC.

Pigott, T. A., L'Heureux, F., Dubbert, B., *et al.* (1994). Obsessive compulsive disorder: comorbid conditions. *Journal of Clinical Psychiatry*, **55** (suppl.), 15–32.

Rasmussen, S. A. and Eisen, J. L. (1990). Epidemiology of obsessive compulsive disorder. *Journal of Clinical Psychiatry*, **51**, 10–13.

Rasmussen, S., Hackett, E., Duboff, E., *et al.* (1997). A 2-year study of sertraline in the treatment of obsessive-compulsive disorder. *International Clinical Psychopharmacology*, **12**, 309–16.

Ravizza, L., Maina, G., Bogetto, F., *et al.* (1998). Long term treatment of obsessive compulsive disorder. *CNS Drugs*, **10**, 247–55.

Ravizza, L., Albert, U., and Ceregato, A. (2001). Venlafaxine in OCD. Presented at the *International obsessive compulsive disorder conference*, Sardinia, Italy.

Reynghe de Voxrie, G. V. (1968). Anafranil (G34586) in obsessive neurosis. *Acta Neurologia Belgica*, **68**, 787–92.

Riddle, M. A., Scahill, L., King, R. A., *et al.* (1992). Double-blind crossover trial of fluoxetine and placebo in children and adolescents with obsessive compulsive disorder. *Journal of the American Academy of Child and Adolescent Psychiatry*, **31**, 1062–9.

Riddle, M. A., Reeve, E. A., Yaryura-Tobias, J., *et al.* (2001). Fluvoxamine for children and adolescents with obsessive compulsive disorder; a randomised, controlled multicentre trial. *Journal of the American Academy of Child and Adolescent Psychiatry*, **40**, 222–9.

Robins, L. N., Helzer, J. E., Weissman, M. M., *et al.* (1984). Lifetime prevalence of specific psychiatric disorders in three sites. *Archives of General Psychiatry*, **41**, 949–58.

Romano, S., Goodman, W. K., Tamura, R., *et al.* (2001). Long-term treatment of obsessive-compulsive disorder after an acute response: a comparison of fluoxetine versus placebo. *Journal of Clinical Psychopharmacology*, **21**, 46–52.

Rosenbaum, J. F., Fava, M., Hoog, S., Ascroft, R. C., and Krebs, W. B. (1998). Selective serotonin reuptake inhibitor discontinuation syndrome; a randomised clinical trial. *Biological Psychiatry*, **44**, 77–87.

Rouillon, F. (1998). A double-blind comparison of fluvoxamine and clomipramine in OCD. *European Neuropsychopharmacology*, **8** (suppl.), 260–1.

Sevincok, L. and Topuz, A. (2003). Lack of efficacy of low dose quetiapine addition in refractory obsessive compulsive disorder. *Journal of Clinical Psychopharmacology*, **23**, 448–50.

Sheehan, D. V., Harnett-Sheehan, K., and Raj, B. A. (1996). The measurement of disability. *International Clinics in Psychopharmacology*, **11** (suppl.), 89–95.

Smeraldi, E., Ergovesi, S., and Bianchi, L. (1992). Fluvoxamine versus clomipramine treatment in obsessive compulsive disorder: a preliminary study. *New Trends in Experimental and Clinical Psychiatry*, **8**, 63–5.

Stein, D. J., Spadaccini, E., and Hollander, E. (1995). Meta-analysis of pharmacotherapy trials of obsessive compulsive disorder. *International Clinical Psychopharmacology*, **10**, 11–18.

Stein, D., Montgomery, S. A., Kasper, S., and Tanghoj, P. (2001). Predictors of response to pharmacotherapy with citalopram in obsessive compulsive disorder. *International Clinical Psychopharmacology*, **16**, 357–61.

Szegedi, A., Wetzel, H., Leal, M., Hartter, S., and Hiemke, C. (1996). Combination treatment with clomipramine and fluvoxamine: drug monitoring, safety and tolerability data. *Journal of Clinical Psychiatry*, **57**, 257–64.

Tenney, N. H., Denys, D. A., Van Megen, H. J. G. M., Glas, G., and Westenberg, H. G. M. (2003). Effect of a pharmacological intervention on quality of life in patients with obsessive-compulsive disorder. *International Clinical Psychopharmacology*, **18**, 29–33.

Thoren, P., Asberg, M., Cronholm, B., Jornestedt, L., and Traskman, L. (1980). Clomipramine treatment and obsessive compulsive disorder. *Archives of General Psychiatry*, **37**, 1281–5.

Tollefson, G., Rampey, A., Potvin, J., *et al.* (1994). A multicenter investigation of fixed-dose fluoxetine in the treatment of obsessive compulsive disorder. *Archives of General Psychiatry*, **51**, 559–67.

Ushijima, S., Kamijima, K., Asai, M., *et al.* (1997). Clinical evaluation of sertraline hydrochloride, a selective serotonin reuptake inhibitor, in the treatment of obsessive-compulsive disorder: a double blind placebo-controlled trial. *Japanese Journal of Neuropsychopharmacology*, **19**, 603–23.

Vallejo, J., Olivares, J., Marcos, T. I., Bulbena, A., and Menchon, J. M. (1992). Clomipramine versus phenelzine in obsessive compulsive disorder: a controlled clinical trial. *British Journal of Psychiatry*, **161**, 665–70.

Volavka, J., Neziroglu, F., and Yaryura-Tobias, J. A. (1985). Clomipramine and imipramine in obsessive compulsive disorder. *Psychiatry Research*, **14**, 85–93.

Wagner, K. D., March, J., and Landau, P. (1999). Safety and efficacy of sertraline in long-term paediatric OCD treatment: a multicentre study. Presented at the 39th annual meeting of the New Clinical Drug Evaluation Unit, Florida, USA.

Weissman, M. M., Bland, R. C., Canino, G. J., *et al.* (1994). The cross national epidemiology of obsessive compulsive disorder. *Journal of Clinical Psychiatry*, **55** (suppl.), 5–10.

Wheadon, D., Bushnell, W., and Steiner, M. (1993). A fixed dose comparison of 20, 40 or 60 mg paroxetine to placebo in the treatment of obsessive compulsive disorder. Poster presented at annual meeting of the American College of Neuropsychopharmacology. Honolulu, Hawaii, USA.

Wilens, T. E., Biederman, J., March, J., *et al.* (1999). Absence of cardiovascular and adverse effects of sertraline in children and adolescents. *Journal of American Academy of Child and Adolescent Psychiatry*, **38**, 573–7.

Wood, A., Tollefson, G. D., and Burkitt, M. (1993). Pharmacotherapy of obsessive compulsive disorder: experience with fluoxetine. *International Clinical Psychopharmacology*, **8**, 301–6.

Yaryura-Tobias, J. A. and Neziroglu, F. A. (1996). Venlafaxine in obsessive compulsive disorder. *Archives of General Psychiatry*, **53**, 653–4.

Yaryura-Tobias, J. A., Neziroglu, F. A., and Bergman, L. (1976). Clomipramine for obsessive-compulsive neurosis – an organic approach. *Current Therapeutic Research*, **20**, 541–8.

Zohar, J. and Judge, R. (1996). Paroxetine versus clomipramine in the treatment of obsessive compulsive disorder. *British Journal of Psychiatry*, **169**, 468–74.

9

Evidence-based pharmacotherapy of eating disorders

Martine F. Flament,[1] Claudia Furino,[1] and
Nathalie Godart[2]

[1] University of Ottawa Institute of Mental Health Research, Ottawa, Canada
[2] Institut Mutualiste Montsouris, Paris, France

Introduction

The eating disorders (EDs) are widespread, disabling, and often chronic psychiatric disorders that occur preponderantly in adolescent girls and young adult women. Although a wide range of psychological, familial, cultural, and biological determinants have been proposed to explain their onset and maintenance (for review, see Fairburn and Harrison, 2003), the core etiology of these disorders remains largely unknown.

Both anorexia nervosa (AN) and bulimia nervosa (BN) share an unusual morbid preoccupation with weight and shape, yet distinctive patterns of feeding behavior and weight regulation lead to distinct clinical pictures. AN is characterized by a refusal to maintain a minimally normal body weight, and an ego syntonic restriction of food intake culminating in profound emaciation (Russell, 2000). The typical eating pattern in BN consists of recurring disinhibition of restraint, resulting in cycles of binge eating and compensatory behaviors to prevent weight gain, including self-induced vomiting, abuse of laxative/diuretics, extreme exercise, and restricting; thus, most individuals with BN maintain an average body weight (Fairburn, 2000). The restricting and bulimic forms of EDs may co-occur or alternate in the same person. This has led to the identification, in the *Diagnostic and Statistical Manual, 4th edition* (DSM IV: American Psychiatric Association, 1994) of two diagnostic types of AN: (1) a restricting type, in which weight loss is achieved primarily through dieting and excessive exercise; and (2) a binge-eating/purging type, in which binge eating and/or self-induced vomiting or the misuse of laxatives, diuretics, and enemas also occurs. For BN, the DSM IV specifies two diagnostic types, purging and non-purging, depending on whether or not the person regularly engages in the above purging behaviors.

Binge-eating disorder (BED) is another form of ED included in the Appendix of DSM IV as a diagnosis requiring further study. It is characterized by recurrent binge-eating episodes accompanied by a sense of distress, loss of control, and feelings of disgust, depression, or guilt (Spitzer *et al.*, 1991). In contrast to BN, individuals with BED do not regularly attempt to prevent weight gain by engaging in purging behaviors, excessive exercise, or fasting. Consequently, most are obese and often seek treatment for weight loss rather than for disturbed eating behaviors. However, the psychopathology of persons with BED seems to bear a closer resemblance to that of those with BN than that of obese subjects who do not binge (Dingemans *et al.*, 2002).

The EDs represent a serious public health concern. AN and BN affect an estimated 0.3–0.7% and 1.5–2.5%, respectively, of young females in the general population (Hoek *et al.*, 1995; Tamburrino and McGinnis, 2002). Among referred cases, 9 out of 10 are women (Kirkpatrick and Caldwell, 2000). The prevalence of BED, which affects men and women almost equally and has a larger age range, has been estimated at between 2% and 3.3% (Spitzer *et al.*, 1993; Hay, 1998). In young people, the EDs profoundly affect physical, emotional, and psychosocial development. In both adolescents and adults, psychiatric complications include social isolation, major depression, severe anxiety, and suicide (Ratnasuriya *et al.*, 1991; Keller *et al.*, 1992), and medical complications include cardiac problems, osteopenia, neurological impairments, and infertility (Bradley *et al.*, 1997; Mitchell *et al.*, 1997). The mortality among youths with an ED has been estimated at up to 20% (Strober *et al.*, 1997). Research indicates that the longer disordered eating symptoms persist, the more difficult they are to treat (Steinhausen *et al.*, 1993). Furthermore, the impact of ED on the health care delivery systems is enormous (McKenzie and Joyce, 1992; Agras, 2001).

The objective of this chapter is to review currently available scientific evidence for the efficacy and safety of pharmacotherapy in adolescents and adults with an ED. We will consider successively AN, BN, and BED, and the review will focus on several aspects of pharmacological treatment: rationale for the choice of agents, short-term efficacy and safety, long-term efficacy (when data are available), comparison or combination with psychological treatment (when available), and current perspectives for clinical management and future research.

We conducted a computer search of MEDLINE and PsychInfo databases for all controlled trials of medication for the treatment of AN, BN, or BED published between 1960 and 2004. We examined already published literature reviews and meta-analyses on the efficacy of pharmacotherapy in the EDs, for any additional information or reference. For drugs for which no controlled study has been published, case series or open trials in patients with an ED were retrieved.

Based on their main pharmacological mode of action, we classified medications which have been tested for the treatment of an ED in the following categories: antipsychotics, tricyclic antidepressants, selective serotonin reuptake inhibitors (SSRIs), monoamine oxidase inhibitors (MAOIs), mood stabilizers, anxiolytics, prokinetic agents (medications that improve gastric emptying), opiate antagonists, and other medications.

Controlled randomized studies are summarized in Tables 9.1–9.3. Open studies and case reports are described in the text. Valid comparisons between pharmacotherapy and psychotherapy, and/or their combination, and meta-analyses of pharmacological trials were only found for the treatment of BN; they are presented in specific sections of the text.

Pharmacotherapy of eating disorders

Treatment strategies that have been tried in the EDs are based on intervention paradigms previously used in psychiatric disorders that frequently co-occur with AN and BN, such as depression, anxiety, impulse disorders, and substance use disorders. The first therapeutic model, viewing the ED as a variant of an affective disorder, comes from: (1) clinical studies showing that up to 80% of ED patients, and at least 15% of their first-degree relatives, have had a major depressive disorder (Lilenfeld *et al.*, 1998; Godart *et al.*, 2004); (2) biological investigations, including response to the dexamethasone suppression test, cerebrospinal fluid concentrations of neurotransmitter metabolites, and pharmacological challenge studies, demonstrating close similarities between patients with an ED and those with major depression (for review, see Jimerson *et al.*, 1996). However, the content of depression in persons with an ED is not univocal, melancholia has rarely been described in anorexic or bulimic patients, and recent studies have failed to demonstrate that, as hypothesized, anorexia–bulimia was an equivalent of bipolar disorder (Swift *et al.*, 1985).

Another theoretical model for the treatment of EDs postulates that, in adults, body weight tends towards a relatively stable value, which implies a mechanism of weight homeostasis. Regulation of body weight is located in the medioventral hypothalamus, with afferent and efferent pathways under the control of both the serotonergic and the noradrenergic system. Serotonin controls satiety and therefore regulates eating behaviors (Glennon, 1990). It also has a global effect on food selection and caloric intake, as part of the complex regulation of glucose absorption (Wurtman and Wurtman, 1981). Dysfunction of the serotonergic system has been proposed as an etiological factor in AN (Kaye *et al.*, 1999a) and BN (Jimerson *et al.*, 1988; Brewerton *et al.*, 1990), as well as in some affective disorders and in impulse control disorders, both of which share common psychopathological features with the EDs.

Other proposed mechanisms of action for pharmacological compounds that have been tried in the treatment of an ED will be briefly described under each class of psychotropic medication.

Pharmacotherapy of anorexia nervosa

Antipsychotics

It was once argued that patients with AN should be treated with antipsychotic medication, because their obsessions regarding weight and body shape seemed to resemble delusions. Chlorpromazine, pimozide, and sulpiride have been tried in early controlled randomized trials (Table 9.1). In the past decade, the increasing use of novel atypical antipsychotics, with a much more favorable side-effect profile, that often includes impressive weight gain, and with a greater serotonin-to-dopamine blockade ratio than traditional antipsychotics, has restored the idea that this class of medication could be effective for the treatment of AN. However, only case reports and open treatment series are as yet available for these compounds.

Over 40 years ago in the UK, Dally and Sargant (1960, 1966) used very high doses of chlorpromazine (1600 mg/day), often in combination with insulin and bed rest, in a group of 30 inpatients with AN. These patients gained weight at a faster rate and were discharged from hospital sooner than 27 placebo-treated patients hospitalized on the same unit. However, those treated with chlorpromazine also experienced significant side-effects, including seizures and increased purging behaviors, and the long-term outcome was not improved in that group.

Twenty years later, two double-blind, placebo-controlled crossover studies were conducted in Belgium, using pimozide (4–6 mg/day) for 3 weeks (Vandereycken and Pierloot, 1982), or sulpiride (300–400 mg/day) for 6 weeks (Vandereycken, 1984). There was only a trend for higher weight gain on pimozide, and no advantage for either drug on eating attitudes and eating behaviors. Thus, given their potential for short- and long-term side-effects, and the fact that weight gain in anorexics tends not to persist if not accompanied by changes in attitudes towards eating and body shape, the treatment of AN with traditional antipsychotics is no longer recommended today. Since 1999, there have been six reports on the use of olanzapine, at a dosage ranging from 5 to 12.5 mg, from 22 days to 9 months, on a total of 52 subjects (Hansen, 1999; Jensen and Mejlhede, 2000; La Via et al., 2000; Powers et al., 2002; Malina et al., 2003; Boachie et al., 2003). Since 1996, three case reports (3 patients) and one retrospective chart series (15 patients) have been published on the use of risperidone, at a dosage of 0.5–1.5 mg/day, from 44.7 days to 12 months (Fisman et al., 1996; Newman-Toker, 2000; Carver et al., 2002). While many of the patients described in these publications suffered from severe illness that was previously resistant to treatment, including with other

Table 9.1 Controlled pharmacological trials with antipsychotics in anorexia nervosa (AN)

Authors, year, country	*n* (drug/placebo): ITT *Completers* Diagnostic criteria	Study design and duration	Treatment (daily dose)	Results: drug versus placebo	Follow-up duration results	Conclusion and comments
Dally and Sargant (1966), UK	30 (a) /27 (b) /8 (c) AN Authors' criteria	Parallel As required for weight gain	(a) Chlorpromazine (maximum 1600 mg) + insulin versus (b) bed rest versus (c) insulin alone	Average time in hospital: 36 days (a) versus 44 days (b) versus 59 days (c) Average weight gain per week: 2.1 kg (a) versus 1.0 kg (b) versus 1.1 kg (c)	Within 2-year follow-up, one-third of each group required readmission because of further weight loss	Early study No other measure than weight Limited short-term effect and risk of adverse events
Vandereycken and Pierloot (1982), Belgium	Total *n*: 18 *Total n: 17* AN DSM-III	Crossover 3 weeks	Pimozide (4–6 mg) versus placebo	Trend for higher weight gain on pimozide Marginal influence of pimozide on the Anorectic Behavior Scale for Inpatient Observation	NA	Small sample size All patients initially involved in contingency management program Findings are small and inconsistent
Vandereycken (1984), Belgium	Total *n*: 18 *Total n: 18* AN DSM-III	Crossover 6 weeks	Sulpiride (300–400 mg) versus placebo	No significant difference for weight gain No difference on the Anorectic Behavior Scale for Inpatient Observation, EAT, and BAT scores	NA	No direct effect of sulpiride on behavioral observation scales Inconsistent advantage of sulpiride regarding weight gain

ITT, intent-to-treat; DSM-III, *Diagnostic and Statistical Manual*, 3rd edn; NA, not applicable; EAT, Eating Attitudes Test; BAT, Body Attitudes Test.

drugs, all seemed to have experienced, when treated with olanzapine or risperidone, a positive effect on weight gain, and symptomatic improvement of anxiety/agitation, obsessive thoughts, paranoid ideation, and compulsive hyperenergetic activity (for review, see Mitchell *et al.*, 2003). Reported adverse reactions were limited to initial sedation. In some cases, the atypical agents were terminated after weight regain, with continued symptom remission.

Since case reports always tend to be biased toward reporting of positive effects, the first open-label study of olanzapine, at a dose of 10 mg/day in a group of 20 anorexic patients, of either restricting or binge-eating/purging type, for 10 weeks is of interest (Powers *et al.*, 2002). No cognitive-behavioral treatment was allowed and no new therapy could be initiated during the study. Fourteen patients completed the study, 10 gained weight (mean ± SD 3.98 ± 4.14 kg (8.75 ± 9.1 lb), and 4 lost weight (mean ± SD 1.02 ± 0.45 kg (2.25 ± 1.0 lb). For completers who gained weight only, a significant improvement was reported on the Hamilton Depression Rating Scale, the Eating Disorder Inventory-2 (EDI-2), and the Positive and Negative Symptom Scale (PANSS). Sedation was the most common side-effect and diminished over 2 weeks.

However, two negative reports on the use of atypical antipsychotics in AN patients are cited in the review by Mitchell *et al.* (2003): an open-label olanzapine series published as a newsletter (Gaskill *et al.*, 2001), and a risperidone retrospective chart review presented at a meeting (Carver *et al.*, 2002). Thus, further evaluation of atypical antipsychotics in the acute treatment of AN is warranted, and controlled trials are required to determine whether or not these drugs hold promise for individuals with AN.

Tricyclic antidepressants

Due to the possible relationship between AN and depression, the tricyclic antidepressants were seen, 30 years ago, as the most promising drug treatment for AN. Unfortunately, findings from subsequent controlled randomized studies (Table 9.2) have been disappointing.

The first controlled trial, in 1985, aimed at evaluating the effectiveness of amitriptyline in 11 anorexic patients versus 14 assigned to placebo; a third group consisted of 18 anorexic patients who refused to be treated with medication (Biederman *et al.*, 1985). No significant difference emerged between the three groups, whether for weight gain, body image, or mood ratings; the only marked difference was the increased occurrence of side-effects in patients receiving medication. Crisp *et al.* (1987) studied the effect of a low dose of clomipramine on weight gain in anorexic patients, and found no significant difference between 8 patients receiving medication and 8 receiving placebo. Halmi *et al.* (1986) compared amitriptyline to placebo and cyproheptadine (see below), and found no major benefit for

Table 9.2 Controlled pharmacological trials with tricyclic antidepressants in anorexia nervosa (AN)

Authors, year, country	*n* (drug/placebo): ITT / *Completers* / Diagnostic criteria	Study design and duration	Treatment (daily dose)	Results: drug versus placebo	Follow-up duration and results	Conclusion and comments
Biederman *et al.* (1985), USA	11/14 / *11/14* AN / DSM III	Parallel 5 weeks	Amitriptyline (mean 115 mg, maximum 175 mg) versus placebo	No significant difference for weight gain or change in other symptoms. No significant difference on SADS-C, HSCL, EAT, CGI-S, and CGI-I scores	NA	High refusal rate to enter the study. All patients also received behavior therapy. Amitriptyline dose is low. Amitriptyline treatment is associated with substantial discomfort and adverse affects
Lacey and Crisp (1980); Crisp *et al.* (1987), UK	8/8 / *6/7* AN / Authors' criteria	Parallel 9 weeks	Clomipramine (50 mg) versus placebo	No significant difference for weight gain or change in other symptoms. Significant advantage of clomipramine for first 2 weeks on analog scale for hunger. No significant differences on six other analog scales on mood and appetite	At 1-year and 4-year follow-up, no significant difference in body weight between the two groups	All patients also received behavior therapy. Clomipramine dose is low. No impact of clomipramine on short- or long-term outcome
Halmi *et al.* (1986), USA	23 (AMI) / 24 (CYP) / 25 (Placebo) AN / DSM III	Parallel 4 weeks	AMI (maximum 160 mg) versus CYP (maximum 32 mg) versus placebo	No significant difference for weight gain. Reduction in number of hospital days to reach weight target: 32 ± 17 days (AMI) versus 36 ± 20 days (CYP) versus 45 ± 18 days (placebo). No significant group difference on BDI and HSCL-90 scores	NA	All patients also received psychotherapy and refeeding. AMI may increase rate of weight gain, but has more complicating side-effects than CYP

ITT, intent-to-treat; DSM III, *Diagnostic and Statistical Manual*, 3rd edn; SADS-C, Schedule for Affective Disorders and Schizophrenia-Change version; HSCL, Hopkins Symptom Checklist; EAT, Eating Attitudes Test; CGI-S, Clinical Global Impression – Severity; CGI-I, Clinical Global Impression – Improvement; NA, not applicable; AMI, amitriptyline; CYP, cyproheptadine; BDI, Beck Depression Inventory.

amitriptyline, except for a significant reduction in the number of days to reach target weight.

Given, on the one hand, the limited evidence and/or lack of adequate trials and, on the other, the potential for arrhythmia at low body weight, the lethal risk with overdose, and the possible concerns about tricyclic antidepressant use and sudden death in the younger age group, this class of medication is no longer recommended in underweight patients with AN.

Selective serotonin reuptake inhibitors

For the last two decades, SSRIs have been increasingly used to treat patients with AN, but only two compounds have been tested in controlled trials (Table 9.3). Fluoxetine was not superior to placebo in a study involving inpatients with AN also receiving behavioral therapy (Attia *et al.*, 1998). However, fluoxetine appeared effective in preventing relapse in AN patients who had been successful in gaining weight due to inpatient treatment: over 1 year, women receiving fluoxetine had a significantly lower rate of relapse than those treated with placebo (Kaye *et al.*, 2001). Bergh *et al.* (1996) treated two groups of undernourished anorexic outpatients, one with psychotherapy alone, and the other with a combination of psychotherapy and citalopram. It was found that patients treated with psychotherapy alone did better than those receiving the combined treatment, and that 8 of 30 subjects treated with citalopram had an alarming drop in body weight (mean of 5.4 kg).

Thus, the research on treatment of AN with SSRIs has not been particularly promising. When using these agents, clinicians and researchers should monitor patients' weight closely. Additional research is needed to establish the possible efficacy of the SSRIs in preventing relapse in weight-restored anorexics.

Mood stabilizers

Like antipsychotic medication, lithium is known to induce weight gain. Several case reports, and one 4-week double-blind, placebo-controlled study of lithium in patients with AN (Gross *et al.*, 1981) can be found in the literature. In the controlled trial (Table 9.4), despite the small sample size, the average weight gain in the group treated with lithium was greater than that in the placebo group, particularly during the last 2 weeks. However, caution is required in the use of lithium in anorexic patients, because sodium and fluid depletion may lead to reduced lithium clearance, resulting in increased potential toxicity. At present the use of mood-stabilizing medication, such as lithium, is not recommended in patients with AN.

Medications that improve gastric emptying (prokinetic agents)

Common complaints of anorexic patients have been feelings of fullness, early satiety, bloating and, although psychological factors have been proven to influence

Table 9.3 Controlled pharmacological trials with specific serotonin inhibitors in anorexia nervosa (AN)

Authors, year, country	n (drug/placebo): ITT *Completers* Diagnostic criteria	Study design and duration	Treatment (daily dose)	Results: drug versus placebo	Follow-up duration and results	Conclusion and comments
Attia *et al.* (1998), USA	15/16 *11/12 AN* DSM IV	Parallel 7 weeks	Fluoxetine (mean 56 mg) versus placebo	No significant difference for weight gain or change in other symptoms No differences in improvement on CGI, ABS, BDI, BSQ, EAT, SCL-90, Y-BOCS-ED scores	NA	All patients also received behaviorally based inpatient treatment Fluoxetine did not add significant benefit to inpatient treatment of AN
Kaye *et al.* (2001), USA	16/19 *10/3 AN-R and AN-B* DSM IV back to normal weight	Relapse prevention after inpatient treatment. Parallel 52 weeks	Fluoxetine (20–60 mg) versus placebo	More study completers in fluoxetine group (63%) than in placebo group (16%) Reduced relapse rate on fluoxetine as determined by significant increase in weight (% ABW) and reduction in HDRS, HARS, Y-BOCS, Y-BOCS-ED scores		Fluoxetine may be useful in improving outcome and preventing relapse in AN patients after weight restoration Study did not control for drug dose or other treatments received during study period

ITT, intent-to-treat; DSM IV, *Diagnostic and Statistical Manual*, 4th edn; NA, not applicable; CGI, Clinical Global Improvement; ABS, Anorexic Behavior Scale; BDI, Beck Depression Inventory; BSQ, Body Shape Questionnaire; EAT, Eating Attitudes Test; SCL-90, Symptom Checklist-90; Y-BOCS-ED, Yale-Brown Obsessive-Compulsive Scale-Eating Disorders; ABW, average body weight; HDRS, Hamilton Depression Rating Scale; HARS, Hamilton Anxiety Rating Scale; Y-BOCS, Yale-Brown Obsessive-Compulsive Scale; AN-R, anorexia nervosa – restricting type; AN-B, anorexia nervosa – binge eating/purging type.

Table 9.4 Controlled pharmacological trial with mood stabilizers in anorexia nervosa (AN)

Authors, year, country	n (drug/placebo): ITT _Completers_ Diagnostic criteria	Study design and duration	Treatment (daily dose)	Results: drug versus placebo	Follow-up duration and results	Conclusion and comments
Gross et al. (1981), USA	8/8 _8/8_ AN Feighner research criteria	Parallel 4 weeks	Lithium (flexible dose) versus placebo	At baseline, lithium group was consuming more calories and weighing more than placebo group Average ($\pm$ SD) weight gain was 6.8 ($\pm$ 0.4) kg on lithium versus 5.2 ($\pm$ 0.1) kg on placebo No significant group difference for scores on most subscales of HSCL-90, GAAQ, SDS, PRS	NA	Treatment also included behavior modification Further studies of longer duration and larger sample size are needed

ITT, intent-to-treat; HSCL, Hopkins Symptom Checklist; GAAQ, Goldberg Anorexic Attitude Questionnaire; SDS, Goldberg Situational Discomfort Scale; PRS, Psychiatric Rating Scale; NA, not applicable.

patients' perceptions of fullness (Garfinkel *et al.*, 1978), it has also been found that biological measures of gastric motility may be abnormal in anorexic patients (Stacher *et al.*, 1986). A number of prokinetic agents, such as metoclopramide, bethanechol, cisapride, and domperidone, have been suggested as possible adjuvants to help anorexic patients eat. However, some of these drugs have a depressant central nervous system effect, and only cisapride has been studied in a controlled fashion (Table 9.5). Compared to placebo, cisapride had minimal effects on weight gain, but appeared to relieve significantly symptoms of fullness, therefore permitting the patients to increase their food intake in one study (Stacher *et al.*, 1993); in the other, no significant differences were reported in terms of weight gain or gastric emptying time (Szmukler *et al.*, 1995). Cisapride has been removed from the US market because of concerns about potentially fatal cardiac effects. It is not currently considered as an acceptable treatment for AN.

Opiate antagonists

Anorexic patients often characterize their behavior as being addictive, and there are similarities between the EDs and substance use disorders (Marrazzi and Luby, 1986). Animal studies have demonstrated that the opioid peptide system helps to modulate appetite and feeding behaviors (Morley and Levine, 1980; Sanger, 1981), and disturbance in the opioid function has been shown in patients with AN (Baranowska *et al.*, 1984; Kaye *et al.*, 1986). Consequently, opiate antagonists, such as naltrexone, have been considered as a treatment option for AN (Table 9.6). In a small crossover study, Marrazzi *et al.* (1995) assessed the efficacy of 200 mg/day of naltrexone in 6 anorexic or bulimic patients. Although the amount of weight gain was not reported, the clinical symptoms of patients taking naltrexone significantly improved compared to those receiving placebo. Additional research is needed to determine the possible value of opiate antagonists in the treatment of AN.

Appetite enhancers

Cyproheptadine, a serotonin and histamine antagonist noted to produce weight gain in the treatment of children with asthma, has been tested in controlled trials for women with AN (Table 9.7). In two studies, using 12 mg/day for one, and up to 32 mg/day for the other, no significant difference in weight gain emerged between patients receiving the active drug and the placebo (Vigersky and Loriaux, 1977; Halmi *et al.*, 1986). In a third study that had a larger sample, the drug only induced significant weight gain in patients who had the most severe form of illness (Goldberg *et al.*, 1979). Cyproheptadine is not currently recommended for AN.

Because of its appetite-stimulating and antiemetic properties, the active compound of cannabis, tetrahydrocannabinol (THC), has been considered as a treatment possibility for AN. However, in a 4-week, randomized, double-blind crossover

Table 9.5 Controlled pharmacological trials with prokinetic agents in anorexia nervosa (AN)

Authors, year, country	n (drug/placebo): ITT / *Completers* / Diagnostic criteria	Study design and duration	Treatment (daily dose)	Results: drug versus placebo	Follow-up duration and results	Conclusion and comments
Stacher et al. (1993), Austria	6/6 *6/6* AN DSM III-R	Parallel 6 weeks then open treatment with cisapride for 6 weeks	Cisapride (30 mg) versus placebo	Mean weight gain: 7.3% on cisapride versus 1.7% on placebo. Cisapride significantly aided in relief of symptoms of fullness (EDI). No significant effect of cisapride on BDI and STAI scores	NA	Cisapride removed from US market because of potentially fatal cardiac effects
Szmukler et al. (1995), Australia	Total n: 34 *13/16* AN DSM III-R	Parallel 8 weeks	Cisapride (30 mg) versus placebo	No significant difference for weight gain. Significant improvement on cisapride for rating of hunger on VAS. No significant effect of cisapride on BDI	NA	Cisapride removed from US market because of potentially fatal cardiac effects

ITT, intent-to-treat; DSM III-R, *Diagnostic and Statistical Manual*, 3rd edn (revised); NA, not applicable; EDI, Eating Disorders Inventory; BDI, Beck Depression Inventory; STAI, Stait–Trait Anxiety Inventory; VAS, Visual Analogue Scale.

Table 9.6 Controlled pharmacological trials with opiate antagonists in anorexia nervosa (AN)

Authors, year, country	*n* (drug/placebo): ITT *Completers* Diagnostic criteria	Study design and duration	Treatment (daily dose)	Results: drug versus placebo	Follow-up duration and results	Conclusion and comments
Marrazzi *et al.* (1995), USA	Total *n*: 6 AN and BN DSM III-R	Crossover 6 weeks	Naltrexone (200 mg) versus placebo	Clinically significant symptomatic improvement on naltrexone Binge/purge frequency significantly reduced on trexone Amount and rate of weight gain not analyzed	NA	Very small sample Associated weekly psychotherapy

ITT, intent-to-treat; BN, bulimia nervosa; NA, not applicable; DSM III-R, *Diagnostic and Statistical Manual*, 3rd edn (revised).

study evaluating the effects of oral THC versus diazepam in 11 anorexic patients (Table 9.7), no significant effect of THC was found on caloric intake or daily weight gain, while significant negative side-effects were reported, including sleep disturbance, paranoia, and dysphoria (Gross *et al.*, 1983). For all these reasons, THC is not recommended as a treatment for AN.

Other medications

Individuals with zinc deficiency seem to exhibit similar symptoms to anorexic patients, i.e., weight loss, depression, appetite and taste changes, and amenorrhea (Zhu and Walsh, 2002). Given the nutritional deprivation in anorexic patients, a possible zinc deficiency in AN and a potential role for zinc supplementation have been suggested. Three controlled studies have been conducted in children and adolescents (Table 9.8). One reported a decrease in depressive symptoms and anxiety, but no effect on weight gain (Katz *et al.*, 1987). In contrast, Birmingham *et al.* (1994) reported a faster increase in body mass index (BMI) among anorexic inpatients that had been randomly assigned to receive zinc gluconate as opposed to placebo. Lask *et al.* (1993) did not find evidence of efficacy of supplementation with zinc sulfate in 26 hospitalized children with AN. At present, results are obviously mixed, and the role of zinc deficiency in the pathogenesis of AN is still controversial.

Table 9.7 Controlled pharmacological trials with appetite enhancers in anorexia nervosa (AN)

Authors, year, country	n (drug/placebo): ITT Completers Diagnostic criteria	Study design and duration	Treatment (daily dose)	Results: drug versus placebo	Follow-up duration and results	Conclusion and comments
Vigersky and Loriaux (1977), USA	Total n: 24 AN Authors' criteria	Parallel 8 weeks	Cyproheptadine (12 mg) versus placebo	No significant difference in weight gain or change in other symptoms	NA	Low dose of cyproheptadine may have contributed to lack of response
Goldberg et al. (1979), UK	39/42 39/42 AN Authors' criteria	Parallel Not reported	Cyproheptadine (12–32 mg) versus placebo	No overall difference for weight gain Cyproheptadine significantly effective in inducing weight gain in a subgroup of patients with greatest percentage weight loss	NA	Subgroup with more severe form of illness also had a history of birth delivery complications
Gross et al. (1983), USA	Total n: 11 Total n: 8 AN Feighner criteria	Crossover 4 weeks	Tetrahydrocannabinol (THC) (7.5–30 mg) versus diazepam (3–15 mg)	No significant difference for weight gain Significantly higher scores on THC for somatization, sleep disturbance, and interpersonal sensitivity scales of HSCL-90 THC associated with significant psychic disturbance	NA	Associated inpatient treatment with behavior therapy THC not a useful agent in treatment of AN
Halmi et al. (1986), USA (see Table 1.2)	24 (CYP) / 23 (AMI) / 25 (placebo) AN DSM III	Parallel 4 weeks	CYP (maximum 32 mg) versus AMI (maximum 160 mg) versus placebo	No differences for weight gain Significant decrease on HDRS score with CYP CYP significantly increased treatment efficacy for restricting anorexics but significantly decreased treatment efficacy for bulimic anorexics	NA	All patients also received psychotherapy and refeeding CYP relatively free of serious side-effects Authors comment that differential effect of CYP on AN subtypes supports their validity

ITT, intent-to-treat; NA, not applicable; HSCL-90, Hopkins Symptom Checklist-90; CYP, cyproheptadine; AMI, amitriptyline; DSM III, *Diagnostic and Statistical Manual*, 3rd edn; HDRS, Hamilton Depression Rating Scale.

Table 9.8 Controlled pharmacological trials of other medications in anorexia nervosa (AN)

Authors, year, country	*n* (drug/placebo): ITT *Completers* Diagnostic criteria	Study design and duration	Treatment (daily dose)	Results: drug versus placebo	Follow-up duration and results	Conclusion and comments
Katz *et al.* (1987), USA	7/7 *6/7* AN adolescents DSM III	Parallel 6 months	Zinc sulfate (50 mg) versus placebo	No significant difference for weight gain Zinc supplementation associated with significant decrease of ZSRDS and STAI scores	NA	Mean zinc intake of AN patients calculated as half of recommended daily allowance for adolescents
Lask *et al.* (1993), USA	Total *n*: 26 AN *9–14 year-olds* DSM III-R	Crossover 6 weeks	Zinc sulfate (50 mg) versus placebo	No significant difference in rate of weight gain	NA	Zinc levels correlated with degree of malnutrition and returned to normal with refeeding
Birmingham *et al.* (1994), Canada	26/28 *16/19* AN DSM III-R	Parallel As needed to achieve 10% increase in BMI	Zinc glucomate (100 mg) versus placebo	Rate of BMI increase in zinc-supplemented group was twice that in placebo group	NA	Findings consistent with previous case studies and open trials
Hill *et al.* (2000), USA	Total *n*: 15 AN *adolescents* DSM IV	Parallel 6 weeks	Recombinant human growth hormone (0.05 mg/kg sc)	No difference in weight gain or duration of hospitalization Growth hormone group achieved cardiovascular stability significantly faster than placebo group (17 versus 37 days)	NA	In addition, refeeding program and usual care No current clinical applicability

ITT, intent-to-treat; DSM III, *Diagnostic and Statistical Manual*, 3rd edn; NA, not applicable; ZSRDS, Zung Self-Rated Depression Scale; STAI, Stait–Trait Anxiety Inventory; BMI, body mass index; s.c., subcutaneously.

Although this does not have any current clinical applicability, let us mention a controlled trial comparing recombinant human growth hormone with placebo (Table 9.8), that found no significant different in weight gain, or duration of hospitalization; the medication group did, however, achieve cardiovascular stability at a faster rate than the placebo group (Hill *et al.*, 2000).

Pharmacotherapy of bulimia nervosa

Although BN is a much more recent diagnostic entity (identified in Russell, 1979) than AN, many more psychological and pharmacological interventions have been proposed and empirically tested in this indication.

Tricyclic antidepressants

Starting with the initial report by Pope *et al.* (1983) of the efficacy of imipramine on binge frequency and other self-rated eating behaviors in a small group of bulimic patients, seven double-blind placebo-controlled studies have been published on the use of tricyclic antidepressants for treatment of BN (two with imipramine, four with desipramine, one with amitriptyline) (Table 9.9). In all but one study, the active drug led to a mean reduction in frequency of binge eating (range, 47–91%) significantly superior to that on placebo. Agras *et al.* (1987) reported that 16 weeks of treatment with imipramine (300 mg/day) reduced by 72% the frequency of both binge and purge episodes (versus 43% and 35%, respectively, on placebo).

Desipramine, a tricyclic antidepressant with relatively specific noradrenergic effects, has been the most studied agent from this class. In a 6-week controlled trial, binge frequency was reduced by more than 90% among subjects who took desipramine (200 mg/day), compared to 19% increase in those on placebo, and two-thirds of patients treated with desipramine achieved full remission at termination of treatment (Hughes *et al.*, 1986). In a larger-size 6-week crossover study, Barlow *et al.* (1988) reported more improvement during the active drug period than the placebo period.

McCann and Agras (1990) conducted one of the rare studies in non-purging bulimics: desipramine (100–300 mg) was significantly superior to placebo, with 63% reduction in binge eating and 60% abstinence rate in desipramine-treated patients, compared to 16% and 15%, respectively, for those on placebo. Unfortunately, within 4 weeks of discontinuing the medication, relapse to baseline levels of binge eating occurred. Similarly, the findings reported by Walsh *et al.* (1991) suggest that even though desipramine was effective in the acute treatment of BN, the long-term effects were limited. Amitriptyline has not been found effective in a controlled study, failing to show significant group differences for eating behaviors, although amitriptyline improved depression in those bulimics who were initially depressed (Mitchell and Groat, 1984).

Table 9.9 Controlled pharmacological trials with tricyclic antidepressants in bulimia nervosa (BN)

Authors, year, country	n (drug/placebo): ITT / *Completers* / Diagnostic criteria	Study design and duration	Treatment (daily dose)	Results: drug versus placebo	Follow-up duration and results	Conclusion and comments
Pope et al. (1983), USA	11/11 *9/10* BN DSM III	Parallel 6 weeks	Imipramine (50–200 mg) versus placebo	Higher decrease on imipramine (P < 0.05) for binge frequency, self-reported global ratings on eating behaviors, and HRSD	1– 8-month subsequent open treatment with imipramine and/or other antidepressant 18/20 patients displayed moderate/marked reduction of binge eating	Early study No standardized rating scale for BN
Mitchell and Groat (1984), USA	21/17 *16/16* BN DSM III	Parallel 10 weeks	Amitriptyline (150 mg) versus placebo	No difference in decrease of binge or purge frequency Higher decrease on amitriptyline for HDRS score (P < 0.005) In the whole group, lower decrease in binge and purge frequency in depressed versus non-depressed patients	NA	Associated behavioral treatment, and clinical improvement in both groups Depressed bulimics improved for depressive but not bulimic symptoms
Hughes et al. (1986), USA	10/12 *7/9* BN DSM III	Parallel 6 weeks + 6 weeks' open treatment with desipramine for initial placebo receivers	Desipramine (200 mg) versus placebo	91% decrease binge frequency on desipramine versus 19% increase on placebo Improvement on ZSRDS for subjects receiving desipramine Subjects on placebo first subsequently improved on desipramine 15/22 patients attained complete abstinence from binge eating and purging at treatment termination	1-month follow-up Persistence of benefits initially attained	Small sample size No standardized rating scale for BN

Study	Sample (ITT)	Design	Drug/dose	Results	Maintenance/discontinuation	Comments
Agras et al. (1987), USA	10/12 / *10/12* / BN DSM-III	Parallel 16 weeks	Imipramine (300 mg) versus placebo	Decrease in binge frequency: 72% versus 43%. Decrease in purge frequency: 72% versus 35%. Abstinence rate at treatment termination: 30% versus 10%	NA	Imipramine likely to be of some benefit to the majority of patients with BN and of great benefit to a few
Barlow et al. (1988), Canada	Total *n*: 47 / *Total n: 24* / Normal weight BN DSM III	Crossover 15 weeks: 6-week drug / 3-week no drug / 6-week placebo (or reverse)	Desipramine (150 mg) versus placebo	Higher decrease on desipramine for binge and vomiting frequency, and fatigue scale of POMS. No effect of desipramine on EDI and SCL-90R scores	NA	High dropout rate. Modest clinical effect. Desipramine antibulimic effect is not associated with alleviation of depressive symptoms
McCann and Agras (1990), USA	10/13 / 5/11 / BN-NP DSM-III-R	Parallel 12 weeks	Desipramine (100–300 mg) versus placebo	63% decrease in binge frequency on desipramine versus 16% increase on placebo. Abstinence at treatment termination: 60% versus 15%. Significant effect of desipramine on the three factors of TFED (disinhibition, hunger, restraint). No difference on BDI or weight	Relapse to baseline levels of binge eating within 4 weeks of discontinuing desipramine	First study with BN-NP patients. Suggesting similar effects as those in BN-P patients. However, small sample size and high dropout rate limit generalization of the findings
Walsh et al. (1991), USA	41/39 / 40/38 / Normal weight BN DSM III-R	Three-phase protocol: 1. Initiation: 8-week parallel trial. 2. Maintenance: 16-week open DMI treatment. 3. Discontinuation: 6-month DMI or placebo	DMI (200–300 mg) versus placebo	1. Initiation phase: Decrease in binge frequency: 47% versus 7%. Significant advantage of desipramine on: vomiting frequency, EAT, BSQ, SCL-90R, weight (decrease on drug). No significant effect of desipramine on BDI, HRSD, STAI-S, and SAS scores	2. Maintenance phase: 21/29 patients entered, 11 completed with no further improvement. 3. Discontinuation phase: not enough patients (5 versus 4)	Short-term beneficial effect of desipramine. Limited improvement and considerable relapse with continued treatment

ITT, intent-to-treat; BN, bulimia nervosa; DSM III, *Diagnostic and Statistical Manual*, 3rd edn; HRSD, Hamilton Rating Scale for Depression; NA, not applicable; ZSRDS, Zung Self-Rated Depression Scale; POMS, Profile of Mood States; EDI, Eating Disorder Inventory; SCL-90, Symptom Checklist-90; BN-NP, bulimia nervosa, non-purging type; TFED, Three-Factor-Eating Questionnaire; BDI, Deck Depression Inventory; DMI, desipramine; EAT, Eating Attitude Test; BSQ, Body Shape Questionnaire; STAI-S, State–Trait Anxiety Inventory – State; SAS, Social Assessment Scale; CGI, Clinical Global Impression.

Thus, existing trials using the tricyclic antidepressants indicate positive short-term effects for desipramine and imipramine. However, because the tricyclic antidepressants often cause unpleasant side-effects and have the potential to be fatal in overdose, this class of medication is not considered as a first-line treatment for BN.

Monoamine oxidase inhibitors

Concerns have been raised regarding the use of MAOIs, because of the potential fatal interactions with certain other medications (cough, cold, and sinus medications, commonly used anesthetics, various other antidepressants) (Blackwell, 1991), as well as frequent adverse reactions, such as insomnia, tremor, hypotension, and weight gain, requiring patients receiving MAOIs to follow severe dietary restrictions, such as a tyramine-restricted diet (Fallon *et al.*, 1991), which might be particularly difficult for bulimic subjects.

Nevertheless, three controlled studies using MAOIs have been published (two phenelzine, one brofaromine) in patients with BN (Table 9.10). In the study by Walsh *et al.* (1988), phenelzine (60–90 mg/day) was superior to placebo for both reduction of binge frequency (64% versus 5%) and the total number of bulimics achieving remission after 10 weeks (35% versus 4%); however, follow-up data collected at 6 months indicated that all the initial responders had relapsed during the follow-up period. Fallon *et al.* (1991) followed the same group of patients up to 4 years, and reported that 3 out of 15 (20%) had experienced severe hypertensive episodes, including one with a fatal outcome. A later study using phenelzine (75 mg/day) in 18 depressed bulimic patients resulted in significant reduction of both bulimic and depressive symptoms (Rothschild *et al.*, 1994). Brofaromine is a reversible MAOI reported as somewhat effective in individuals suffering from BN (Kennedy *et al.*, 1993), but is not commercially available in the USA.

Overall, because of the various adverse reactions and the potential for dangerous effects, MAOIs are not a first-line treatment for BN.

Selective serotonin reuptake inhibitors

As in AN, fluoxetine is the SSRI that has been most studied in BN. It is the only medication approved by the Food and Drug Administration for the treatment of BN in the USA. Fluvoxamine has also been studied in one open-label and two controlled trials, with mixed results (Table 9.11).

After fluoxetine had been shown to produce weight loss in obese (Ferguson and Feighner, 1987) and depressed patients (Cohn and Wilcox, 1985), it was investigated in a large multicenter study including 387 DSM III-R bulimic women (Fluoxetine Bulimia Nervosa Collaborative Study Group, 1992). Fluoxetine, administered at 60 mg/day for 8 weeks in one group of patients, was superior to placebo for reduction of binge frequency (in endpoint analysis, the median reduction was 67% on

Table 9.10 Controlled pharmacological trials with monoamine oxidase inhibitors (MAOIs) in bulimia nervosa (BN)

Authors, year, country	n (drug/placebo): ITT Completers Diagnostic criteria	Study design and duration	Treatment (daily dose)	Results: drug versus placebo	Follow-up duration and results	Conclusion and comments
Walsh et al. (1988), USA	31/31 23/27 BN DSM III	Parallel 10 weeks	Phenelzine (maximum 90 mg) versus placebo	Significant advantage of phenelzine on: • decrease in binge frequency: 64% versus 5% • decrease on CGI, EAT, BDI, HDRS, and SCL-90 scores • abstinence rate at termination: 35% versus 4% • 9/31 patients randomized to phenelzine dropped out due to side-effects (orthostatic hypotension, sedation) but no hypertensive reaction	6-month follow-up of 36/42 patients participating in the controlled trial or on open treatment 27/36 rated by their psychiatrist as much improved during treatment 24/27 responders discontinued medication (13 due to side-effects) All initial responders relapsed after treatment discontinuation	Significant therapeutic effects of phenelzine Depressed patients did worse than non-depressed but effect of phenelzine on binge reduction was not related to being depressed Side-effects are problematic and limit usefulness of phenelzine in this population
Kennedy et al. (1993), Canada	19/17 15/13 BN DSM III-R	Parallel 8 weeks	Brofaromine (maximum 200 mg) versus placebo	No significant difference in decrease of binge or purge frequency At termination, 19% versus 13% abstained from binging, 44% versus 20% abstained from purging No significant difference in decrease of EAT-26, EDI, HDRS, HARS scores Significantly higher percentage of patients on brofaromine lost weight	NA	Reversible MAOI with safer adverse effects profile Symptomatic decrease but most patients remained clinically ill Subjects treated with brofaromine reported eating fewer non-binge meals at end of treatment, suggesting reduced hunger or increased satiety signals Brofaromine not marketed in the USA
Rothschild et al. (1994), USA	8/10 8/10 BN DSM III	Parallel 6 weeks	Phenelzine (75 mg) versus placebo	Significant reduction in bulimic and depressive symptoms	NA	Data suggest a link between depression and bulimia in atypical depressives

ITT, intent-to-treat; DSM III, *Diagnostic and Statistical Manual*, 3rd edn; CGI, Clinical Global Improvement; EAT, Eating Attitudes Test; BDI, Beck Depression Inventory; HARS, Hamilton Anxiety Rating Scale; NA, not applicable; SCL-90, Symptom Checklist-90; EDI, Eating Disorder Inventory; HDRS, Hamilton Depression Rating Scale; MAOI, monoamine oxidase inhibitors.

Table 9.11 Controlled pharmacological trials with specific serotonin reuptake inhibitors in bulimia nervosa (BN)

Authors, year, country	n (drug/placebo): ITT *Completers* Diagnostic criteria	Study design and duration	Treatment (daily dose)	Results: drug versus placebo	Follow-up duration and results	Conclusion and comments
Freeman and Hampson (1987)	Total n = 40 BN DSM III-R	Parallel 6 weeks	Fluoxetine (60 mg) versus placebo	51% reduction in binge frequency on fluoxetine versus 17% in the placebo group Significant difference for reduction of EDI score Weight loss significantly greater on fluoxetine in "compliers," but not ITT analysis	NA	Fluoxetine showed a modest effect Side-effects were mild to moderate More positive (and significant) results were seen in "compliers" analysis (as determined by plasma levels of fluoxetine)
The Fluoxetine Bulimia Nervosa Collaborative Study Group (1992), USA	129 (FLX 20 mg) / 129 (FLX 60 mg) / 129 (placebo) 89 *(FLX 20 mg)* / 98 *(FLX 60 mg)* / 79 *(placebo)* BN DSM III-R	Parallel 8 weeks	FLX (20 mg) versus FLX (60 mg) versus placebo	Significantly greater reduction in binge (median frequency decreased by 67% versus 33%) and purge frequency (median decreased by 56% versus 5%) for FLX 60 mg group versus placebo Intermediate effect of FLX 20 mg Significant improvement with FLX (60 mg and, on some measures, 20 mg) for: depression, carbohydrate craving, eating attitudes 27% of FLX 60 mg group and 14% of FLX 20 mg group had complete binge remission at termination Side-effects (insomnia, nausea, fatigue, tremors) most frequent with 60 mg fluoxetine but no group difference for dropout rate	NA	Short-term treatment with fluoxetine appears relatively effective and well tolerated The high therapeutic dose of FLX in BN (60 mg) is at variance with studies in depressed patients, but not with previous study in obese patients The study failed to find pretreatment predictors of outcome

Reference	Sample	Design	Medication	Results	Comments
Flament et al. (1994), France, Belgium, Netherlands	53/50 38/39 BN DSM III-R	Placebo run-in period: 3 weeks part 1 Parallel trial 8 weeks part 2 Drug-free period 4 weeks	Fluvoxamine (range 150–300 mg, mean 233 mg) versus placebo	Part 1: No significant difference for reduction of binge (median 33% versus 28%) and purge frequency No change in weight in either group No significant difference for change on BITE, EDI, CGI-S, CGI-I, BINGE, and HDRS scores Responder rate: 27% on both fluvoxamine and placebo Most common side-effects on fluvoxamine: nausea, insomnia, somnolence, asthenia, headache 24 patients discontinued treatment due to adverse reactions Part 2: Higher rate of relapse in the group previously treated with fluoxetine (5/7) compared to placebo (2/10) No group difference for change in BINGE, BITE, EDI, and HDRS scores	Based on plasma concentration of fluvoxamine, compliance was satisfactory, and adverse events were not dose-related Fluvoxamine did not prove to be efficacious, relative to placebo, in reducing either the frequency or the intensity of any aspect of bulimic behavior or symptomatology
Goldstein et al. (1995), USA	296/102 229/62 BN DSM III-R	Parallel 16 weeks	Fluoxetine (60 mg) versus placebo	Significantly larger decrease in binge (50% versus 18%) and purge frequency (50% versus 21%) on fluoxetine compared to placebo Greater improvement on fluoxetine in other outcome measures: EDI, CGI, patient global impression Remission rate at week 16: 19% on fluoxetine versus 12% on placebo	Drug was effective and safe in patients with BN for up to 16 weeks Clinical efficacy was limited No long-term follow-up NA
Fichter et al. (1996), Germany, Belgium	37/35 23/30 BN DSM III-R	Parallel 15 weeks (3 weeks inpatient then 12 weeks outpatient)	Fluvoxamine (maximum 300 mg) versus placebo	In both ITT and completer analysis, significantly larger decrease of binge and purge frequency, and of scores on EDI-bulimia, SIAB total score with fluvoxamine compared to placebo In completer analysis, significantly larger decrease of EDI total score and SIAB-bulimia with fluvoxamine compared to placebo Dropout rate: 38% versus 14%	Positive effects of fluvoxamine in maintaining improvement achieved by intensive inpatient psychotherapy on most but not all outcome variables High number of subjects discontinued treatment due to side-effects Research has not established a dose-response course for fluvoxamine in BN Very short follow-up At 1-month follow-up, no effect of drug discontinuation (no rebound or withdrawal symptom)

ITT, intent-to-treat; DSM III-R, *Diagnostic and Statistical Manual*, 3rd edn (revised); EDI, Eating Disorder Inventory; NA, not applicable; FLX, fluoxetine; BITE, Bulimia Investigatory Test Edimburg; CGI-S, Clinical Global Impression – Severity; CGI-I, Clinical Global Impression – Improvement; BINGE, Severity Index of Bulimic Condition; HDRS, Hamilton Depression Rating Scale; SIAB, Structured Interview for Anorexia and Bulimia nervosa.

fluoxetine versus 33% on placebo, the difference being statistically significant at week 7 but not at week 8), and vomiting frequency (median reduction, 56% versus 5%, $P < 0.001$). In another group of patients, fluoxetine at 20 mg/day had an intermediate effect (median reduction of 45% for binge and 29% for purge frequency). At termination of treatment, 27% of bulimics receiving 60 mg of fluoxetine versus 14% of those receiving 20 mg or a placebo had achieved complete binge remission. Fluoxetine at 60 mg also improved depression, carbohydrate binges, and eating attitudes scores on the Eating Attitudes Test and the EDI. Side-effects (insomnia, nausea, fatigue, tremor) were most frequent on fluoxetine 60 mg. There was a mean weight loss of 1.7 kg on the higher dosage of fluoxetine.

Another multicenter placebo-controlled trial with a large sample (10 sites, 389 DSM III-R bulimics) reported similar findings (Goldstein *et al.*, 1995): compared with subjects who received placebo, those who were given 60 mg/day of fluoxetine showed superior improvement in binge (50% versus 18% reduction) and purge behaviors (50% versus 21% reduction); however, the full remission rate after 16 weeks of treatment was only 19% for fluoxetine and 12% for placebo. Fluvoxamine is a potent and specific serotonin reuptake inhibitor, with little or no effect on the noradrenergic system, and no monoamine oxidase-inhibiting action. One open study (Ayuso-Gutierrez *et al.*, 1994), including 20 patients with BN treated with daily doses of 50–150 mg fluvoxamine for 8 weeks, reported a significant improvement from baseline on EDI total score, Clinical Global Impression, and binge frequency.

A larger multicenter controlled study, aiming at measuring the efficacy of fluvoxamine (150–300 mg/day) and the relapse rate upon discontinuation of treatment, included 117 adolescent and adult women with DSM III-R BN, and at least 3 months' duration of the disorder (Flament *et al.*, 1994). A single-blind placebo run-in period of 3 weeks preceded the actual 8-week double-blind study, in order to exclude placebo responders (14 subjects). The remaining 103 patients were randomized to either fluvoxamine or placebo: 81% were of normal weight, 19% were non-purging bulimics, and 13% had a comorbid major depressive disorder. Fluvoxamine (mean dose during last 4 weeks of treatment, 233 mg/day) did not prove to be efficacious, relative to placebo, in reducing the frequency or intensity of any aspect of bulimic behavior or symptomatology, neither in the total sample, nor in separate analyses for purgers and non-purgers. On average, the key symptoms of bulimia nervosa were unaltered by treatment. Seventy-seven patients completed the first part of the study and were eligible for the subsequent 4-week discontinuation phase; of those, only 17 had been responders (score of 1 or 2 on Clinical Global Impression – Improvement scale), and 5/7 patients who had responded to fluvoxamine, compared to 2/10 of placebo responders, relapsed during the month following treatment discontinuation.

Table 9.12 Controlled pharmacological trials with mood stabilizers in bulimia nervosa (BN)

Authors, year, country	*n* (drug/ placebo): ITT *Completers* Diagnostic criteria	Study design and duration	Treatment (daily dose)	Results: drug versus placebo	Follow-up duration and results	Conclusion and comments
Hsu *et al.* (1991), USA	47/44 *38/30* BN DSM III	Parallel 8 weeks	Lithium (300 mg) versus placebo	No difference in decrease of binge or purge frequency No difference in decrease on EDI, EAT, HDRS, BDI, and SCL-90 scores Significant improvement on lithium only in depressed bulimic patients	NA	Lithium not more effective than placebo Relatively low plasma concentrations of lithium Depression and other symptoms decreased with improvement in bulimic behavior

ITT, intent-to-treat; DSM III, *Diagnostic and Statistical Manual*, 3rd edn; EDI, Eating Disorders Inventory; EAT, Eating Attitudes Test; HDRS, Hamilton Depression Rating Scale; BDI, Beck Depression Inventory; SCL-90, Symptom Checklist-90; NA, not applicable.

Fluvoxamine was also tested in a double-blind placebo-controlled trial assessing its efficacy to maintain improvement in 54 female BN patients following discontinuation of intensive inpatient psychotherapy (Fichter *et al.*, 1996). Fluvoxamine (mean daily dose, 188 mg) had several statistically significant effects in preventing relapse or deterioration of eating behaviors, both on patient's and expert's ratings; however, it had no effect on the course of attitudes towards slimness and figure consciousness. The positive effects of fluvoxamine in maintaining improvement achieved by intensive inpatient psychotherapy were shown on 1/3 primary efficacy variables and 6/9 secondary efficacy variables. Of note was the relatively high number of patients discontinuing treatment in the fluvoxamine group, including 9 because of unpleasant (although not serious) side-effects.

Mood stabilizers

Hsu *et al.* (1991) examined whether bulimic patients treated with lithium for 8 weeks demonstrated better results than those treated with placebo (Table 9.12). Lithium

Table 9.13 Controlled pharmacological trials with opiate antagonists in bulimia nervosa (BN)

Authors, year, country	*n* (drug/placebo): ITT *Completers* Diagnostic criteria	Study design and duration	Treatment (daily dose)	Results: drug versus placebo	Follow-up duration and results	Conclusion and comments
Jonas and Gold (1988), USA	Total *n*: 16 BN DSM III-R	Parallel 6 weeks	Naltrexone 50–100 mg (low dose) versus 200–300 mg (high dose)	Significant reduction for the amount of days binge eating (mean reduction:1.9, SD: 3.0) and purging (mean: 2.0, SD: 2.9) in the naltrexone high-dose group only	NA	More research is needed

ITT, intent-to-treat; DSM III-R, *Diagnostic and Statistical Manual*, 3rd edn; NA, not applicable.

resulted in significant improvement only in depressed bulimic patients; however, plasma concentrations of lithium were relatively low. Anticonvulsants have been anecdotally tried in BN: patients treated with either phenytoin or carbamazepine reported modest benefits, but no significant effects were demonstrated (Wermuth *et al.*, 1977; Kaplan *et al.*, 1983).

Opiate antagonists

Despite preliminary work indicating that intravenous opiate antagonists decreased the duration and quantity of food eaten during a binge meal (Mitchell *et al.*, 1986), naltrexone first appeared ineffective in BN (Mitchell *et al.*, 1989). Subsequent research (Jonas and Gold, 1988) demonstrated some positive results: in a 6-week controlled trial, modest improvement was reported in 16 bulimic patients who received high doses (200–300 mg/day) of naltrexone (Table 9.13).

Other medications (Table 9.14)

Mianserin, a tetracyclic antidepressant acting on presynaptic alpha$_2$-adrenergic receptors, was studied in a controlled trial including 50 bulimics, but failed to show a significant difference from placebo (Sabine *et al.*, 1983). Horne *et al.* (1988) conducted a controlled trial in 81 BN patients using the norepinephrine (noradrenaline) dopamine reuptake inhibitor (NDRI) bupropion; although it was found superior to placebo, bupropion was also associated with the unexplained occurrence of seizures in 4 patients. The serotonin-2 antagonist/reuptake inhibitor (SARI) trazodone was superior to placebo in a double-blind, placebo-controlled study conducted by

Table 9.14 Controlled pharmacological trials with other medications in bulimia nervosa (BN)

Authors, year, country	n (drug/placebo): ITT / Completers / Diagnostic criteria	Study design and duration	Treatment (daily dose)	Results: drug versus placebo	Follow-up duration and results	Conclusion and comments
Sabine et al. (1983), UK	20/30 / 14/22 / BN / DSM III	Parallel 8 weeks	Mianserin (60 mg) versus placebo	No significant difference for binge or purge frequency	NA	Further studies are needed
Horne et al. (1988), USA	55/26 / 37/12 / BN (no current major depression) / DSM III	Parallel 8 weeks	Bupropion (maximum, 450 mg) versus placebo	Significant advantage of bupropion for decrease in binge and purge frequency Little change on HDRS score Side-effects on bupropion generally minimal, except for 4 subjects with grand mal seizures	NA	Drug not recommended for bulimic patients because of (unexplained) high frequency of seizures
Hudson et al. (1989), USA	20/22 / 20/22 / BN / DSM III-R	Parallel 6 weeks subsequent open treatment with trazodone and/or 2 days or 3 days antidepressant	Trazodone (200–400 mg) versus placebo	Higher percentage of change for binge and purge frequency with trazodone compared to placebo 10% patients abstinent and 30% improved on trazodone versus 0% improved on placebo Few bothersome side-effects (drowsiness, dizziness)	9–19-month follow-up of 36/42 subjects Most still on trazodone alone (2 patients) and/or other antidepressant 26/36 (72%) with continued improvement 18/36 (50%) had achieved remission (of those, 65% were still on medication)	Trazodone was safe and moderately effective Useful addition to pharmacological options for BN Long-term response in BN may require several trials of antidepressant compounds
Faris et al. (2000), USA	14/12 / 13/12 severe BN (>= 7 binges/week) / DSM IV	Parallel 4 weeks	Odansetron (24 mg) versus placebo	Significant advantage of odansetron for time spent engaging in bulimic behaviors and number of normal eating episodes per week On odansetron, mean weekly binge/purge frequency decreased from 12.8 to 6.5	NA	Findings indicate normalization of physiological mechanisms controlling meal termination and satiety Symptom improvement may result from pharmacological correction of abnormal vagal neurotransmission

ITT, intent-to-treat; DSM III, *Diagnostic and Statistical Manual*, 3rd edn; NA, not applicable; HDRS, Hamilton Depression Rating Scale.

Hudson *et al.* (1989) on 42 bulimic women. Trazodone showed a net reduction in binge-eating frequency of 50%, and data collected at 9–19 months' follow-up (most subjects were still on trazodone or had been switched to another antidepressant) indicated that 72% of subjects were still improved, and 50% were abstinent. Ondansetron, a 5-HT$_3$-antagonist, was administered to severely bulimic patients, at a dosage of 24 mg/day (Faris *et al.*, 2000). After 4 weeks of treatment, it appeared to reduce the mean weekly binge/purge frequency from 12.8 to 6.5, whereas no significant change occurred in patients receiving placebo. It was suggested that the drug might normalize physiological mechanisms controlling meal termination and satiety. Treatment with ondansetron has also been associated with an increase in frequency of normal meals and decrease in time occupied by bulimic behaviors (Roerig *et al.*, 2002).

Medication versus psychotherapy versus combined treatment in bulimia nervosa

Cognitive-behavioral therapy (CBT) is the psychological treatment of choice for BN. The therapeutic model developed by Fairburn in 1985 and reviewed in 1993 (Fairburn *et al.*, 1993) rests on five major points of emphasis: (1) self-monitoring of food intake as well as of the thoughts and feelings that trigger binge and purge episodes; (2) regular weighing; (3) specific recommendations to normalize eating behavior and reduce dieting; (4) cognitive restructuring directed at countering persistence of the disorder; and (5) prevention of relapse.

Four small sample size studies (Mitchell *et al.*, 1990; Agras *et al.*, 1992; Leitenberg *et al.*, 1994; Goldbloom *et al.*, 1997) have compared the use of antidepressant medication (desipramine, imipramine, or fluoxetine) with standard-length CBT. Three studies compared CBT alone, medication alone, and the combination, and one compared CBT/placebo, medication alone, and the combination. All found CBT or CBT/placebo to be superior to medication alone, and not significantly different from the combination. In a longer-term study, Pyle *et al.* (1990) divided 68 bulimic patients into three groups treated with imipramine alone, intensive group psychotherapy plus placebo, or combined treatment. Overall, 47% of subjects responded to treatment during the acute phase of the study and were included in a 4-month maintenance phase. Relapse rate was high (30%), but those patients receiving group psychotherapy alone or combined with imipramine were the least likely to relapse.

Walsh *et al.* (1997) randomized 120 women with BN to 4 months of individual CBT or supportive psychotherapy (SPT) plus antidepressant medication (200–300 mg/day of desipramine for 8 weeks, switched, if not effective, to 60 mg/day of fluoxetine) or placebo, or a medication-alone condition. CBT was superior to

SPT in reducing the frequency of binge eating and vomiting. Patients receiving active medication in combination with psychological treatment experienced greater improvement in binge eating and depression than did patients receiving placebo and psychological treatment. CBT plus active medication was superior to medication alone, whereas SPT plus active medication was not. A second article on the same study (Wilson *et al.*, 1999) indicated that a high baseline frequency of binge eating or vomiting, as well as a positive history of substance abuse or dependence, were negative predictors of treatment response.

In a multicenter study by Mitchell *et al.* (2002), 194 patients were initially treated with CBT; then those treated unsuccessfully ($n = 62$) were randomized to treatment with interpersonal psychotherapy (IPT) or medication management (fluoxetine starting at 60 mg/day, switched if not effective after 8 weeks to 50–300 mg/day of desipramine); 37 patients completed treatment, and 25 dropped out or were withdrawn. The abstinence rate for subjects assigned to treatment with IPT was 16% and, for those assigned to medication management, it was 10%. No significant difference emerged between medication and IPT, in either the intent-to-treat or the completer analysis.

Meta-analyses on the efficacy of pharmacotherapy or combined pharmacological–psychological treatment for bulimia nervosa

We reviewed three meta-analyses on pharmacotherapy of BN: (1) a meta-analysis by Whittal *et al.* (1999), including nine double-blind, placebo-controlled medication trials (a total of 870 subjects) and 26 randomized psychosocial studies using either CBT or behavior therapy (460 subjects); (2) a multidimensional meta-analysis conducted by Nakash-Eisikovits *et al.* (2002) aggregating data from 16 studies involving a pharmacological treatment condition on a total of 918 subjects (9/16 studies also included a combined pharmacotherapy/psychotherapy condition); (3) the meta-analysis by Bacaltchuk *et al.* (2000), following a Cochrane review by the same authors (Batalchuk *et al.*, 1998), aiming at evaluating the efficacy of several antidepressant medications. Since the three meta-analyses were conducted within a few years from each other, and include similar or complementary analyses, we will summarize their findings together.

Inclusion and completion rates

An unusual though useful calculation included in the meta-analysis of Nakash-Eisikovits *et al.* (2002) concerns the rate of potential participants rejected from research trials due to specific exclusion criteria (e.g., medical condition, suicidality, substance use, comorbid AN, obesity, major depressive disorder, obsessive-compulsive disorder, and psychosis). In the average study, approximately

50% of potential participants were excluded, yielding inclusion rates ranging from 64% for SSRIs to 29% for MAOIs. Among those subjects who actually entered the study, the percentage of completers was high (73% on average), and only 10% dropped out because of side-effects. For the combined pharmacotherapy/psychotherapy studies, inclusion and completion rates were 54% and 76%, respectively.

Effect size for short-term pharmacological treatment

Whittal *et al.* (1999) calculated the effect size (ESs) of medication as the magnitude of change from pre- to posttreatment weighted for sample size. For nine medication trials, the pooled ESs were 0.66 for binge frequency, 0.39 for purge frequency, 0.73 for depression, and 0.71 for eating attitudes (self-reported restraint, weight/shape concern). In the meta-analysis of Nakash-Eisikovits *et al.* (2002), the average ES for short-term drug treatment, using Cohen's *d* (mean outcome score of treatment group minus mean of placebo group divided by pooled posttest standard deviation), was moderate ($d = 0.6$) for both binge and purge episodes. Pre- and posttreatment ESs were larger, averaging 1.0 for binges and 0.7 for purges.

In the systematic Cochrane review by Bacaltchuk *et al.* (1998) of 16 trials comparing remission rate in 1300 patients treated exclusively with antidepressants or placebo, the pooled relative risk (RR) was 0.88 (95% confidence interval = 0.83–0.94; $P < 0.0001$) favoring active drugs, and no differential effect regarding efficacy and tolerability among the various classes of antidepressants could be demonstrated.

Short-term efficacy of pharmacotherapy versus cognitive-behavioral therapy versus combined treatment

In the meta-analysis of Whittal *et al.* (1999), the relative effectiveness of medication (nine trials) versus CBT (26 trials) was calculated on all outcome measures, yielding superiority for CBT on each of the constructs: ESs = 1.28 versus 0.66 for binge frequency, 0.22 versus 0.39 for purge frequency, 0.31 versus 0.73 for depression, and 1.35 versus 0.71 for eating attitudes. For effectiveness of combined treatment with CBT and medication (four trials), the pooled ESs were 1.77 for binge frequency, 1.33 for purge frequency, 0.88 for depression, and 1.27 for eating attitudes. Combined treatment (based on three trials) was significantly better than medication alone (binge frequency: 1.77 versus 0.66; purge frequency: 1.33 versus 0.39) and significantly better than CBT alone for binge frequency (1.77 versus 1.28) but not purge frequency (1.33 versus 1.22). The dropout rate in medication trials was higher (25.4%) compared to CBT studies (18.6%), but the difference was not significant; both treatments were fairly well tolerated. The meta-analysis of Nakash-Eisikovits *et al.* (2002) demonstrated a small advantage for combined treatment over medication alone for binge episodes, and a moderate advantage for purging episodes ($d = 0.2$ and 0.5, respectively, with d referring to the difference between the standardized effects of combined treatments over medication alone). There was a small to moderate advantage of combined treatments over psychotherapy alone ($d = 0.3$ for binges and 0.3 for purges).

One objective of the meta-analysis of Bacaltchuk *et al.* (2000) was to evaluate the efficacy of the combination of antidepressant medication (desipramine, fluoxetine, or imipramine) with psychological treatment for BN. Two types of trials were included: single antidepressant treatment versus combination (five studies, 247 patients), and single psychological approaches versus combination (seven studies, 343 patients). Although dropout rates were high (41% for patients receiving single antidepressant treatment and 34% for those receiving the combination), patients receiving both treatments had a better outcome than those receiving either antidepressant treatment alone or psychological treatment alone. Remission rates were 23% for antidepressant treatment versus 42% for the combination ($P = 0.06$), and 36% for psychological treatment versus 49% for the combination ($P = 0.03$). Thus, the efficacy of combined treatments was superior to single approaches.

Improvement and recovery rate

Nakash-Eisikovits *et al.* (2002) computed the overall improvement and/or recovery rate at the end of treatment. In completer analysis (including only patients who terminated treatment), studies using tricyclic medication showed higher improvement/recovery rate (94% for binge episodes) than did studies using SSRIs (54%), MAOIs (41%), or atypical antidepressants (48%). In intent-to-treat analysis (including all subjects who had started treatment), the recovery rate after pharmacotherapy was 25% for remission of both binge and purge episodes, 17% for remission of bingeing episodes only, and 23% for remission of purging episodes only. The overall remission rate of bingeing episodes among completers was higher after treatment with MAOIs (35%) than with SSRIs (19%), or atypical antidepressants, such as trazodone or bupropion (20%). At termination of combined drug and pharmacological treatment, the percentage of subjects who had stopped bingeing and purging was 55% in completer analysis, and 39% in intent-to-treat analysis.

Posttreatment symptoms

Based on 10 controlled medication trials, Nakash-Eisikovits *et al.* (2002) also calculated the rate of posttreatment symptoms, as the mean frequency of binge and purge episodes at termination of treatment: across all types of medication, bulimic patients still binged, on average, 4.3 times per week, and still purged, on average, 6.2 times per week, at termination of treatment. For bulimic patients receiving both pharmacotherapy and psychotherapy, the average rates (based on nine studies) were 2.5 for both binge and purge frequency. Thus, although these data point to substantial improvement over conditions before treatment, they do not constitute a return to mental health, i.e., according to DSM IV criteria, the average patient still has BN, even after an adequate trial of drug or combined treatment.

Long-term efficacy

All meta-analyses conclude that evidence-based data on long-term efficacy of pharmacotherapy for BN are mostly lacking. The longest follow-up period is 12–18 months in the study by Agras (1997), in which 30% of completers reached and maintained recovery, and binge frequency averaged 4.1 per week at the end of follow-up. Walsh and colleagues (1991) continued treatment for 4 months after termination of a controlled trial in improved BN patients: of the 40 initially enrolled, only 13% improved and remained improved through the maintenance phase. Pyle and coworkers (1990) had planned a 6-month maintenance trial for treatment responders (9 out of 31 initial inclusions), but only 2 patients completed this phase! No data are available to date on pharmacotherapy combined with long-term psychotherapy, although this combination of treatments would seem likely to reduce relapse.

Pharmacotherapy of binge-eating disorder

The pharmacological literature on BED is still limited. A small number of controlled trials have been published and, of those, most are of short duration and use relatively narrow outcome measures.

Tricyclic antidepressants

Alger *et al.* (1991) compared the effectiveness of imipramine (150 mg/day), naltrexone (100–150 mg/day), and placebo in a controlled trial including 41 obese binge eaters and 28 normal-weight DSM III bulimics (Table 9.15). The mean reduction in binge-eating frequency after 8 weeks was 90% and 78% for the groups treated with imipramine and naltrexone, respectively, versus 70% for the group on placebo, with no statistically significant difference. Because of the high placebo response, the results are difficult to interpret. The only significant effect of imipramine was to reduce binge duration in obese bingers, but weight did not change in any group.

Selective serotonin reuptake inhibitors (Table 9.16)

Fluvoxamine was the first SSRI to be studied for treatment of BED. After the open-label study of Gardiner *et al.* (1993), including 10 non-vomiting bingeing women and reporting a significant reduction in binge-eating frequency over 8 weeks, Hudson *et al.* (1998) conducted a 9-week multicenter, placebo-controlled trial in 85 patients with DSM IV-defined BED. Fluvoxamine (50–300 mg/day) was associated with a statistically significant reduction in the frequency of binge-eating

Table 9.15 Controlled pharmacological trials with tricyclic antidepressants in binge-eating disorder (BED)

Authors, year, country	*n* (drug/placebo) ITT *Completers* Diagnostic criteria	Study design and duration	Treatment (daily dose)	Results: drug versus placebo	Follow-up duration and results	Conclusion and comments
Alger *et al.* (1991), USA	Obese binge eaters: 12 (IMI) / 10 (NAL) / 11 (placebo) Bulimics: 7 (IMI) / 8 (NAL) / 7 (placebo) Obese binge eaters: BES score ≥ 25 BN: DSM III and BULIT score ≥ 102	Parallel 8 weeks	IMI (150 mg) versus NAL (100–150 mg) versus placebo	Mean reduction in binge eating frequency: 90% (IMI) versus 78% (NAL) versus 70% (placebo) Compared to placebo, IMI significantly reduced binge duration in obese bingers but not bulimics No significant weight reduction in any treatment group No group difference for decrease in BDI score	NA	Results are difficult to interpret because of high placebo response and incomplete report of pre- and posttreatment group scores Imipramine significantly reduced binge duration in obese bingers

ITT, intent-to-treat; IMI, imipramine; NAL, naltrexone; BES, Gormally Binge-Eating Scale; DSM III, *Diagnostic and Statistical Manual*, 3rd edn; BDI, Beck Depression Inventory; NA, not applicable; BULIT, The Bulimia Test.

Table 9.16 Controlled pharmacological trials with specific serotonin reuptake inhibitors in binge-eating disorder (BED)

Authors, year, country	n (drug/placebo) ITT Completers Diagnostic criteria	Study design and duration	Treatment (daily dose)	Results: drug versus placebo	Follow-up duration and results	Conclusion and comments
Hudson et al. (1998), USA	42/43 29/38 BED DSM IV	Parallel 9 weeks	Fluvoxamine (50–300 mg) versus placebo	Fluvoxamine better for reduction of binge-eating frequency and BMI 45% subjects stopped binge eating and 28% improved with fluvoxamine (versus 24% and 24% with placebo) On fluvoxamine, significantly greater decrease of CGI severity and greater increase on CGI improvement score No group effect for decrease on HDRS score	NA	According to most outcome measures, fluvoxamine was effective in the acute treatment of BED Greater proportion of patients receiving fluvoxamine than placebo dropped out due to adverse events
McElroy et al. (2000), USA	18/16 13/13 BED DSM IV	Parallel 6 weeks	Sertraline (50–200 mg) versus placebo	Significant advantage of sertraline for reduction of binge frequency, CGI severity score, and BMI Non-significantly higher response rate for sertraline compared to placebo No significant difference for incidence of adverse events	NA	Brief report showing that sertraline was effective and well tolerated for the acute treatment of BED
Ricca et al. (2001), Italy	Total n: 108 21 (FLX) / 22 (FLV) / 20 (CBT) / 22 (CBT + FLX) / 23 (CBT + FLV) BED DSM IV	Parallel 24 weeks	FLX (60 mg) versus FLV (300 mg) versus CBT versus CBT + FLX (60 mg) versus CBT + FLV (300 mg)	At treatment termination, significant reduction of BMI and EDE score in CBT, CBT + FLX, and CBT + FLV groups, not in FLX and FLV groups Significantly greater reduction of EDE score for CBT + FLV group, compared to CBT or CBT + FLX groups	At 1-year follow-up, BMI was higher than at termination, but still significantly lower than at baseline in CBT and CBT + FLV groups EDE scores remained unchanged in all groups	CBT more effective than FLX or FLV in the treatment of BED Addition of FLV (but not FLX) enhanced effects of CBT on eating behaviors Modification of eating behaviors maintained at 1 year, although weight lost was partially regained

ITT, intent-to-treat; DSM IV, *Diagnostic and Statistical Manual*, 4th edn; BMI, body mass index; CGI, Clinical Global Improvement; HDRS, Hamilton Depression Rating Scale; NA, not applicable. FLX, Fluoxetine; FLV, Fluvoxamine; CBT, cognitive-behavioral therapy; EDE, Eating Disorders Examination.

episodes, decrease in BMI, overall clinical improvement, and a higher remission rate than placebo (45% versus 24%).

In a 12-day challenge study, Greeno and Wing (1996) examined whether fluoxetine reduced energy consumption and body weight in 38 women with BED and 32 age- and weight-matched healthy women, randomly assigned to receive, after a 6-day baseline, 60 mg/day of fluoxetine or placebo for 6 days. Compared to placebo, fluoxetine lowered the overall energy intake, decreasing the energy consumed at each eating episode; however, the frequency of episodes was unaffected, suggesting that fluoxetine affects satiety, not hunger. Subsequently, Ricca *et al.* (2001) conducted a long-term treatment study including 108 patients (64 females, 44 males) with BED, randomly assigned to one of five groups for 24 weeks: (1) fluoxetine (60 mg/day); (2) fluvoxamine (300 mg/day); (3) CBT; (4) CBT + fluoxetine; (5) CBT + fluvoxamine. At termination of treatment, both the BMI and the score on the Eating Disorder Examination (EDE) were significantly reduced in the three groups treated by CBT, with or without medication, and the group receiving fluvoxamine was superior to the other two groups for reduction of the EDE score. At 1-year follow-up, the BMI was significantly higher than at treatment endpoint, but still significantly lower than at baseline, in the three groups that had received CBT, while the EDE score had remained unchanged in all groups. Thus, the addition of fluvoxamine seemed to have enhanced the effects of CBT on eating behaviors, and the treatment effects were maintained at 1 year posttreatment.

Sertraline has been tested in a 6-week, double-blind controlled trial including 34 patients with DSM IV BED (McElroy *et al.*, 2000). Compared with placebo, sertraline was associated with a significantly greater reduction of binge frequency, and a greater decrease of the Clinical Global Severity score and the BMI. Paroxetine has only been studied in an open-label trial including 9 patients with BED, resulting in a significant reduction in frequency of binge eating after 16 weeks (Prats *et al.*, 1994).

Other medications (Table 9.17)

In the study by Alger *et al.* (1991), described above, the opioid antagonist naltrexone (100–150 mg/day) produced, similar to imipramine, a substantial reduction in binge-eating frequency, without significant difference from placebo; naltrexone significantly reduced binge duration in bulimics, but not in obese subjects with BED.

d-Fenfluramine has been used for 30 years as an appetite-suppressant medication. It inhibits the reuptake of serotonin, and its main metabolite increases presynaptic release of serotonin and acts on postsynaptic receptors. The net effect is to enhance serotonin transmission in the neural pathways mediating satiety, leading to decreased food intake and body weight (McTavish and Heel, 1992). After

Table 9.17 Controlled pharmacological trials with other medications in binge-eating disorder (BED)

Authors, year, country	*n* (drug/placebo) ITT *Completers* Diagnostic criteria	Study design and duration	Treatment (daily dose)	Results: drug versus placebo	Follow-up duration and results	Conclusion and comments
Alger et al. (1991), USA (see Table 3.1)	Obese binge eaters: *12 (IMI) / 10 (NAL) / 11 (placebo)* Bulimics: *7 (IMI) / 8 (NAL) / 7 (placebo)* Obese binge eaters: BES score ≥ 25BN; DSM III and BULIT score ≥ 102	Parallel 8 weeks	IMI (150 mg) versus NAL (100–150 mg) versus placebo	Mean reduction in binge-eating frequency: 90% for IMI versus 78% for NAL versus 70% for placebo Compared to placebo, NAL significantly reduced binge duration in bulimics, but not obese bingers	NA	NAL significantly reduced binge duration in bulimics but not obese binge eaters Four subjects dropped from NAL group because of side-effects (headache, nausea, agitation, diaphoresis)
Stunkard et al. (1996), USA	50 (placebo lead-in) *d*-FEN / placebo: *14/14* *12/12 BED* DSM IV	Placebo lead-in period (4 weeks) then parallel study 8 weeks	*d*-FEN (15–30 mg) versus placebo	Linear regression analysis showed that rate of binge eating in the *d*-FEN group fell three times more rapidly than in placebo group (significant statistical and clinical result)	At 1- and 4-month follow-up, no significant difference between the drug and placebo groups At 4-month follow-up, binge frequency in the *d*-FEN group was back to pretreatment level	*d*-FEN has been withdrawn from the market
McElroy et al. (2003), USA	30/31 *24/28 BED* DSM IV-TR	Parallel 14 weeks	Topiramate (50–600 mg, mean 212 mg/day) versus placebo	Significantly greater decrease on topiramate than placebo for: weekly binge frequency (94% versus 46%), binge day frequency (93% versus 46%), weight loss (mean 5.9 versus 1.2 kg) Most common reasons for discontinuing topiramate: headache (*n* = 3), paresthesias (*n* = 2)	NA	Topiramate was efficacious and relatively well tolerated in the acute treatment of BED associated with obesity Mechanisms by which topiramate affects food intake and energy expenditure remain unknown Comparative studies with other active compounds needed

ITT, intent-to-treat; IMI, imipramine; NAL, naltrexone; BES, Gormally Binge-Eating Scale; BN, bulimia nervosa; DSM III, *Diagnostic and Statistical Manual*, 3rd edn; BULIT, the Bulimia Test; NA, not applicable; *d*-FEN, *d*-fenfluramine.

a 4-week placebo lead-in period including 50 severely obese women with DSM IV BED, Stunkard *et al.* (1996) randomized the 28 placebo non-responders to 8 weeks of *d*-fenfluramine (15–30 mg/day) or placebo. The rate of binge eating in the *d*-fenfluramine group fell three times more rapidly than that in the placebo group, a result considered by the authors as both statistically and clinically significant; however, relapse to baseline levels of binge-eating frequency occurred within 4 months of medication discontinuation. Because of an increased rate of valvular abnormalities, *d*-fenfluramine was withdrawn from the market in 1997.

Topiramate is a structurally novel antiepileptic medication which has been found to induce weight loss in patients with seizure disorder (Langtry *et al.*, 2003); its pharmacological mechanisms of action include blockade of glutamate receptors shown to influence food intake in animal studies (Stanley *et al.*, 1993). McElroy *et al.* (2003) conducted a 14-week, flexible-dose parallel study comparing topiramate (50–600 mg/day) to placebo in 61 obese outpatients (53 women, 8 men) with BED. Topiramate was associated with a significantly higher reduction of weekly binge frequency and binge day frequency, and a significantly greater weight loss. No serious adverse medical events were reported, but 5 patients discontinued topiramate due to headache or paresthesias.

Methodological considerations

Research on the pharmacological – and psychological – treatment of AN has been hampered by several factors, including the relative rarity of the condition, patients' ambivalence about treatment, and the tenuous medical status of anorexic individuals that usually requires a multiplicity of simultaneous interventions. Data from the few existing controlled studies are further hampered by a variety of methodological shortcomings, including small sample size, significant dropout rate, ceiling effect for additive treatments, and lack of assessment of the durability of gains in preventing relapse.

Many more placebo-controlled double-blind trials, with larger sample size and better methodology, are available for pharmacotherapy of BN. Three studies were found using fluoxetine, on a total of 825 subjects, and two using fluvoxamine on a total of 157 subjects; desipramine has been investigated in four trials (172 patients), imipramine in two (44 subjects), and phenelzine in two (80 subjects). The following compounds have each been studied once: lithium (91 subjects); bupropion (81 subjects); mianserin (50 subjects); trazodone (42 subjects); amitriptyline (38 subjects); brofaromine (36 subjects); odansetron (26 subjects); and naltrexone (16 subjects). Treatment duration has ranged from 6 to 16 weeks, with an average of 6–8 weeks.

However, as discussed in Anderson and Maloney's (2001) review on psychological treatment of the disorder, the five core symptoms of BN (binge eating, purging, restrictive eating, concerns with shape and weight, and self-esteem) are rarely all addressed in the choice of outcome treatment measures. Only few studies provide data on restrictive eating and self-esteem, although these may be crucial in the stability of initial treatment gains. Another limitation of available treatment studies is that, although the DSM IV specifies two subtypes of BN, the vast majority of studies have included only (or mainly) participants who meet criteria for the purging type. We found only one small ($n = 23$) study specifically investigating the efficacy of pharmacotherapy (desipramine) for non-purging BN patients. Whether the results of the other studies are applicable to non-purging BN has not been established.

Pharmacological treatment research on BED has been initiated recently. Several studies have shown a high placebo response rate, which, in addition to small sample size and short duration of treatment, makes it difficult to assess the clinical significance of results. Furthermore, treatment expectancies of individuals with BED are often twofold – regulation of eating behavior and decrease in weight – but reduction of binge eating does not necessarily lead to relevant weight loss.

Short-term efficacy of pharmacotherapy

Given the clinical symptoms associated with AN, including depression, anxiety, and appetite disturbance, all of which overlap with symptoms seen in other psychiatric conditions that are responsive to a range of medications, drug treatment appears singularly ineffective in the acute management of AN. The lack of efficacy of antidepressants in anorexic patients may be related to poor intake of the dietary precursors for neurotransmitter synthesis, and/or other neurochemical disturbances associated with starvation (Kaye *et al.*, 1998). This points to the importance of weight restoration as a first and essential step to help AN patients normalize both their biological and their psychological condition.

To date, no psychopharmacological agent has clearly been established to be of benefit in the treatment of the primary symptoms of AN. Antidepressant medication may be considered as an adjunct to a multifaceted treatment approach, especially when there is evidence of a comorbid mood or anxiety disorder. Due to their superior side-effect profile, the SSRIs are currently the preferred class of agents. Yet, for reasons mentioned above, it is often prudent to defer the consideration of a medication trial until significant weight gain has taken place. There is no strong evidence that other medications, including food supplements or prokinetic agents, may be of benefit in the acute management of AN.

The most promising finding to date may be preliminary evidence that antidepressant medication can help prevent relapse in AN patients who have returned to normal weight (on the basis of one study using fluoxetine for a year, in 35 weight-restored anorexic patients, of whom only 13 completed the trial).

The empirical literature on drug treatment for BN includes at least one positive randomized controlled trial for imipramine, desipramine, fluoxetine, trazadone, and ondansetron. However, treatment results are often mixed and can be summarized as follows:

1. Pharmacotherapy yields a moderate initial effect: subjects demonstrate a reduction in binge and/or purge frequency anywhere from 22% to 92%.
2. At termination of most drug studies, residual symptoms tend to be the norm, and the average patient continues to meet diagnostic criteria for BN.
3. In patients who passed a series of exclusion criteria to enter treatment studies rigorous enough to exclude roughly half of eligible subjects, recovery rate is low (0–68%, mean 24%), which is of concern when one considers that abstinence at the end of treatment may predict long-term outcome.
4. In most studies, there is no relationship between concurrent major depressive diagnosis and the effectiveness of various antidepressants, although it is clear that depressive symptoms do improve with treatment.
5. The relapse risk during continuation therapy may be higher than that typically observed in studies of continuation therapy, for example in depression.
6. How long to continue treatment once binge eating abates, to protect maximally against the risk of relapse or recurrence, is a question that remains unanswered.

Because of overlapping eating patterns and psychopathological features between BN and BED, medication that has been shown helpful in patients with BN is often proposed to those with BED, although there is much less empirical evidence for their efficacy in this indication. Two positive studies have been published to date regarding the use of SSRIs, with short-term effects of fluvoxamine and sertraline for reduction of binge-eating frequency, and initial decrease in weight. One study with topiramate, a novel antiepileptic drug also used as a mood stabilizer, demonstrated similar effects. Clearly, these promising results need to be supported by more data, and the utility of other classes of drugs (e.g., weight-loss agents such as sibutramine) are still to be explored.

Combined pharmacological and psychological treatment

Only in BN have pharmacological and psychological treatments been compared to each other and to their combination, and the question of whether or not combination therapy with CBT and antidepressant medication truly has additive or synergistic effects remains unsettled. Several relatively small studies have found CBT, or CBT plus placebo, superior to medication alone (desipramine, imipramine, or fluoxetine), and one study suggested that the combined treatment may carry an advantage over CBT alone for reduction of binge eating and depression; however, in all studies, the incremental benefit was modest at best. When data from all available studies are combined, the three meta-analyses reviewed support: (1) the superiority of CBT over medication alone; (2) the superiority of the combined treatment over medication alone; (3) to a lesser extent, the superiority of the combined treatment over CBT alone. Again, the advantage for one condition over another is statistically and clinically small to moderate, and no long-term data are available to compare stability of results across the different treatment conditions/combination. In BED, only one study over 24 weeks indicates that CBT might be more effective than pharmacotherapy, and that fluvoxamine could enhance the effects of psychological treatment on eating behaviors.

Predictors of response to pharmacotherapy

The prognostic indicators of outcome in pharmacotherapy of BN have rarely been investigated, and findings remain inconsistent. As reviewed by Peterson and Mitchell (1999), identified predictors of poor response in some (but not in other) studies have been symptoms of cluster B personality disorders (that is, borderline, narcissistic, histrionic, antisocial), impulsive traits, and low self-esteem. The findings are mixed for the duration and severity of symptoms before treatment. The majority of studies have not found an association between depression, a history of AN, age at onset of illness, and outcome. Residual symptoms at the end of treatment have been associated with a greater likelihood of relapse (Maddocks *et al.*, 1992). The paucity and small sample size of controlled pharmacological trials for AN and BED did not permit the search for possible predictors of treatment response in those patients.

Long-term pharmacotherapy

Treatment interventions shown to date to have value in the acute management of the EDs do not guarantee long-term maintenance of gains. For patients with BN or BED, this is reflected in the difficulty of achieving complete remission of illness with either psychosocial (Garner *et al.*, 1993) or pharmacological therapies (Walsh *et al.*, 1991, Mitchell *et al.*, 2003), and the frequent relapse during continuation therapy with antidepressants (Walsh *et al.*, 1991). In a review of the long-term outcome of medication in BN, Agras (1997) reported that the use of an antidepressant resulted in the recovery of an average of 25% of patients entering treatment, although over time about one-third of these patients relapsed, leading to a sustained recovery rate of about 15%. The frequency with which anorexic patients lose weight after hospital discharge, and the protracted course of their full recovery, have also been recurrent findings (Strober *et al.*, 1997). How to reduce the risk of relapse in weight-restored patients with AN is currently being investigated by several groups.

It is possible that ED patients have difficulty achieving robust and persisting clinical improvement with treatment, because of underlying long-term patho-physiological processes (Peterson and Mitchell, 1999). Both behavioral symptoms and altered serotonergic neurotransmission persist after recovery from AN or BN. Whether such persisting phenomena have etiological relevance, are scars of illness, or compensatory adaptational effects, remains unknown. Issues currently debated in the long-term treatment of other chronic relapsing illnesses may be informative for the EDs: unipolar (Keller and Boland, 1998) and bipolar affective patients (Coryell *et al.*, 1995) who recover and become fully asymptomatic have a lower risk of recurrence, compared to patients who improve but have continuing residual symptoms.

Treatment guidelines

In the acute treatment of AN, weight gain is a critical element (see above) and often requires a combined treatment approach including psychological support, nutritional remediation, and cognitive-behavioral elements, to restore body weight and normalize distorted thinking about food and body shape. Family interventions are particularly important for children and adolescents with the disorder. A small series of randomized controlled studies examined the efficacy of various types of psychological therapies in promoting weight gain in acutely ill patients (Channon *et al.*, 1989; Crisp *et al.*, 1991; Treasure *et al.*, 1995), or in preventing relapse after restoration of normal body weight (Russell *et al.*, 1987). Overall, the results indicate that substantial improvement in body mass, and general psychosocial adjustment, can be achieved using psychoeducative interventions. The American Psychiatric Association's (2000) guidelines for EDs acknowledge that:

psychotropic medications should not be used as the sole or primary treatment for AN . . . Medication therapy should not be used routinely during the weight restoration period. The role for antidepressants is usually best assessed following weight gain, when the psychological effects of malnutrition are resolving . . . These medications should be considered to prevent relapse among weight-restored patients or to treat associated features . . . such as depression or obsessive-compulsive problems.

To date, medication alone is an imperfect treatment option for BN and combined pharmacotherapy and short-term psychotherapy appear to produce better results, although most patients continue to show symptoms at termination. The American Psychiatric Association's guidelines (2000) state that, in the treatment of BN:

the antidepressants are effective as one component of an initial treatment program for most patients . . . They may be especially helpful for patients with substantial symptoms of depression, anxiety, or obsessions, or certain impulse disorder symptoms, or for patients who have failed or had a suboptimal response to previous attempts at appropriate psychosocial therapy. Dose levels of . . . antidepressants for treating BN are similar to those used to treat depression; practitioners should try to avoid prescribing tricyclics to patients who may be suicidal and MAOIs to patients with chaotic binge eating and purging.

Several experts in the field of EDs (S. Agras, D. Jimerson, T. Walsh) recommend that pharmacotherapy should last at least 6 months and be flexible, since patients who do not respond to one drug may respond to dosage adjustments, the addition of a new drug, or a switch to a new medication.

No guidelines have yet been published for the treatment of BED. In a recent review, Mitchell *et al.* (2003) concluded that medication alone generally seems inferior to psychotherapy in the short-term management of BED, but that antidepressant treatment may increase the amount of weight loss when combined with psychotherapy, and benefit associated symptoms such as depression.

Directions for future research

Despite significant progress over the past two decades, pharmacotherapeutic – and psychotherapeutic – research for the EDs still has a long way to go towards more effective treatment/treatments for the majority of individuals with these disorders. The following directions may be suggested.

- Methodological improvements are needed in treatment trials, notably to include a more comprehensive assessment of the cognitive and emotional disturbance in individuals with EDs, to obtain both objective and subjective measures, to assess dietary restraint and non-purging as well as purging methods of weight control.
- Novel pharmacological compounds should be investigated for specific therapeutic effect not only in suppressing dietary restraint or binge eating, but also in altering perseverative, obsessionally driven weight- and shape-related cognitions.
- New trials should include patients with BN and severe comorbid conditions, such as depression, substance abuse, or impulse disorders, frequently seen in clinical settings, as well as non-purging BN.
- More research should be done on treatment of BN during adolescence, in order to prevent chronicity and the numerous psychosocial consequences of the disorder.
- A new generation of clinical trials in the EDs should investigate the comparative efficacy of strategies differing in the type and intensity of various treatment combinations (including somatic and psychological approaches, pharmacological associations, combined or sequential treatments), to achieve complete

recovery and reduce the long-term risk of relapse and recurrence; integrative research paradigms should incorporate the expertise of a broad array of disciplines.

- Research into the factors (historical, clinical, biological) differentiating ED patients who achieve full remission during acute treatment from those who remain partially or fully symptomatic will provide clues to treatment resistance, and help define best clinical practices using pharmacotherapy and/or psychotherapy.
- Cost-effectiveness assessment should, ideally, be incorporated in efficacy studies.
- The consequences of starvation, and also malnutrition, on the efficacy of (or resistance to) both somatic and psychological therapies should be further investigated and possibly corrected.
- The possible relevance to the EDs of the models of kindling and stress sensitization proposed in the affective disorders to study treatment responsivity and illness course (Post and Weiss, 1997) might lead to integrative models of research, wherein treatment and behavioral neurobiology are viewed in a dynamic, temporal framework.

Conclusions

Although considerable progress has been made in the understanding and treatment of AN, BN, and BED, a substantial proportion of people with these disorders still have a limited response to treatment, and are subjected to a high risk of chronicity, likely to pose a great burden on the life of most young sufferers. Short- and long-term treatment of EDs still remains a challenge for the clinician, and is an issue of immense clinical and public health importance. Only with improved and continued therapeutic research, dwelling on better knowledge of factors responsible for the onset but also the maintenance of an ED, will the scientific community be able to state clearly which drugs should or should not be used as first-line treatment for AN, BN, or BED, what are the alternatives in case of treatment resistance, and how long treatment should be continued to maximize the chance of a person's complete and stable return to physical and mental health.

REFERENCES

Agras, W. S. (1997). Pharmacotherapy of bulimia nervosa and binge eating disorder: longer-term outcomes. *Psychopharmacology Bulletin*, **33**, 433–6.

  (2001). Treatment of binge-eating disorder. In: *Treatment of Psychiatric Disorders*, 3rd edn, ed. G. O. Gabbard. Washington, DC: American Psychiatric Press, pp. 2209–19.

Agras, W. S., Dorian, B., and Kirkley, B. G. (1987). Imipramine in the treatment of bulimia: a double-blind controlled study. *International Journal of Eating Disorders*, **6**, 29–38.

Agras, W. S., Rossiter, E. M., Arnow, B., *et al.* (1992). Pharmacologic and cognitive-behavioral treatment for bulimia nervosa: a control comparison. *American Journal of Psychiatry*, **149**, 82–7.

Alger, S. A., Schwalberg, M. D., Bigaouette, J. M., Michalek, A. V., and Howard, L. J. (1991). Effect of a tricyclic antidepressant and opiate antagonist on binge-eating behavior in normoweight bulimic and obese, binge-eating subjects. *American Journal of Clinical Nutrition*, **53**, 865–71.

American Psychiatric Association (1994). *Diagnostic and Statistical Manual of Mental Disorders*, 4th edn. Washington, DC: American Psychiatric Association.

  (2000). Practice guideline for eating disorders. *American Journal of Psychiatry*, **157**, 1–39.

Anderson, D. A. and Maloney, K. C. (2001). The efficacy of cognitive-behavioral therapy on the core symptoms of bulimia nervosa. *Clinical Psychology Review*, **21**, 971–88.

Attia, E., Haiman, C., and Walsh, B. T. (1998). Does fluoxetine augment the inpatient treatment of anorexia nervosa. *American Journal of Psychiatry*, **155**, 144–51.

Ayuso-Gutierrez, J. L., Palazon, M., and Ayuso-Mateos, J. L. (1994). Open trial of fluvoxamine in the treatment of bulimia nervosa. *International Journal of Eating Disorders*, **15**, 245–9.

Bacaltchuk, J. B., Hay, P., Trefiglio, R., and Mari, J. J. (1998). *Antidepressants for the treatment of bulimia nervosa*. Paper presented at the Sixth International Cochrane Colloquium, Baltimore, Maryland.

Bacaltchuk, J., Trefiglio, R. P., Oliveira, I. R., *et al.* (2000). Combination of antidepressants and psychological treatments for bulimia nervosa: a systematic review. *Acta Psychiatrica Scandinavica*, **101**, 256–64.

Baranowska, B., Rozbicka, G., Jeske, W., *et al.* (1984). The role of endogenous opiates in the mechanism of inhibited luteinizing hormone (LH) secretion in women with anorexia nervosa: the effect of endorphin secretion. *Journal of Clinical Endocrinology and Metabolism*, **59**, 412–16.

Barlow, J., Blouin, J., and Blouin, A. (1988). Treatment of bulimia nervosa with desipramine: a double-blind crossover study. *Canadian Journal of Psychiatry*, **33**, 129–33.

Bergh, C., Eriksson, M., Lindberg, G., and Sodersten, P. (1996). Selective serotonin reuptake inhibitors in anorexia. *Lancet*, **348**, 1459.

Biederman, J., Herzog, D. B., Rivinus, T. M., *et al.* (1985). Amitriptyline in the treatment of anorexia nervosa: a double-blind, placebo-controlled study. *Journal of Clinical Psychopharmacology*, **5**, 10–16.

Birmingham, C. L., Goldner, E. M., and Bakan, R. (1994). Controlled trial of zinc supplementation in anorexia nervosa. *International Journal of Eating Disorders*, **15**, 251–5.

Blackwell, B. (1991). Monoamine oxidase inhibitor interactions with other drugs. *Journal of Clinical Psychopharmacology*, **11**, 55–9.

Boachie, A., Goldfield, G. S., and Spettigue, W. (2003). Olanzapine use as an adjunctive treatment for hospitalized children with anorexia nervosa: case reports. *International Journal of Eating Disorders*, **33**, 98–103.

Bradley, S. J., Taylor, M. J., Rovet, J. F., *et al.*. (1997). Assessment of brain function in adolescent anorexia nervosa before and after weight gain. *Journal of Clinical and Experimental Neuropsychology*, **19**, 20–33.

Brewerton, T. D., Brandt, H. A., Lessem, M. K., Murphy, K. L., and Jimerson, D. C. (1990). Serotonin in eating disorders. In: *Serotonin in Major Psychiatric Disorders*, ed. E. F. Coccaro and D. L. Murphy. Washington, DC: American Psychiatric Association, pp. 155–184.

Carver, A. E., Miller, S., Hagman, J., and Sigel, E. (2002). The use of risperidone for the treatment of anorexia nervosa. Presented at the Academy of Eating Disorders Annual Meeting, Boston, Massachusetts.

Channon, S., DeSilva, P., Hensley, D., and Perkins, K. (1989). A controlled trial of cognitive-behavioral and behavioral treatment of anorexia nervosa. *Behavior Research Therapy*, **27**, 529–35.

Cohn, J. B. and Wilcox, R. R. (1985). A comparison of fluoxetine, imipramine, and placebo in patients with major depressive disorders. *Journal of Clinical Psychiatry*, **46**, 26–31.

Coryell, W., Endicott, J., Maser, J. D., *et al.* (1995). The likelihood of recurrence in bipolar affective disorder: the importance of episode recency. *Journal of Affective Disorders*, **33**, 201–6.

Crisp, A. H., Lacey, J. H., and Crutchfield, M. (1987). Clomipramine and "drive" in people with anorexia nervosa. *British Journal of Psychiatry*, **150**, 355–8.

Crisp, A. H., Norton, K., Gowers, S., *et al.* (1991). A controlled study of the effect of therapies aimed at adolescent and family psychopathology in anorexia nervosa. *British Journal of Psychiatry*, **159**, 325–33.

Dally, P. and Sargant, W. (1960). A new treatment of anorexia nervosa. *British Medical Journal*, **1**, 1770–3.

(1966). Treatment and outcome of anorexia nervosa. *British Medical Journal*, **2**, 793–5.

Dingemans, A. E., Bruna, M. J., and van Furth, E. F. (2002). Binge eating disorder: a review. *International Journal of Obesity*, **26**, 299–307.

Fairburn, F. G. (1985). Cognitive-behavioural treatment for bulimia. In: *Handbook of Psychotherapy for Anorexia Nervosa and Bulimia*, ed. D. M. Gardner and P. E. Garfinkel. New York: Guilford Press, pp. 160–92.

(2000). Bulimia nervosa. In: *New Oxford Textbook of Psychiatry*, vol. 1, sections 1–4 and index, ed. M. G. Gelder, J. J. Lopez-Ibor Jr., and N. C. Andreasen. New York: Oxford University Press, pp. 856–67.

Fairburn, C. G. and Harrison, P. J. (2003). Eating disorders. *Lancet*, **361**, 407–16.

Fairburn, C. G., Marcus, M. D., and Wilson, G. T. (1993). Cognitive-behavioural therapy for binge eating and bulimia nervosa: a comprehensive treatment manual. In: *Binge Eating: Nature, Assessment and Treatment*, ed. C. G. Fairburn and G. T. Wilson. New York: Guilford Press, pp. 361–404.

Fallon, B. A., Walsh, B. T., Sadik, C., Saoud, J. B., and Lukasik, V. (1991). Outcome and clinical course in inpatient bulimic women: a 2-to-9-year follow-up study. *Journal of Clinical Psychiatry*, **52**, 272–8.

Faris, P. L., Kim, S. W., Meller, W. H., *et al.* (2000). Effect of decreasing afferent vagal activity with odansetron on symptoms of bulimia nervosa: a randomized double-blind trial. *Lancet*, **355**, 792–7.

Ferguson, J. M. and Feighner, J. P. (1987). Fluoxetine-induced weight loss in overweight non-depressed humans. *International Journal of Obesity*, **11** (suppl. 3), 163–70.

Ferguson, C. P. and Pigott, T. A. (2000). Anorexia and bulimia nervosa: neurobiology and pharmacotherapy. *Behavior Therapy*, **31**, 237–63.

Fichter, M. M., Leibl, K., Rief, W., *et al.* (1991). Fluoxetine versus placebo: a double blind study with bulimic inpatients undergoing intensive psychotherapy. *Pharmacology*, **24**, 1–7.

Fichter, M. M., Kruger, R., and Rieg, W. (1996). Fluvoxamine in prevention of relapse in bulimia nervosa: effects on eating-specific psychopathology. *Journal of Clinical Psychopharmacology*, **16**, 9–18.

Fisman, S., Steele, M., Short, J., Byrne, T., and Lavallée, C. (1996). Case study: anorexia nervosa and autistic disorder in an adolescent girl. *Journal of the American Academy of Child and Adolescent Psychiatry*, **35**, 937–40.

Flament, M. F., Corcos, M., Igoin, L., Jeammet, P., and Apfelbaum, M. (1994). *Treatment of normal-weight bulimia nervosa with fluvoxamine: negative results from a controlled double-blind study with 103 outpatients.* Presented at the European Regional Symposium of the World Psychiatric Association, Developmental Issues in Psychiatry, Lisbon.

Fluoxetine Bulimia Nervosa Collaborative Study Group (1992). Fluoxetine in the treatment of bulimia nervosa: a multicenter, placebo-controlled, double-blind trial. *Archives of General Psychiatry*, **49**, 139–47.

Freeman, C. P. and Hampson, M. (1987). Fluoxetine as a treatment for bulimia nervosa. *International Journal of Obesity*, **2** (suppl. 3), 171–7.

Gardiner, H. M., Freeman, C. P. L., and Jesinger, D. K. (1993). Fluvoxamine: an open pilot study in moderately obese female patients suffering from atypical eating disorders and episodes of bingeing. *International Journal of Obesity*, **11** (suppl. 3), 171–7.

Garfinkel, P. E., Moldofsky, H., and Garner, D. M. (1978). The stability of perceptual disturbances in anorexia nervosa. *Psychological Medicine*, **9**, 703–8.

Garner, D. M., Rockert, W., Davis, R., *et al.* (1993). Comparison of cognitive-behavioral and supportive-expressive therapy for bulimia nervosa. *American Journal of Psychiatry*, **150**, 37–46.

Gaskill, J. A., Treat, T. A., McCabe, E. B., and Marcus, M. D. (2001). Does olanzapine affect the rate of weight gain among patients with eating disorders? *Eating Disorders Review*, **12**, 1–2.

Glennon, R. A. (1990). Serotonin receptors: clinical implications. *Neuroscience and Biobehavioral Reviews*, **14**, 35–47.

Godart, N. T., Perdereau, F., Curt, F., *et al.* (2004). Are mood disorders more frequent in eating disorder patients than in the general populations? (in press).

Goldberg, S. C., Halmi, K. A., Eckert, E. D., Casper, R. C., and Davis, J. M. (1979). Cyproheptadine in anorexia nervosa. *British Journal of Psychiatry*, **134**, 67–70.

Goldbloom, D. S., Olmstead, M., Davis, R., *et al.* (1997). A randomized controlled trial of fluoxetine and cognitive behavioral therapy for bulimia nervosa: short-term outcome. *Behavior Research Therapy*, **35**, 803–11.

Goldstein, D. J., Wilson, M. G., and Thompson, V. L. (1995). Long-term fluoxetine treatment of bulimia nervosa. Fluoxetine Bulimia Nervosa Research Group. *British Journal of Psychiatry*, **166**, 660–6.

Greeno, C. G. and Wing, R. R. (1996). A double-blind, placebo-controlled trial of the effect of fluoxetine on dietary intake in overweight women with and without binge-eating disorder. *American Journal of Clinical Nutrition*, **64**, 267–73.

Gross, H. A., Ebert, M. H., Faden, V. B., *et al.* (1981). A double-blind controlled trial of lithium carbonate in primary anorexia nervosa. *Journal of Psychopharmacology*, **1**, 376–81.

Gross, H. A., Ebert, M. H., Faden, V. B., *et al.* (1983). A double-blind trial of delta9-tetrahydrocannabinol in primary anorexia nervosa. *Journal of Clinical Psychopharmacology*, **3**, 165–71.

Halmi, K. A., Eckert, E., LaDu, T. J., and Cohen, J. (1986). Anorexia nervosa: treatment efficacy of cyproheptadine and amitriptyline. *Archives of General Psychiatry*, **43**, 177–81.

Hansen, L. (1999). Olanzapine in the treatment of anorexia nervosa. *British Journal of Psychiatry*, **175**, 592.

Hay, P. (1998). The epidemiology of eating disorder behaviors: an Australian community-based survey. *International Journal of Eating Disorders*, **23**, 371–82.

Hill, K., Bucuvalas, J., McClain, C., *et al.* (2000). Pilot study of growth hormone administration during the refeeding of malnourished anorexia nervosa patients. *Journal of Child and Adolescent Psychopharmacology*, **10**, 3–8.

Hoek, H. W., Bartelds, A. I., Bosveld, J. J., *et al.* (1995). Impact of urbanization on detection rates of eating disorders. *American Journal of Psychiatry*, **152**, 1272–8.

Horne, R. L., Ferguson, J. M., Pope, Jr., H. G., *et al.* (1988). Treatment of bulimia with bupropion: a multicenter controlled trial. *Journal of Clinical Psychiatry*, **49**, 262–6.

Hsu, L. K. G., Clement, L., Santhouse, R., and Jun, E. S. Y. (1991). Treatment of bulimia nervosa with lithium carbonate: a controlled study. *Journal of Nervous and Mental Disease*, **179**, 351–5.

Hudson, J. I., Pope, Jr., H. G., Keck, Jr., P. E., and McElroy, S. L. (1989). Treatment of bulimia nervosa with trazodone: short-term response and long-term follow-up. *Clinical Neuropharmacology*, **12** (suppl. 1), S38–46.

Hudson, J. I., McElroy, S. L., Raymond, N. C., *et al.* (1998). Fluvoxamine in the treatment of binge-eating disorder: a multicenter placebo-controlled, double-blind trial. *American Journal of Psychiatry*, **155**, 1756–62.

Hughes, P. L., Weslls, L. A., Cuningham, C. J., and Ilstrup, D. M. (1986). Treating bulimia with desipramine: a double-blind, placebo-controlled study. *Archives of General Psychiatry*, **43**, 182–6.

Jensen, V. S. and Mejlhede, A. (2000). Anorexia nervosa: treatment with olanzapine. *British Journal of Psychiatry*, **177**, 177–87.

Jimerson, D. C., Lessem, M. D., Kaye, W. H., and Brewerton, T. D. (1988). Symptom severity and neurotransmitter studies in bulimia. *Psychopharmacology*, **96** *(suppl.)*, 124.

Jimerson, D. C., Wolfe, B. E., Brotman, W. W., and Metzger, E. D. (1996). Medications in the treatment of eating disorders. *Psychiatric Clinics of North America*, **19**, 739–54.

Jonas, J. M. and Gold, M. S. (1988). The use of opiate antagonists in treating bulimia: a study of low-dose versus high-dose naltrexone. *Psychiatry Research*, **24**, 195–9.

Kaplan, A. S., Garfinkel, P. E., Darby, P. L., and Garner, D. M. (1983). Carbamazepine in treatment of bulimia. *American Journal of Psychiatry*, **140**, 1225–6.

Katz, R. L., Keen, C. L., Litt, I. F., *et al.* (1987). Zinc deficiency in anorexia nervosa. *Journal of Adolescent Health Care*, **8**, 400–6.

Kaye, W. H., Berrettini, W. H., Gwirtsman, H. E., *et al.* (1986). Alterations of CSF, CRH, and POMC in anorexia nervosa. Presented at the American Psychiatric Association 139th Annual Meeting, Washington, DC.

Kaye, W. H., Greenco, C. G., Moss, H., *et al.* (1998). Alterations in serotonin activity and psychiatric symptoms after recovery from bulimia nervosa. *Archives of General Psychiatry*, **55**, 927–35.

Kaye, W., Strober, M., Stein, D., and Gendall, K. (1999a). New directions in treatment research of anorexia and bulimia nervosa. *Biological Psychiatry*, **45**, 1285–92.

Kaye, W. H., Frank, G. K., and McConaha, C. (1999b). Altered dopamine activity after recovery from restricting-type anorexia nervosa. *Neuropsychopharmacology*, **21**, 503–6.

Kaye, W. H., Nagata, T., Weltzin, T. E., *et al.* (2001). Double-blind placebo-controlled administration of fluoxetine in restricting and restricting-purging type anorexia nervosa. *Biological Psychiatry*, **49**, 644–52.

Keller, M. B. and Boland, R. J. (1998). Implications of failing to achieve successful long-term maintenance treatment of recurrent unipolar major depression. *Biological Psychiatry*, **44**, 348–60.

Keller, M. B., Herzog, D. B., Lavori, P. W., Bradburn, I. S., and Mahoney, E. M. (1992). The naturalistic history of bulimia nervosa: extraordinarily high rates of chronicity, recurrence, and psychosocial morbidity. *International Journal of Eating Disorders*, **12**, 1–9.

Kennedy, S. H., Goldbloom, D. S., and Ralevski, E. (1993). Is there a role for selective monoamine oxidase inhibitor therapy in bulimia nervosa? A placebo-controlled trial of brofaromine. *Journal of Clinical Psychopharmacology*, **13**, 415–22.

Kirkpatrick, J. and Caldwell, P. (2000). *Eating Disorders: Anorexia Nervosa, Bulimia, Binge Eating and Others*. Toronto: Key Porter Books.

Lacey, I. H. and Crisp, A. H. (1980). Hunger, food intake and weight: the impact of clomipramine on a refeeding anorexia nervosa population. *Postgraduate Medical Journal*, **56** (suppl. 1), 79–85.

Langtry, H. D., Gillis, J. C., and Davis, R. (2003). Topiramate: a review of its pharmacodynamic and pharmacokinetic properties and clinical efficacy in the management of epilepsy. *Drugs*, **54**, 752–73.

La Via, M. C., Gray, N., and Kaye, W. H. (2000). Case reports of olanzapine treatment of anorexia nervosa. *International Journal of Eating Disorders*, **27**, 363–6.

Lask, B., Fosson, A., Rolfe, U., and Thomas, S. (1993). Zinc deficiency and childhood-onset anorexia nervosa. *Journal of Clinical Psychiatry*, **54**, 63–6.

Leitenberg, H., Rosen, J. C., Wolf, J., *et al.* (1994). Comparison of cognitive-behavioral therapy and desipramine in the treatment of bulimia nervosa. *Behavior Research Therapy*, **32**, 37–45.

Lilenfeld, L. R., Kaye, W. H., Greeno, C. G., *et al.* (1998). A controlled family study of anorexia nervosa and bulimia nervosa: psychiatric disorders in first-degree relatives and effects of proband comorbidity. *Archives of General Psychiatry*, **55**, 603–10.

Maddocks, S., Kaplan, A. S., Woodside, D. B., Langdon, L., and Piran, N. (1992). Two-year follow-up of bulimia nervosa: the importance of abstinence as the criterion of outcome. *International Journal of Eating Disorders*, **12**, 133–41.

Malina, A., Gaskill, J., McConaha, C., *et al.* (2003). Olanzapine treatment of anorexia nervosa: a retrospective study. *International Journal of Eating Disorders*, **33**, 234–7.

Marrazzi, M. A. and Luby, E. D. (1986). An auto-addiction opioid model of chronic anorexia nervosa. *International Journal of Eating Disorders*, **5**, 191–208.

Marrazzi, M. A., Bacon, J. P., Kinzie, J., *et al.* (1995). Naltrexone use in the treatment of anorexia nervosa and bulimia nervosa. *International Journal of Clinical Psychopharmacology*, **10**, 163–72.

McCann, U. D. and Agras, W. S. (1990). Successful treatment of nonpurging bulimia nervosa with desipramine: a double-blind, placebo-controlled study. *American Journal of Psychiatry*, **147**, 1509–13.

McElroy, S. L., Casuto, L. S., Nelson, E. B., *et al.* (2000). Placebo-controlled trial of sertraline in the treatment of binge eating disorder. *American Journal of Psychiatry*, **157**, 1004–6.

McElroy, S. L., Arnold, L. M., Shapira, N. A., *et al.* (2003). Topiramate in the treatment of binge eating disorder associated with obesity: a randomized, placebo-controlled trial. *American Journal of Psychiatry*, **160**, 255–68.

McKenzie, J. M. and Joyce, P. R. (1992). Hospitalization for anorexia nervosa. *International Journal of Eating Disorders*, **11**, 235–41.

McTavish, D. and Heel, R. C. (1992). Dexfenfluramine: a review of its pharmacological properties and therapeutic potential in obesity. *Drug Evaluation*, **43**, 713–33.

Mitchell, J. E. and Groat, R. (1984). A placebo-controlled, double-blind trial of amitriptyline in bulimia. *Journal of Clinical Psychopharmacology*, **4**, 186–93.

Mitchell, J. E., Laine, D. E., Morley, J. E., and Levine, A. S. (1986). Naloxone but not CCK-8 may attenuate binge eating behavior in patients with the bulimia syndrome. *Biological Psychiatry*, **21**, 1399–406.

Mitchell, J. E., Pyle, R. L., Eckert, E. D., *et al.* (1989). Response to alternative antidepressants in imipramine nonresponders with bulimia nervosa. *Journal of Clinical Psychopharmacology*, **9**, 291–3.

Mitchell, J. E., Pyle, R. L., Eckert, E. D., *et al.* (1990). A comparison study of antidepressants and structured group therapy in the treatment of bulimia nervosa. *Archives of General Psychiatry*, **47**, 149–57.

Mitchell, J. E., Maki, D. D., Adson, D. E., Ruskin, B. S., and Crow, S. (1997). The selectivity of inclusion and exclusion criteria in bulimia nervosa treatment studies. *International Journal of Eating Disorders*, **22**, 243–52.

Mitchell, J. E., Halmi, K., Wilson, G. T., *et al.* (2002). A randomized secondary treatment study of women with bulimia nervosa who fail to respond to CBT. *International Journal of Eating Disorders*, **32**, 271–81.

Mitchell, J. E., de Zwann, M., and Roerig, J. L. (2003). Drug therapy for patients with eating disorders. *CNS and Neurological Disorders*, **2**, 17–29.

Morley, J. E. and Levine, A. S. (1980). Stress-induced eating is mediated through endogenous opiates. *Science*, **209**, 1259–61.

Nakash-Eisikovits, O., Dierberger, A., and Westen, D. (2002). A multidimensional meta-analysis of pharmacotherapy for bulimia nervosa: summarizing the range of outcomes in controlled clinical trials. *Harvard Review of Psychiatry*, **10**, 193–211.

Newman-Toker, J. (2000). Risperidone in anorexia nervosa. *Journal of the American Academy of Child and Adolescent Psychiatry*, **39**, 941–2.

Peterson, C. B. and Mitchell, J. E. (1999). Psychosocial and pharmacological treatment of eating disorders: a review of research findings. *Psychotherapy in Practice*, **55** , 685–97.

Pope, H. G., Hudson, J. I., Jonas, J. M., and Yurgelun-Todd, D. (1983). Bulimia treated with imipramine: a placebo-controlled, double-blind study. *American Journal of Psychiatry*, **140**, 554–8.

Post, R. M. and Weiss, S. R. (1997). Emergent properties of neural systems: how focal molecular neurobiological alterations can affect behavior. *Development and Psychopathology*, **9**, 907–29.

Powers, P. S., Santana, C. A., and Bannon, Y. S. (2002). Olanzapine in the treatment of anorexia nervosa: an open label trial. *International Journal of Eating Disorders*, **32**, 146–54.

Prats, M., Diez-Quevedo, C., Avila, C., and Planell, L. S. (1994). Paroxetine treatment for bulimia nervosa and binge eating disorder. Abstract no. 308. Presented at the Sixth International Conference on Eating Disorders, New York.

Pyle, R., Mitchell, J., Eckert, E., and Hatsukami, D. (1990). Maintenance treatment and 6 month outcome for bulimic patients who respond to initial treatment. *American Journal of Psychiatry*, **147**, 871–5.

Ratnasuriya, R. H., Eisler, I., Szmukler, G. I., and Russell, G. F. (1991). Anorexia nervosa: outcome and prognostic factors after 20 years. *British Journal of Psychiatry*, **158**, 495–502.

Ricca, V., Mannucci, E., Mezzani, B., *et al.* (2001). Fluoxetine and fluvoxamine combined with individual cognitive-behaviour therapy in binge eating disorder: a one-year follow-up study. *Psychotherapy and Psychosomatics*, **70**, 298–306.

Roerig, J. L., Mitchell, J. E., Cook Myers, T., and Glass, J. B. (2002). Pharmacotherapy and medical complications of eating disorders in children and adolescents. *Child and Adolescent Psychiatric Clinics*, **11**, 365–85.

Rothschild, R., Quitkin, H. M., and Quitkin, F. M. (1994). A double-blind placebo controlled comparison of phenelzine and imipramine in the treatment of bulimia in atypical depressives. *International Journal of Eating Disorders*, **15**, 1–9.

Russell, G. (1979). Bulimia nervosa: an ominous variant of anorexia nervosa. *Psychological Medicine*, **9**, 429–48.

  (2000). Disorders of eating. In: *New Oxford Textbook of Psychiatry*, vol. 1, sections 1–4 and index, ed. M. G. Gelder, J. J. Lopez-Ibor Jr., and N. C. Andreasen. New York: Oxford University Press, pp. 835–55.

Russell, G., Szmukler, G. I., Dare, C., and Eisler, I. (1987). An evaluation of family therapy in anorexia and bulimia nervosa. *Archives of General Psychiatry*, **44**, 1047–56.

Sabine, E. J., Yonace, A., and Farrington, A. J. (1983). Bulimia nervosa: a placebo-controlled double-blind therapeutic trial of mianserin. *British Journal of Clinical Pharmacology*, **15**, 195S-202S.

Sanger, D. J. (1981). Endophinergic mechanisms in the control of food and water intake. *Appetite*, **2**, 193–208.

Spitzer, R. L., Devlin, M. J., Walsh, B. T., *et al.* (1991). Binge eating disorder : to be or not to be in DSM-IV. *International Journal of Eating Disorders*, **10**, 627–9.

Spitzer, R. L., Yanovski, S. Z., Wadden, T., and Wing, R. (1993). Binge eating disorder: its further validation in a multisite study. *International Journal of Eating Disorders*, **13**, 137–53.

Stacher, G., Kiss, A., Wiesnagrotzki, S., *et al.* (1986). Oesophageal and gastric motility disorders in patients categorized as having primary anorexia nervosa. *Gut*, **27**, 1120–6.

Stacher, G., Abatzi-Wenzel, T.-A., Wiesnagrotzki, S., *et al.* (1993). Gastric emptying, body weight and symptoms in primary anorexia nervosa: long-term effects of cisapride. *British Journal of Psychiatry*, **162**, 398–402.

Stanley, B. G., Ha, L. H., Spears, L. C., and Dee, M. G. II (1993). Lateral hypothalamic injections of glutamate, kainic acid, D, L-alpha-amino-3-hydroxy-5-methyl-isoxazole propionic acid or *N*-methyl-D-aspartic acid rapidly elicit intense transient eating in rats. *Brain Research*, **613**, 88–95.

Steinhausen, H. C., Rauss-Masson, C., and Seidal, R. (1993). Short-term and intermediate term outcome in adolescent eating disorders. *Acta Psychiatrica Scandinavica*, **88**, 169–73.

Strober, M., Freeman, R., DeAntonio, M., Lampert, C., and Diamond, J. (1997). Does adjunctive fluoxetine influence posthospital course of anorexia nervosa? A 24-month perspective, longitudinal follow-up and comparison with historical controls. *Psychopharmacology Bulletin*, **33**, 425–31.

Stunkard, A., Berkowitz, R., Tanrikut, C., Reiss, E., and Young, L. (1996). D-fenfluramine treatment of binge eating disorder. *American Journal of Psychiatry*, **153**, 1455–9.

Swift, W. J., Kalin, N. H., and Wambold, F. (1985). Depression in bulimia at 2 to 5 years follow up. *Psychiatric Research*, **16**, 111–22.

Szmukler, G. I., Young, G. P., Miller, G., Lichtenstein, M., and Binns, D. S. (1995). A controlled trial of cisapride in anorexia nervosa. *International Journal of Eating Disorders*, **17**, 347–57.

Tamburrino, M. B. and MacGinnis, R. A. (2002). Anorexia nervosa: a review. *Panminerva Medica*, **44**, 301–11.

Treasure, J., Todd, G., Brolly, M., *et al.* (1995). A pilot study of a randomized trial of cognitive behavioural therapy vs educational behavioural therapy for adult anorexia nervosa. *Behavioural Research Therapy*, **33**, 363–7.

Vandereycken, W. (1984). Neuroleptics in the short-term treatment of anorexia nervosa: a double-blind placebo-controlled trial with sulpiride. *British Journal of Psychiatry*, **144**, 288–92.

Vandereycken, W. and Pierloot, R. (1982). Pimozide combined with behavior therapy in the short-term treatment of anorexia nervosa: a double-blind placebo-controlled crossover study. *Acta Psychiatrica Scandinavica*, **66**, 445–50.

Vigersky, R. A. and Loriaux, D. L. (1977). The effect of cyproheptadine in anorexia nervosa. In: *Anorexia Nervosa*, ed. R. A. Vigersky. New York: Raven Press, pp. 349–56.

Walsh, B. T., Gladis, M., and Roose, S. P. (1988). Phenelzine vs placebo in 50 patients with bulimia. *Archives of General Psychiatry*, **45**, 471–5.

Walsh, B. T., Hadigan, C. M., Devlin, M. J., Gladis, M., and Roose, S. P. (1991). Long-term outcome of antidepressant treatment for bulimia nervosa. *American Journal of Psychiatry*, **148**, 1206–12.

Walsh, B. T., Wilson, G. T., Lobe, K. L., *et al.* (1997). Medication and psychotherapy in the treatment of bulimia nervosa. *American Journal of Psychiatry*, **154**, 523–31.

Wermuth, B. M., Davis, K. L., Hollister, E., and Stunkard, A. J. (1977). Phenytoin treatment of the binge-eating syndrome. *American Journal of Psychiatry*, **134**, 1249–53.

Whittal, M. L., Agras, W. S., and Gould, R. A. (1999). Bulimia nervosa: a meta-analysis of psychosocial and pharmacological treatments. *Behavior Therapy*, **30**, 117–35.

Wilson, G. T., Loeb, K. L., Labouvie, E., *et al.* (1999). Psychological versus pharmacological treatments of bulimia nervosa: predictors and processes of change. *Journal of Consulting and Clinical Psychology*, **67**, 451–9.

Wurtman, J. J. and Wurtman, R. J. (1981). Fenfluramine suppresses snack intake among carbohydrate cravers but not among non carbohydrate cravers. *International Journal of Eating Disorders*, **6**, 687–9.

Zhu, A. J. and Walsh, B. T. (2002). Pharmacologic treatment of eating disorders. *Canadian Journal of Psychiatry*, **47**, 227–34.

10

Evidence-based pharmacotherapy of attention-deficit hyperactivity disorder

Joseph Biederman, Thomas Spencer, and Timothy Wilens

Massachusetts General Hospital and Harvard University, Boston, MA, USA

Attention-deficit hyperactivity disorder

Attention-deficit hyperactivity disorder (ADHD) is defined in *Diagnostic and Statistical Manual*, 4th edition (DSM-IV) as a behavioral disorder of childhood onset (by the age of 7 years) characterized by symptoms of inattentiveness and impulsivity/hyperactivity. Based on the type of symptoms that predominate, DSM-IV recognizes a combined type in which both inattention and hyperactivity/impulsivity symptoms are present, a predominantly inattentive subtype and a predominantly hyperactive/impulsive subtype. In addition, DSM-IV also recognizes the category of ADHD not otherwise specified (NOS) for individuals presenting with atypical features.

ADHD is one of the major clinical and public health problems in the USA in terms of morbidity and disability in children and adolescents. It is estimated to affect at least 5% of school-age children. Its impact on society is enormous in terms of financial cost, stress to families, impact on schools, and damaging effects on self-esteem.

The pathophysiology of ADHD

ADHD is a heterogeneous disorder of unknown etiology. An emerging neuro-psychological and neuroimaging literature suggests that abnormalities in frontal networks or frontostriatal dysfunction are the disorder's underlying neural substrate, and catecholamine dysregulation is its underlying pathophysiological substrate. The pattern of neuropsychological deficits found in ADHD children implicates executive functions and working memory; this pattern is similar to what has been found among adults with frontal lobe damage, which suggests that the frontal cortex or regions projecting to the frontal cortex are dysfunctional in at least some ADHD subjects.

Recent studies using magnetic resonance imaging (MRI) of the brain indicate that there are subtle anomalies in caudate and corpus callosum size and shape or possible reductions in the right frontal area in ADHD (Castellanos *et al.*, 1996). These data are consistent with a positron emission tomography (PET) study that identified abnormalities of cerebral metabolism in the prefrontal and premotor areas of the frontal lobe in ADHD adults who had ADHD children (Zametkin *et al.*, 1990). Thus, the emerging neuroimaging literature points to abnormalities in frontal networks in ADHD (frontostriatal dysfunction) and it is these networks that control attention and motor intentional behavior. Zametkin and Rapoport (1987) postulated "inhibitory influences of frontal cortical activity, predominantly noradrenergic acting on lower (striatal) structures that are driven by . . . dopamine agonists . . .". The frontosubcortical pathways are rich in catecholamines and catecholamines are also implicated in ADHD because of the mechanism of action of stimulants. Yet human studies of the catecholamine hypothesis of ADHD have produced conflicting results, perhaps due to the insensitivity of peripheral measures.

Data from family-genetic, twin, and adoption studies as well as segregation analysis suggest a genetic origin for some forms of the disorder (Biederman *et al.*, 1992). Although their results are still tentative, molecular genetic studies suggest that some genes may increase the susceptibility to ADHD – the D4 dopamine receptor gene, the dopamine transporter gene, and the D2 dopamine receptor gene (Faraone, 2000). Studies of environmental adversity have implicated pregnancy and delivery complications, marital distress, family dysfunction, and low social class (Biederman *et al.*, 1994; Milberger *et al.*, 1997b).

Data from follow-up studies indicate that children with ADHD are at risk for maintaining and developing new psychiatric disorders in adolescence and adulthood, including antisocial and substance use disorders (tobacco, alcohol, and drugs). Follow-up data also document that the disorder persists into adulthood in a substantial number of children and that it may be a common adult diagnosis (Spencer *et al.*, 1998b). In recent years there has been an increasing recognition that ADHD is highly heterogeneous, with high levels of psychiatric (disruptives (conduct and oppositional defiant disorders), mood (unipolar and bipolar), and anxiety disorders), cognitive (learning disability) and social (social disability, non-verbal learning disability) disorders. Neuroimaging studies identified subtle anomalies in the frontal cortex and in projecting subcortical structures (Faraone and Biederman, 1999) and dysregulation of catecholamine neurotransmission has been posited to underlie its pathophysiology (Zametkin and Rapoport, 1987).

Adult ADHD

While it was originally thought that individuals with ADHD inevitably outgrew the disorder, converging evidence has revealed that the majority of children with ADHD continue to have significant ADHD-associated impairment as adults. Because disruptive outward manifestations of ADHD like hyperactivity decrease with age, adult ADHD has remained somewhat hidden and underdiagnosed. However with systematic investigation, adults have been shown to have the "look and feel" of ADHD children. In addition, the subthreshold diagnosis in adults has been demonstrated to correlate with considerable functional impairment. Like child ADHD, adult ADHD runs in families and shows neuropsychological deficits and neuroimaging abnormalities consistent with the idea that catecholaminergic hypoactivity in frontal subcortical circuits underlies the disorder. Notably, in both childhood and adulthood, ADHD symptoms respond favorably to drugs that block either the dopamine transporter or the norepinephrine (noradrenaline) transporter. (see below)

What is the first-line pharmacotherapy of ADHD?

Stimulant treatments

Stimulant drugs are the first class of compounds reported as effective in the treatment of the behavioral disturbances that are evident in children with ADHD. Stimulants are sympathomimetic drugs structurally similar to endogenous catecholamines. The most commonly used compounds in this class include methylphenidate (Ritalin), D-amfetamine (Dexedrine), a mixed amfetamine product (Adderall), and magnesium pemoline (Cylert). These drugs are thought to act in both the central nervous system and peripherally by enhancing dopaminergic and noradrenergic neurotransmission. Since the various stimulants have somewhat different mechanisms of action, some patients may respond preferentially to one or another (Greenhill *et al.*, 1998).

An extensive literature has clearly documented the short-term efficacy of methylphenidate treatment, mostly in latency-age Caucasian boys (Spencer *et al.*, 1997). A much more limited literature exists for stimulants at other ages, for females, and for ethnic minorities. Despite small numbers, the few studies of stimulants in adolescents reported rates of response highly consistent with those seen in latency-age children. In contrast, the few studies on preschoolers appear to indicate that young children respond less well to stimulant therapy, suggesting that ADHD preschoolers may be more treatment-refractory. The literature clearly documents that treatment with stimulants not only improves abnormal behaviors of ADHD but also self-esteem, cognitive, social, and family function, supporting the importance of treating ADHD patients beyond school or work hours to include evenings, weekends, and vacations. Three recent controlled clinical trails documented the efficacy of methylphenidate, Adderall, and pemoline in adults with ADHD (Spencer *et al.*, 1995; Wilens *et al.*, 1999c). It is remarkable that these trials documented not only a highly clinically and statistically significant separation from placebo, but also that the magnitude of effects was consistent with pediatric trials.

Treatment with stimulants improves a wide variety of cognitive abilities (Barkley, 1977; Klein, 1987; Rapport *et al.*, 1988), increases school-based productivity (Famularo and Fenton, 1987), and improves performance in academic testing (Abikoff *et al.*, personal communication) (Table 10.1). However, despite these beneficial cognitive effects, it is important to be aware that patients with ADHD may manifest additional learning disabilities that are not responsive to pharmacotherapy (Bergman *et al.*, 1991; Faraone *et al.*, 1993) but respond to educational remediation.

The early concern that optimal clinical efficacy is attained at the cost of impaired learning ability has not been confirmed (Gittelman-Klein, 1987). In fact, recent studies indicate that both behavior and cognitive performance improve with stimulant treatment in a dose-dependent fashion (Klein, 1987; Pelham *et al.*, 1985; Rapport *et al.*, 1987, 1989a, 1989b; Douglas *et al.*, 1988; Kupietz *et al.*, 1988; Tannock *et al.*, 1989). The literature on the association between clinical benefits in ADHD and plasma levels of stimulants has been equivocal and complicated by large inter- and intraindividual variability in plasma levels at constant oral doses (Gittelman-Klein, 1987).

Usual daily dose ranges from 0.3 to 2 mg/kg per day for methylphenidate and approximately half that for amfetamine compounds, since they are roughly twice as potent as methylphenidate. Due to their short half-life, the short-acting stimulants (methylphenidate and dextroamfetamine) are given in divided doses throughout the day, typically 4 h apart. The starting dose is generally 2.5–5 mg/day, given in the morning, with the dose being increased if necessary every few days by 2.5–5 mg in a divided-dose schedule. Due to the anorexogenic effects of the stimulants, it may be beneficial to administer the medicine after meals. A longer half-life agent, magnesium pemoline, typically lasts through the school period. For full-day coverage pemoline is typically given twice daily (such as 0800 h and 1400 h) in doses ranging from 1 to 3 mg/kg per day (pemoline is approximately three times less potent than methylphenidate). The typical starting dose of pemoline is 18.75–37.5 mg with increments of 18.75 mg every few days thereafter until desired effects occur or side-effects preclude further increments. Although magnesium pemoline is a longer-acting compound, its potential for severe hepatotoxicity has relegated its use to third-line treatment. Similarly, Adderall (a mixed amfetamine salt), with its longer half-life, lasts through most or all of the school day but for full coverage it is typically given twice daily (such as 0800 h and 1400 h) in doses ranging from 1 to 1.5 mg/kg per day. Typically, stimulants have a rapid onset of action so that clinical response will be evident when a therapeutic dose has been obtained.

The most commonly reported side-effects associated with the administration of stimulant medication are appetite suppression and sleep disturbances. The sleep disturbance that is commonly reported is delay of sleep onset, and it usually

Table 10.1 Major drug classes used in the pharmacotherapy of attention-deficit hyperactivity disorder (ADHD)

Drug	Daily dose (mg/kg)	Daily dosage schedule	Main indications and duration of behavioral effect	Common adverse effects and comments
Stimulants				
Dextroamfetamine (Dexedrine)	0.3–1.0	Twice or three times	ADHD MR + ADHD	Insomnia, decreased appetite, weight loss, depression, psychosis (rare, with very high doses)
	0.5–1.5	Once–twice	Adjunct treatment in refractory depression	Increase in heart rate and blood pressure (mild)
				Possible reduction in growth velocity with long-term use Withdrawal effects and rebound phenomena
Mixed salts of levo- and dex-troamfetamine (Adderall)	1.0–2.0	Twice or three times		Adderall 6 h of action
Methylphenidate (Ritalin, Methylin, Focalin)	0.5–1.0			
Magnesium pemoline (Cylert)	1.0–2.5	Once–twice		Pemoline has rare serious hepatotoxicity Pemoline requires monitoring of liver function tests
New long-acting stimulants				
Methylphenidate Concerta	1.0–2.0	Once–twice	10–12 h	Ascending profile, OROS technology Capsules with immediate release (IR) and delayed release (DR) beads
Ritalin LA			8–9 h	50:50 ratio (IR:DR)
Metadate CD			8–9 h	30:70 ratio (IR:DR)
Mixed salts of levo- and dex-troamfetamine	0.5–1.5	Once–twice	10–12 h	Capsule with IR and DR beads
Adderall XR				50:50 ratio (IR:DR)

(*cont.*)

Table 10.1 (*cont.*)

Drug	Daily dose (mg/kg)	Daily dosage schedule	Main indications and duration of behavioral effect	Common adverse effects and comments
Noradrenergic specific-reuptake inhibitors (NSRI)				
Atomoxetine	0.5–1.4 mg/kg per day	Once or twice	ADHD ± comorbidity	Mechanism of action: noradrenergic specific reuptake inhibitor
				Mild/moderate appetite decrease
			? Enuresis	Gastrointestinal symptoms
			? Tic disorder	
			? Depression	Mild initial weight loss
			? Anxiety disorders	Cardiovascular (mild increase) blood pressure, pulse. No ECG conduction or repolarization delays. Not abusable
Tricyclic antidepressants (TCAs)				
Tertiary (imipramine, amitriptyline, clomipramine)	2.0–5.0 (1.0–3.0 for nortripty-line)	Once or twice	ADHD Enuresis Tic disorder	Mixed mechanism of action (noradrenergic/ serotonergic)
Secondary amines (desipramine, nortriptyline)	Dose adjusted according to serum levels (therapeutic window for nortripty-line)		?Anxiety disorders OCD (Clomipramine)	Secondary amines more noradrenergic Clomipramine primarily serotonergic Narrow therapeutic index Overdoses can be fatal Anticholinergic (dry mouth, constipation, blurred vision). Weight loss Cardiovascular (mild increase) diastolic blood pressure and ECG conduction parameters with daily doses >3.5 mg/kg Treatment requires serum levels and ECG monitoring No known long-term side-effects

Table 10.1 (*cont.*)

Drug	Daily dose (mg/kg)	Daily dosage schedule	Main indications and duration of behavioral effect	Common adverse effects and comments
Monoamine oxidase inhibitors (MAOIs)	0.5–1.0 mg/kg	Twice–three times	Atypical depression	Withdrawal effects can occur (severe gastrointestinal symptoms, malaise) Risk of seizures Difficult medicines to use in juveniles Reserved for refractory cases
Phenelzine Tranyl- cypromine			Treatment-refractory depression	Severe dietary restrictions (high-tyramine foods)
Selegiline	0.2–0.4 mg/kg			Drug–drug interactions Hypertensive crisis with dietetic transgression or with certain drugs Weight gain Drowsiness Changes in blood pressure Insomnia Liver toxicity (remote)
Other antidepressants				
Selective serotonin reuptake inhibitors (SSRIs)				Mechanism of action serotonergic Large margin of safety
Fluoxetine, paroxetine, citalopram	0.3–0.9 mg/kg	Once (in the morning)	MD, dysthymia OCD	No cardiovascular effects Irritability
Sertraline	1.5–3.0 mg/kg		Anxiety disorders	Insomnia Gastrointestinal symptoms
Fluvoxamine	1.5–4.5 mg/kg		Eating disorders ? PTSD	Headaches Sexual dysfunction Withdrawal symptoms more common in short-acting Potential drug–drug interactions (P450)

(*cont.*)

Table 10.1 (*cont.*)

Drug	Daily dose (mg/kg)	Daily dosage schedule	Main indications and duration of behavioral effect	Common adverse effects and comments
Bupropion (SR)	3–6 mg/kg	Twice a day	ADHD MD Smoking cessation ? Anticraving effects ? Bipolar depression	Mixed mechanism of action (dopaminergic/ noradrenergic) Irritability Insomnia Drug-induced seizures (in doses > 6 mg/kg) Contraindicated in bulimics
Venlafaxine (XR)	1–3 mg/kg	Once a day	MD Anxiety disorders ? ADHD ? OCD	Mixed mechanism of action (serotonergic/ noradrenergic) Similar to SSRIs Irritability Insomnia Gastrointestinal symptoms Headaches Potential withdrawal symptoms Blood pressure changes
Nefazodone	4–8 mg/kg	Once a day	MD Anxiety disorders ? OCD ? Bipolar depression	Mixed mechanism of action (serotonergic/ noradrenergic) Dizziness Nausea Potential interactions with non-sedating antihistamines, cisapride (cytochrome P450) Rare serious hepatotoxicity ? Less manicogenic
Mirtazapine	0.2–0.9 mg/kg	Once (in the afternoon)	MD Anxiety disorders ? Stimulant-induced insomnia ? Bipolar depression	Mixed mechanism of action (serotonergic/ noradrenergic) Sedation Weight gain Dizziness ? Less manicogenic

Table 10.1 (*cont.*)

Drug	Daily dose (mg/kg)	Daily dosage schedule	Main indications and duration of behavioral effect	Common adverse effects and comments
Noradrenergic modulators				
Alpha$_2$-Agonists Clonidine	0.003–0.010	Twice or three times	Tourette's disorder ADHD Aggression/ self-abuse Severe agitation Withdrawal syndromes	Sedation (very frequent) Hypotension (rare) Dry mouth Confusion (with high dose) Depression Rebound hypertension Localized irritation with transdermal preparation
Guanfacine	0.015–0.05	Once or twice		Same as clonidine. Less sedation, hypotension
Beta-blockers Propranolol	1–7 mg/kg/day	Twice	Aggression/ self-abuse Severe agitation Akathisia	Sedation Depression Risk for bradycardia and hypotension (dose-dependent) and rebound hypertension Bronchospasm (contraindicated in asthmatics) Rebound hypertension on abrupt withdrawal

Note: Doses are general guidelines. All doses must be individualized with appropriate monitoring. Weight corrected doses are less appropriate for obese children. When high doses of antidepressants are used serum levels may be obtained in order to avoid toxicity. MR, mental retardation; ECG, electrocardiogram; OCD, obsessive-compulsive disorder; MD, major depression; PTSD, posttraumatic stress disorder.

accompanies late-afternoon or early-evening administration of stimulant medications. Although less commonly reported, mood disturbances ranging from
increased tearfulness to a full-blown major depression-like syndrome can be associated with stimulant treatment (Wilens and Biederman, 1992). Other infrequent
side-effects include headaches, abdominal discomfort, increased lethargy, and
fatigue.

Although adverse cardiovascular effects of stimulants beyond heart rate and
blood pressure have not been examined, mild increases in pulse and blood pressure
of unclear clinical significance have been observed (Brown *et al.*, 1984). Although

less of a clinical concern in pediatric care, potential increases in blood pressure associated with stimulant drugs may be of greater clinical significance in the treatment of adults with ADHD. A stimulant-associated toxic psychosis has also been very rarely observed, usually in the context of either a rapid rise in the dosage or very high doses. The reported psychosis in children in response to stimulant medications resembles a toxic phenomenon (i.e., visual hallucinosis) and is dissimilar from the exacerbation of the psychotic symptoms present in schizophrenia. The development of psychotic symptoms in a child exposed to stimulants requires careful evaluation to rule out the presence of a preexisting psychotic disorder. Administration of magnesium pemoline has been associated with rare hypersensitivity reactions involving the liver accompanied by elevations in liver function studies (serum glutamic oxaloacetic and pyruvic transaminases) after several months of treatment. Thus, baseline and repeat liver function studies are recommended with the administration of this compound. Because of increasing concerns about hepatotoxicity, the US Food and Drug Administration is now requiring biweekly liver function monitoring when pemoline is used.

Early reports indicated that children with a personal or family history of tic disorders were at greater risk for developing a tic disorder when exposed to stimulants (Lowe *et al.*, 1982). However, recent work has increasingly challenged this view (Comings and Comings, 1988; Gadow *et al.*, 1992, 1995). For example, in a controlled study of 34 children with ADHD and tics, Gadow *et al.* (1995) reported that methylphenidate effectively suppressed ADHD symptoms with only a weak effect on the frequency of tics. In a study of 128 boys with ADHD, Spencer *et al.* (1999) reported no evidence of earlier onset, greater rates, or worsening of tics in the subgroup exposed to stimulants. Although this work is reassuring, clearly more information is needed in larger numbers of subjects over a longer period of time to obtain closure on this issue. Until more is known it seems prudent to weigh risks and benefits in individual cases with appropriate discussion with the child and family about the benefits and pitfalls of the use of stimulants in children with ADHD and tics.

Similar uncertainties remain about the abuse potential of stimulants in ADHD children. Despite the concern that ADHD may increase the risk of abuse in adolescents and young adults (or their associates), to date there is no clear evidence that stimulant-treated ADHD children abuse prescribed medication when appropriately diagnosed and carefully monitored. Moreover, the most common abused substance in adolescents and adults with ADHD has been shown to be marijuana and not stimulants (Biederman *et al.*, 1995b). Furthermore, a recent report provides statistical evidence documenting that the use of stimulants and other pharmacological treatments for ADHD significantly decreased the risk for subsequent substance use disorders in ADHD youth (Biederman *et al.*, 1999).

Although concerns continue on the effect of long-term administration of stimulants on growth, recent work has begun to question this issue. Although stimulants routinely produce anorexia and weight loss, their effect on growth in height is much less certain. While initial reports suggested that there was a persistent stimulant-associated decrease in growth in height in children (Safer *et al.*, 1972; Mattes and Gittelman, 1983), other reports have failed to substantiate this claim (Gross, 1976; Satterfield *et al.*, 1979). Moreover, several studies showed that ultimate height appears to be unaffected if treatment is discontinued in adolescence (Gittelman and Mannuzza, 1988). A recent study suggested that deficits in growth in height may be transient maturational delays associated with ADHD rather than stunting of growth in height in ADHD children (Swanson *et al.*, 2000). If confirmed, this would not support the common practice of drug holidays in ADHD children. However, it seems prudent in children suspected of stimulant-associated growth deficits to provide them with drug holidays or alternative treatment. This recommendation should be carefully weighed against the risk for exacerbation of symptoms due to drug discontinuation. A transient behavioral deterioration can occur upon the abrupt discontinuation of stimulant medications in some children. The prevalence of this phenomenon and the etiology are unclear. Rebound phenomena can also occur in some children between doses, creating an uneven, often disturbing clinical course. In those cases consideration should be given to alternative treatments.

New-generation stimulants

A new generation of highly sophisticated, well-developed, safe, and effective long-acting preparations of stimulant drugs has reached the market and revolutionized the treatment of ADHD. These compounds employ novel delivery systems to overcome acute tolerance, termed "tachyphylaxis." In a number of these medications, an analog classroom paradigm was used to test the fine-grained pharmacodynamic and pharmacokinetic profiles of these medications. Developed by Swanson and colleagues (2000), these settings simulate real-life demands and distractions of a typical classroom. Hour-by-hour ratings consist of trained observers recording frequency counts of behaviors as well as academic production and accuracy. Sequential serum sampling from catheters allows correlation of blood levels to behavioral activity.

The first medication developed was Concerta. Concerta uses an osmotic pump mechanism to create an ascending profile of methylphenidate in the blood to provide effective extended treatment to approximate TID dosing of methylphenidate immediate-release (MPH IR). Concerta is available in 18, 27, 36, and 54 mg to approximate 5, 7.5, 10, and 15 mg TID dosing of MPH IR. A laboratory classroom study of 68 children found that a single morning dose of Concerta was effective for 12 h on social and on task behaviors as well as academic performance (Pelham *et al.*, 2001).

A large multicenter, randomized, clinical trial was used to determine the safety and efficacy of Concerta in an outpatient setting (Wolraich *et al.*, 2001). Two hundred and eighty-two children with ADHD (ages 6–12 years) were randomized to placebo ($n = 90$), MPH IR TID ($n = 97$), or Concerta once a day ($n = 95$) in a double-blind, 28-day trial. Children in the Concerta and MPH IR groups showed significantly greater reductions in core ADHD symptoms than did children on placebo throughout the study. Concerta was well tolerated; there was a mild appetite suppression but no sleep abnormalities. A 1-year follow-up study of 407 children treated with Concerta found no marked effects on weight, height, blood pressure, pulse, or tic exacerbation (Palumbo, 2002; Spencer, 2002; Wilens *et al.*, 2002).

Metadate-CD is a capsule with a mixture of immediate- and delayed-release beads containing methylphenidate. In Metadate-CD, 30% of the beads are immediate-release and 70% delayed, designed to provide effective methylphenidate treatment for 8–9 h. The efficacy and safety of Metadate-CD were tested in a multicenter, randomized, double-blind, placebo-controlled trial conducted at 32 sites with 16 children with ADHD. The trial consisted of a 1-week single-blind, placebo run-in, followed by a 3-week double-blind titration and treatment period. Improvement versus placebo was equally good morning and afternoon as measured by teachers on the Conners' Global Index. The medication was well tolerated with relatively low rates of decreased appetite (9.7% versus 2.5%) and insomnia (7.1% versus 2.5%) in active versus placebo. Metadate-CD is available in 20 mg capsules to approximate 10 mg BID dosing of MPH IR (Greenhill *et al.*, 2002). Recently a study documented that the bioavailability and tolerability of Metadate-CD are not altered when the capsule is opened and the beads are sprinkled on food (Pentikis *et al.*, 2002).

A new extended-release dosage form of Ritalin (Ritalin LA) has been developed to provide effective methylphenidate treatment for 8 h. Ritalin LA uses a bimodal release system that produces pharmacokinetic characteristics that, in single-dose administration, resemble those of two doses of Ritalin tablets administered 4–5 h apart. Ritalin LA consists of a mixture of immediate- and delayed-release beads in a 50:50 ratio. The delayed-release beads are coated with an absorption-delaying polymer. Ritalin LA is available in 20, 30, and 40 mg capsules to approximate 10, 15, and 20 mg BID dosing of MPH IR. Ritalin LA may be used as a sprinkle preparation for children who are unable to swallow pills. The initial analog classroom study evaluated the pharmacodynamic (efficacy) profile, safety, and tolerability of Ritalin LA (Spencer *et al.*, 2000). Single doses of all variants of Ritalin LA were effective relative to placebo in improving classroom behavior and academic productivity over the 9-h period after dosing. Ritalin LA had a rapid onset of effect, and the improvement relative to placebo was statistically significant during both the morning (0–4 h after dosing) and the afternoon (4–9 h after dosing).

Ritalin LA was further tested in a multicenter, double-blind trial of 160 children (Biederman *et al.*, 2002b). There was an initial 2–4-week titration to optimal dose followed by a 1-week placebo washout period. One hundred and thirty-seven subjects with persistent ADHD symptoms during the washout were randomized to Ritalin LA or placebo. Children on Ritalin LA were rated as greatly improved over placebo by teachers and parents on the Conners' ADHD DSM-IV Scale. Improvements were equally robust in the subscales of inattention and hyperactivity. Significant drug-specific improvement was also noted by clinicians on the Clinical Global Impression scale. Ritalin LA was well tolerated with minimal side-effects. Rates of mild appetite suppression and mild insomnia were both low (3.1%).

Adderall XR is a capsule with a 50:50 ratio of immediate- to delayed-release beads designed to release drug content in a time course similar to Adderall, given BID (0 and 4 h). Adderall XR is available in 5, 10, 15, 20, 25, and 30 mg capsules. An analog classroom study compared various doses of Adderall XR to Adderall BID and placebo (McCracken *et al.*, 2000). Behavioral and academic improvement were documented to 12 h postdose. The efficacy and safety of Adderall XR were further tested in a multicenter, randomized, double-blind, placebo-controlled trial conducted at 47 sites (Biederman *et al.*, 2002a). A total of 584 children with ADHD were randomized to receive single-daily morning doses of placebo or Adderall XR 10, 20, or 30 mg for 3 weeks. Continuous, significant improvement was noted in morning and afternoon assessments by teachers and morning, afternoon, and late-afternoon assessments by parents on Conners Global Index Scale for Teachers and Parents. All active treatment groups showed significant dose-related improvement in behavior from baseline. The medication was well tolerated with rates of adverse events similar for active treatments and placebo. A 1-year follow-up of 411 children on Adderall XR examined long-term safety and efficacy (Chandler *et al.*, 2002). Efficacy was maintained for 12 months as measured by the Conners Global Index Scale. The medication was safe and well tolerated, with a low frequency of mild adverse events and no evidence of untoward cardiovascular effects.

Methylphenidate as a secondary amine gives rise to four optical isomers: D-threo, L-threo, D-erythro, and L-erythro. There is stereoselectivity in receptor site binding and its relationship to response. The standard preparation comprises the threo, D,L-racemate as it appears to be the active central nervous system form. Moreover, recent data suggest that the D-methylphenidate isomer is the active form. In a PET study, D-threo-methylphenidate was found to bind specifically to the basal ganglia, rich in dopamine transporter receptors, whereas L-threo-methylphenidate was widely distributed with only non-specific binding (Ding *et al.*, 1995). This has led to the development of a purified D-threo-methylphenidate compound, Focalin. Studies have documented similar pharmacokinetic profiles of D-threo-methylphenidate and D,L-threo-methylphenidate when given in equimolar doses.

Thus the time to maximum concentration (T_{max}), the maximum concentration of D-threo-methylphenidate (C_{max}) and the half-life ($t_{1/2}$) were the same between D and D,L-threo-methylphenidate.

The efficacy of Focalin was established in two controlled studies. In the first trial 132 children and adolescents were randomized to receive D-threo-methylphenidate, D,L-threo-methylphenidate, or placebo at 0800 h and 1200 h for 4 weeks. At week 4, teacher ratings on the Swanson, Nolan, and Pelham (SNAP) questionnaire revealed robust improvement in both active treatments. The average improvement from baseline was equivalent to one standard deviation on the SNAP rating scale, a magnitude of change that is clinically important. Parent ratings on the SNAP revealed superiority of both treatments over placebo 3 h after dosing, but only superiority of D-methylphenidate and not D,L-methylphenidate 6 h after dosing (Conners *et al.*, 2001).

In a second controlled study, investigators tested the specificity of response to D-threo-methylphenidate (West *et al.*, 2002). A total of 116 patients were treated openly with D-threo-methylphenidate to determine the optimal dose. At the end of 6 weeks 75 responders were randomized to blinded treatment with D-threo-methylphenidate or placebo over 2 weeks. Subjects randomized to placebo had a high rate (62%) of relapse compared to those who continued on D-threo-methylphenidate (17%). In addition, the parent SNAP ratings indicated persistent effect of D-threo-methylphenidate 6 h after dosing. In both studies, adverse effects of D-threo-methylphenidate were consistent with those of D,L-threo-methylphenidate. These studies have shown Focalin to be as effective as the racemate at half the dosage. Focalin is available in 2.5, 5, and 10 mg to approximate 5, 10, and 20 mg of D,L-methylphenidate.

Non-stimulants in ADHD

While there is no doubt that the stimulants are effective in the treatment of ADHD, it is estimated that at least 30% of affected individuals do not respond adequately or cannot tolerate stimulant treatment (Barkley, 1977; Gittelman, 1980; Spencer *et al.*, 1996). In addition, stimulants are short-acting drugs that require multiple administrations during the day with their attendant impact on compliance and need to take treatment during school or work hours. While this problem may be offset by the development of an effective long-acting stimulant, this class of drugs often adversely impacts on sleep, making their use in the evening hours difficult when children and adults need the ability to concentrate to help them deal with daily demands and when they interact with family members and friends. In addition to these problems, the fact that stimulants are controlled substances continues to fuel worries in children, families, and in the treating community that further inhibit their use. These fears are based on lingering concerns about the abuse potential of stimulant drugs by the child, family member, or his/her associates, the possibility of diversion, and safety concerns regarding the use of a controlled substance by patients who are impulsive and frequently have antisocial tendencies (Goldman *et al.*, 1998). Similarly, the controlled nature of stimulant drugs poses important medicolegal concerns to the treating community that further increase the barriers to treatment.

Outside the psychostimulants, noradrenergic and dopaminergic active compounds, including monoamine oxidase inhibitors (MAOIs) (Zametkin *et al.*, 1985), secondary amine tricyclic antidepressants (TCAs) (Donnelly *et al.*, 1986; Biederman *et al.*, 1989; Wilens *et al.*, 1993), and bupropion (Casat *et al.*, 1989; Barrickman *et al.*, 1995; Conners *et al.*, 1996) have been found to be superior to placebo in controlled clinical trials. Possible advantages of these compounds over stimulants include a longer duration of action without symptom rebound or insomnia, greater flexibility in dosage, the option of monitoring plasma drug levels (for TCAs), minimal risk of abuse or dependence, as well as the potential treatment of comorbid internalizing symptoms. Although one open-case series reported on the beneficial effects of the selective serotonin reuptake inhibitor (SSRI) fluoxetine in the treatment of ADHD (Barrickman *et al.*, 1991), there is little other clinical or scientific evidence implicating serotonergic systems in the pathophysiology of ADHD.

One of the best established second-line treatments for ADHD are the TCAs. Out of 33 studies (21 controlled, 12 open) evaluating TCAs in children, adolescents ($n = 1139$), and adults ($n = 78$), 91% reported positive effects on ADHD symptoms (Spencer *et al.*, 1997). Imipramine and desipramine are the most studied TCAs followed by a handful of studies on other TCAs. Although most TCA studies (73%) were relatively brief, lasting from a few weeks to several months, nine studies (27%) reported enduring effects for up to 2 years. Outcomes in both short- and long-term studies were equally positive. Although one study (Quinn and Rapoport, 1975), reported a 50% dropout rate after 1 year, it is noteworthy that, in those who remained on imipramine, improvement was sustained. More recent studies using aggressive doses of TCAs reported sustained improvement for up to 1 year with desipramine (> 4 mg/kg) (Gastfriend *et al.*, 1985; Biederman *et al.*, 1986) and nortriptyline (2.0 mg/kg) (Wilens *et al.*, 1993). Although response was equally positive in all the dose ranges, it was more sustained in those studies that used higher doses. A high interindividual variability in TCAs serum levels has been consistently reported for imipramine and desipramine, with little relationship between serum level to daily dose, response, or side-effects. In contrast, nortriptyline appears to have a positive association between dose and serum level (Wilens *et al.*, 1993).

In the largest controlled study of a TCA in children, our group reported favorable results with desipramine in 62 clinically referred ADHD children, most of whom had previously failed to respond to psychostimulant treatment (Biederman *et al.*, 1989). The study was a randomized, placebo-controlled, parallel-design, 6-week clinical trial. Clinically and statistically significant differences in behavioral improvement were found for desipramine over placebo, at an average daily dose of 5 mg/kg. Although the presence of comorbidity increased the likelihood of a placebo response, neither comorbidity with conduct disorder, depression, or anxiety, nor a family history of ADHD yielded differential responses to desipramine treatment. In addition, desipramine-treated ADHD patients showed a substantial reduction in depressive symptoms compared with placebo-treated patients. Similar results were observed in a similarly designed controlled clinical trial of desipramine in 41 adults with ADHD (Wilens *et al.*, 1996b). Desipramine, at an average daily dose of 150 mg (average serum level of 113 ng/ml), was statistically and clinically more effective than placebo. Sixty-eight percent of desipramine treated patients responded, compared with none of the placebo-treated patients ($P < 0.0001$). Moreover, at the end of the study, the average severity of ADHD symptoms was reduced to below the level required to meet diagnostic criteria in patients receiving desipramine. Importantly, while the full desipramine dose was achieved at week 2, clinical response improved further over the following 4 weeks, indicating a latency of response. Response was independent of dose, serum desipramine level, gender, or lifetime psychiatric comorbidity with anxiety or depressive disorders.

In a prospective placebo-controlled discontinuation trial, we recently demonstrated the efficacy of nortriptyline in doses of up to 2 mg/kg daily in 35 school-aged youths with ADHD (Prince *et al.*, 1999). In that study, 80% of youths responded by week 6 in the open phase. During the discontinuation phase, subjects randomized to placebo lost the anti-ADHD effect compared to those receiving nortriptyline, who maintained a robust anti-ADHD effect. ADHD youths receiving nortriptyline were also found to have more modest but statistically significant reductions in oppositionality and anxiety. Nortriptyline was well tolerated, with some weight gain. Weight gain is frequently considered to be a desirable side-effect in this population. In contrast, a systematic study in 14 treatment-refractory ADHD youths receiving protriptyline (mean dose of 30 mg) reported less favorable results. We found that only 45% of ADHD youth responded or could tolerate protriptyline secondary to adverse effects (Wilens *et al.*, 1996a).

Thirteen of the 33 TCA studies (40%) compared TCAs to stimulants. Four studies each reported that stimulants were superior to TCAs (Gittelman-Klein, 1974; Rapoport *et al.*, 1974; Greenberg *et al.*, 1975; Garfinkel *et al.*, 1983), seven studies reported stimulants are equal to TCAs (Huessy and Wright, 1970; Gross, 1973; Kupietz and Balka, 1976; Yepes *et al.*, 1977; Kupietz *et al.*, 1988; Faraone *et al.*, 1993; Rapport *et al.*, 1993), and three studies reported that TCAs were superior to stimulants (Winsberg *et al.*, 1972; Watter and Dreyfuss, 1973; Werry, 1980). Analysis of response profiles indicates that TCAs more consistently improve behavioral symptoms, as rated by clinicians, teachers, and parents, than they impact on cognitive function, as measured in neuropsychological testing (Quinn and Rapoport, 1975; Werry, 1980; Gualtieri and Evans, 1988; Rapport *et al.*, 1993). As noted above, studies of TCAs have uniformly reported a robust rate of response of ADHD symptoms in ADHD subjects with comorbid depression or anxiety (Cox, 1982; Biederman *et al.*, 1993; Wilens *et al.*, 1993, 1995). In addition, studies of TCAs have consistently reported a robust rate of response in ADHD subjects with comorbid tic disorders (Dillon *et al.*, 1985; Hoge and Biederman, 1986; Riddle *et al.*, 1988; Spencer *et al.*, 1993a, 1993b; Singer *et al.*, 1994). For example, in a recent controlled study, Spencer *et al.* (2002a) replicated data from a retrospective chart review indicating that desipramine had a robust beneficial effect on ADHD and tic symptoms. The potential benefits of TCAs in the treatment of ADHD have been clouded by concerns about their safety stemming from reports of sudden unexplained death in four ADHD children treated with desipramine (Abramowicz, 1990), although the causal link between desipramine and these deaths remains uncertain (see below).

The mechanism of action of antidepressant drugs appears to be due to various effects on pre- and postsynaptic receptors impacting the release and reuptake of brain neurotransmitters, including norepinephrine, serotonin, and dopamine. Although these agents have variable effects on various pre- and postsynaptic neurotransmitter systems, their effect and adverse effect profiles differ greatly among the various classes of antidepressant drugs. Since a substantial interindividual variability in metabolism and elimination has been demonstrated in children, dose should always be individualized.

The TCAs include the tertiary (imipramine and amitriptyline) and the secondary (desipramine and nortriptyline) amine compounds. Treatment with a TCA should be initiated with a 10 or 25 mg dose and increased slowly every 4–5 days by 20–30%. When a daily dose of 3 mg/kg (or a lower effective dose) or 1.5 mg/kg for nortriptyline is reached, steady-state serum levels and an electrocardiogram (ECG) should be obtained. Typical dose ranges for the TCAs are 2.0–5.0 mg/kg (1.0–3.0 mg/kg for nortriptyline). Common short-term adverse effects of the TCAs include anticholinergic effects, such as dry mouth, blurred vision, and constipation. However, there are no known deleterious effects associated with chronic administration of these drugs. Gastrointestinal symptoms and vomiting may occur when these drugs are discontinued abruptly, thus slow tapering of these medications is recommended. Since the anticholinergic effects of TCAs limit salivary flow, they may promote tooth decay.

Evaluations of short- and long-term effects of therapeutic doses of TCAs on the cardiovascular systems in children have found TCAs to be generally well tolerated with only minor ECG changes associated with TCA treatment in daily oral doses as high as 5 mg/kg. TCA-induced ECG abnormalities (conduction defects) have been consistently reported in children at doses higher than 3.5 mg/kg (Biederman *et al.*, 1989) (1.0 mg/kg for nortriptyline). Although of unclear hemodynamic significance, the development of conduction defects in children receiving TCA treatment merits closer ECG and clinical monitoring, especially when relatively high doses of these medicines are used. In the context of cardiac disease, conduction defects may have potentially more serious clinical implications. When in doubt about the cardiovascular state of the patient, a more comprehensive cardiac evaluation is suggested, including 24-h ECG, and cardiac consultation, before initiating treatment with a TCA to help determine the risk-versus-benefit ratio of such an intervention. Recently, a controlled study of heart rate variability examined the question of cardiac risk in the use of desipramine in children (Prince *et al.*, unpublished data). Although changes in individual markers of heart rate variability were noted in ADHD youths treated with desipramine, desipramine did not appear adversely to affect the overall balance of sympathetic/parasympathetic input into the myocardium.

Several case reports in the 1980s of sudden death in children being treated with desipramine raised concern about the potential cardiotoxic risk associated with TCAs in the pediatric population (Riddle *et al.*, 1991). Despite uncertainty and imprecise data, an epidemiologic evaluation of this issue (Biederman *et al.*, 1995a) suggested that the risk of desipramine-associated sudden death may be slightly elevated but not much greater than the baseline risk of sudden death in children not on medication. Nevertheless, treatment with a TCA should be preceded by a baseline ECG, with serial ECGs at regular intervals throughout treatment. Because of the potential lethality of TCA overdose, parents should be advised to store the medication carefully in a place that is inaccessible to the children and their siblings.

The mixed dopaminergic/noradrenergic antidepressant bupropion has been shown to be effective for ADHD in children, in a controlled multisite study ($n = 72$) (Casat *et al.*, 1987, 1989; Conners *et al.*, 1996) and in a comparison with methylphenidate ($n = 15$) (Barrickman *et al.*, 1995). In an open study of ADHD adults, sustained improvement was documented at 1 year at an average of 360 mg for 6–8 weeks (Wender and Reimherr, 1990). A double-blind controlled clinical trial of bupropion in adults with ADHD documented superiority over a placebo (Wilens *et al.*, 1999a) with an effect size highly consistent with the pediatric trials.

Bupropion hydrochloride is a novel-structured antidepressant of the amino-ketone class related to the phenylisopropylamines but pharmacologically distinct from known antidepressants. Although its specific site or mechanism of action remains unknown, bupropion seems to have an indirect mixed agonist effect on dopamine and norepinephrine neurotransmission. Bupropion is indicated for depression and smoking cessation in adults (Hunt *et al.*, 1997). Bupropion is rapidly absorbed, with peak plasma levels usually achieved after 2 h, with an average elimination half-life of 14 h (8–24 h). The usual dose range is 4.0–6.0 mg/kg per day in divided doses. Side-effects include irritability, anorexia, and insomnia, and rarely, edema, rashes, and nocturia. Exacerbation of tic disorders has also been reported with bupropion. While bupropion has been associated with a slightly increased risk (0.4%) of drug-induced seizures relative to other antidepressants, this risk has been linked to high doses, a previous history of seizures, and eating disorders. Bupropion has been formulated into a long-acting preparation that can be administered twice daily.

Although a small number of studies suggested that MAOIs may be effective in juvenile and adult ADHD, their potential for hypertensive crisis associated with dietetic transgressions and drug interactions seriously limits their use. The MAOIs include the hydrazines (phenelzine) and non-hydrazines (tranylcypromine) compounds. In adults MAOIs have been found to be helpful in the treatment of atypical depressive disorders with reverse endogenous features and depressive disorders with prominent anxiety features (Quitkin et al., 1991). Daily doses should be carefully titrated based on response and adverse effects, and range from 0.5 to 1.0 mg/kg. Short-term adverse effects include orthostatic hypotension, weight gain, drowsiness, and dizziness. However, major limitations for the use of MAOIs in children and adolescents are the severe dietetic restrictions of tyramine-containing foods (i.e., most cheeses), pressor amines (i.e., sympathomimetic substances), and severe drug interactions (i.e., most cold medicines, amfetamines), which can induce a hypertensive crisis and a serotonergic syndrome. Although not available in the USA, a new family of reversible inhibitors of MAOIs (also known as RIMA) has been developed and used in Europe and Canada, and these medications may be free of these difficulties.

While a single small open study (Barrickman et al., 1991) suggested that fluoxetine may be beneficial in the treatment of ADHD children, the usefulness of SSRIs in the treatment of core ADHD symptoms is not supported by clinical experience (NIMH, 1996). Similarly uncertain is the usefulness of mixed serotonergic/noradrenergic atypical antidepressant venlafaxine in the treatment of ADHD. While a 77% response rate was reported in completers in open studies of ADHD adults, 21% dropped out due to side-effects ($n = 4$ open studies; $n = 61$ adults) (Adler et al., 1995; Hornig-Rohan and Amsterdam, 1995; Reimherr et al., 1995; Findling et al., 1996). Additionally, a single open study of venlafaxine in 16 ADHD children reported a 50% response rate in completers with a 25% dropout rate due to side-effects, most prominently increased hyperactivity (Luh et al., 1996).

Currently available SSRIs include fluoxetine, paroxetine, sertraline, fluvoxamine, and citalopram. At present, expert opinion does not support the usefulness of these serotonergic compounds in the treatment of core ADHD symptoms (NIMH, 1996).

Nevertheless, because of the high rates of comorbidity in ADHD, these compounds are frequently combined with effective anti-ADHD agents (Table 10.1). Since many psychotropics are metabolized by the cytochrome P450 system (Nemeroff *et al.*, 1996) which in turn can be inhibited by the SSRIs, caution should be exercised when combining agents such as the TCAs with SSRIs.

The antidepressants and many other psychotropics are metabolized in the liver by the cytochrome P450 system (Table 10.1) (Nemeroff *et al.*, 1996; DeVane, 1998; Greenblatt *et al.*, 1998). Because of genetic polymorphism, there are slow and rapid metabolizers. In addition, exogenous compounds can dramatically affect the efficacy of these enzymes and lead to drug–drug interactions. The coadministration of TCAs and SSRIs (paroxetine, fluoxetine, and sertraline, fluvoxamine with a weak nefazodone effect) may result in increased levels of the TCAs. High levels of cisapride (propulsid) have been associated with QT prolongation and led to potentially lethal ventricular arrhythmias (torsades de pointes). Thus, great caution should be exercised when using cisapride and the SSRIs that affect cytochrome IIIA4 (fluvoxamine, nefazodone and, to a lesser degree, fluoxetine and sertraline). Citalopram, venlafaxine, and mirtazapine have minimal inhibition of P450 enzymes. Since levels of any drug metabolized by an isoenzyme that is inhibited by another drug can rise to dangerous levels, caution should be exercised when using combination treatments (Nemeroff *et al.*, 1996; DeVane, 1998; Greenblatt *et al.*, 1998).

Atomoxetine

Atomoxetine is a potent, noradrenergic-specific reuptake inhibitor that has been studied in over 1800 children and over 250 adults and recently approved by the Food and Drug Administration. An initial controlled clinical trial in adults documented "proof of concept" in the treatment of ADHD (Spencer *et al.*, 1998c). These initial encouraging results, coupled with extensive safety data in adults, fueled efforts at developing this compound in the treatment of pediatric ADHD. An open-label, dose-ranging study of this compound in pediatric ADHD documented strong clinical benefits with excellent tolerability, including a safe cardiovascular profile, and provided dosing guidelines for further controlled studies (Spencer *et al.*, 2001).

There are two acute, randomized, double-blind, placebo-controlled studies (one in children, one in children and adolescents) (Michelson *et al.*, 2001; Spencer *et al.*, 2002b). The Spencer *et al.* study included 291 children aged 7–13 with ADHD who were randomized in two trials (combined: atomoxetine = 129, placebo = 124, and methylphenidate = 38). The acute treatment period was 9 weeks. The stimulant-naive stratum patients were randomized to double-blind treatment with either atomoxetine ($n = 56$), placebo ($n = 53$), or methylphenidate ($n = 38$). Stimulant-prior-exposure stratum (prior exposure to any stimulant) patients were randomized to double-blind treatment with atomoxetine ($n = 73$) or placebo ($n = 71$).

Atomoxetine significantly reduced total scores on an investigator-rated DSM-IV ADHD rating scale. Using a definition of response of $\geq 25\%$ decrease of the ADHD rating scale, the response rates were greater on atomoxetine than placebo (61.4% versus 32.3%, respectively; $P < 0.05$). In the stimulant-naive stratum, 69.1% of atomoxetine patients, 73% of methylphenidate patients, and 31.4% of placebo patients were considered responders. Atomoxetine was well tolerated. Mild appetite suppression was reported in 22% on atomoxetine versus 32% on methylphenidate and 7% on placebo. Compared to methylphenidate there was less insomnia on atomoxetine (7.0% versus 27.0%; $P < 0.05$). Mild increases in diastolic blood pressure and heart rate were noted in the atomoxetine treatment group with no significant differences between atomoxetine and placebo in laboratory parameters and ECG intervals (Spencer *et al.*, 2002b).

In an additional controlled study, 297 children and adolescents were randomized to different doses of atomoxetine or placebo for 8 weeks (Michelson *et al.*, 2001). Atomoxetine was associated with a graded dose response: response was best at 1.2 or 1.8 mg/kg per day and superior to 0.5 mg/kg per day, which was superior to placebo. In close parallel to the dose relationship to lowering ADHD symptoms, this study documented a dose-dependent enhancement of social and family function. The Child Health Questionnaire was used to assess the well-being of the child and family (Landgraf, 1995). Parents of children on atomoxetine reported fewer emotional difficulties and behavioral problems as well as greater self-esteem in their children and less emotional worry and less limitations in their personal time in themselves.

Safety and efficacy data were evaluated in a year-long open follow-up of atomoxetine-treated children and adolescents ($n = 325$) (Kratochvil *et al.*, 2001). Atomoxetine treatment continued to be effective and well tolerated. The acute mild increases in diastolic blood pressure and heart rate persisted, without worsening. Growth in height and weight were normal and there were no significant differences between atomoxetine and placebo in laboratory parameters and ECG intervals.

Alpha-adrenergic agents: clonidine and guanfacine

Clonidine is an imidazoline derivative with alpha-adrenergic agonist properties that has been primarily used in the treatment of hypertension. At low doses, it appears to stimulate inhibitory, presynaptic autoreceptors in the central nervous system. The most common use of clonidine in pediatric psychiatry is the treatment of Tourette's disorder and other tic disorders (Leckman *et al.*, 1991), ADHD, and ADHD-associated sleep disturbances (Hunt *et al.*, 1990; Prince *et al.*, 1996). In addition, clonidine has been reported to be useful in developmentally disordered patients to control aggression to self and others. Clonidine is a relatively short-acting compound with a plasma half-life ranging from approximately 5.5 h (in children) to 8.5 h (in adults). Daily doses should be titrated and individualized. Usual daily dose ranges from 3 to 10 μg/kg given generally in divided doses, BID, TID, and sometimes QID. Therapy is usually initiated at the lowest manufactured dose of a full or half tablet of 0.1 mg depending on the size of the child (approximately 1–2 μg/kg) and increased depending on clinical response and adverse effects. Initial dosage can more easily be given in the evening hours or before bedtime due to sedation.

The most common short-term adverse effect of clonidine is sedation. It can also produce, in some cases, hypotension, dry mouth, depression, and confusion. Clonidine is not known to be associated with long-term adverse effects. In hypertensive adults, abrupt withdrawal of clonidine has been associated with rebound hypertension. Thus, it requires slow tapering when discontinued.

Clonidine should not be administered concomitantly with beta-blockers since adverse interactions have been reported with this combination. Recent reports of death in several children on the combination of methylphenidate and clonidine have generated new concerns about its safety. Although more work is needed to evaluate if an increased risk exists with this combination, a cautious approach is advised, including increased surveillance and cardiovascular monitoring. Recently there has been anecdotal evidence that the more selective alpha$_{2a}$-agonist guanfacine may have a similar spectrum of benefits to those of clonidine with less sedation and longer duration of action (Chappell *et al.*, 1995; Horrigan and Barnhill, 1995; Hunt *et al.*, 1995). Usual daily dose ranges from 42 to 86 μg/kg generally given in divided doses, BID or TID.

Despite its wide use in ADHD children, there have been relatively few studies ($n =$ six studies (four controlled), $n = 292$ children) (Hunt *et al.*, 1985; Hunt, 1987; Gunning, 1992; Steingard *et al.*, 1993; Singer *et al.*, 1994; Kurlan, 2002) supporting the efficacy of clonidine. A recent study compared clonidine to methylphenidate in a sample of children with ADHD and Tourette's syndrome (Kurlan, 2002). The authors reported that clonidine worked as well as methylphenidate on teacher ratings of ADHD, but that clonidine was most helpful for impulsivity and hyperactivity and not as helpful for inattention. Moreover, sedation was a common side-effect, occurring in 28% of subjects. Equally limited is the literature on guanfacine. There are three open studies ($n = 36$ total) and one controlled study ($n = 34$) of guanfacine in children and adolescents with ADHD (Chappell *et al.*, 1995; Hunt *et al.*, 1995; Horrigan and Barnhill, 1995; Scahill *et al.*, 2001). In these studies beneficial effects on hyperactive behaviors and attentional abilities were reported. In the controlled study of children with tic disorders and ADHD, guanfacine improved attention by teacher ratings and performance on a continuous performance test (Scahill *et al.*, 2001). In a study in adults with ADHD ($n = 17$), guanfacine was shown to improve both ADHD symptoms and performance on a cognitive test of response inhibition, as measured by the Stroop test (Taylor, 2000). Several cases of sudden death have been reported in children treated with clonidine plus methylphenidate, raising concerns about the safety of this combination (Wilens and Spencer, 1999). A recent study examined the combination in 33 children and found no evidence of cardiac toxicity (Kurlan, 2002).

Beta-noradrenergic blockers also have been studied for use in ADHD. An open study of propranolol for ADHD adults with temper outbursts reported improvement at daily doses of up to 640 mg/day (Mattes, 1986). Another report indicated that beta-blockers may be helpful in combination with the stimulants (Ratey et al., 1991). In a controlled study of pindolol in 52 ADHD children, symptoms of behavioral dyscontrol and hyperactivity were improved, with less apparent cognitive benefit (Buitelaar et al., 1996). However, prominent adverse effects such as nightmares and paresthesias led to discontinuation of the drug in all test subjects. An open study of nadolol in aggressive, developmentally delayed children with ADHD symptoms reported effective diminution of aggression with little apparent effect on ADHD symptoms (Connor et al., 1997).

A recent open study of 12 ADHD children reported that the non-benzodiazepine anxiolytic buspirone at 0.5 mg/kg per day improved both ADHD symptoms and psychosocial function in ADHD youth (Malhotra and Santosh, 1998). Buspirone has a high affinity to 5-HT1-A-receptors, both pre- and postsynaptic, as well as a modest effect on the dopaminergic system and alpha-adrenergic activity. However, results from a recent multisite controlled clinical trial of transdermal buspirone failed to separate it from placebo in a large sample of children with ADHD (Bristol Myers Squibb, unpublished data). While an old literature suggested that typical antipsychotics were effective in the treatment of children with ADHD, their spectrum of both short-(extrapyramidal reactions) and long-(tardive dyskinesia) term adverse effects greatly limits their usefulness. A recent meta-analysis pooling data from 10 studies provided preliminary evidence that carbamazepine may have activity in ADHD (Silva et al., 1996).

In recent years, evidence has emerged that nicotinic dysregulation may contribute to the pathophysiology of ADHD. This is not surprising considering that nicotinic activation enhances dopaminergic neurotransmission (Westfall et al., 1983; Mereu et al., 1987). Independent lines of investigation have documented that ADHD is associated with an increased risk and earlier age of onset of cigarette smoking (Pomerleau et al., 1996; Milberger et al., 1996), that maternal smoking during pregnancy increases the risk for ADHD in the offspring, and that in utero exposure to nicotine in animals confers a heightened risk for an ADHD-like syndrome in the newborn (Johns et al., 1982; Fung, 1988; Fung and Lau, 1989; Milberger et al., 1996). In non-ADHD subjects, central nicotinic activation has been shown to improve temporal memory (Meck and Church, 1987), attention (Peeke and Peeke, 1984; Wesnes and Warburton, 1984; Jones et al., 1992), cognitive vigilance (Wesnes and Warburton, 1984; Parrott and Winder, 1989; Jones *et al.*, 1992), and executive function (Wesnes and Warburton, 1984).

Support for a "nicotinic hypothesis" of ADHD can be derived from a recent study that evaluated the therapeutic effects of nicotine in the treatment of adults with ADHD (Levin *et al.*, 1996). Although this controlled clinical trial in adults with ADHD documented that commercially available transdermal nicotine patches resulted in a significant improvement of ADHD symptoms, working memory, and neuropsychological functioning (Levin *et al.*, 1996), the trial was very short (2-day) and included only a handful of patients. More promising results supporting the usefulness of nicotinic drugs in ADHD derives from a recent controlled clinical trial of ABT-418 in adults with ADHD (Wilens *et al.*, 1999b). ABT-418 is a central nervous system cholinergic nicotinic activating agent with structural similarities to nicotine. Phase I studies of this compound in humans have indicated its low abuse liability, as well as adequate safety and tolerability in elderly adults (Abbott Laboratories, unpublished data). A double-blind, placebo-controlled, randomized, crossover trial, comparing a transdermal patch of ABT-418 (75 mg/day) to placebo in adults with DSM-IV ADHD showed a significantly higher proportion of ADHD adults to be very much improved while receiving ABT-418 than when receiving placebo (40% versus 13%; $\chi^2 = 5.3$, $P = 0.021$). Although preliminary, these results suggest that nicotinic analogs may have activity in ADHD.

Several other compounds have been evaluated and found to be ineffective in the treatment of ADHD; these include dopamine agonists (amantidine and L-dopa) (Gittelman-Klein, 1987) and amino acid precursors (D,L-phenylalanine and L-tyrosine) (Reimherr *et al.*, 1987). In addition, a controlled study failed to find therapeutic benefits in ADHD for the antiserotonergic, anorexogenic drug fenfluramine (Donnelly *et al.*, 1989).

How long should pharmacotherapy of ADHD continue?

A recent study, the Multimodal Treatment Study for ADHD (MTA) addresses long-term treatment (MTA Cooperative Group, 1999). In this 5-year, six-site project, 579 elementary-age children with ADHD were randomly assigned to one of four 14-month treatment conditions: (1) behavioral treatment; (2) medication management (usually methylphenidate); (3) combined behavioral treatment and medication management; and (4) a community comparison group (most of the children in this last group were receiving medication for ADHD). Key outcome assessment occurred at 9 and 14 months. Children in the behavioral treatment arm received a very intensive combination of predominantly operant treatment ingredients, including school consultation, a classroom aide, an 8-week summer treatment program, and 35 sessions of parent management training. Behavioral treatment was faded prior to the final assessment. By contrast, pharmacotherapy – in both the medication management and combined treatment conditions – was not tapered but rather was ongoing throughout treatment.

Findings in this study document continued treatment effects of all four treatment assignments over the 14 months. In addition, similar to previous findings, medical intervention was significantly more effective than behavioral and community treatments; behavioral treatment only modestly enhanced the effect of medication alone; and behavioral treatment alone was no more effective than the treatment received by children in the community comparison group (MTA Cooperative Group, 1999).

Conclusions

ADHD is a heterogeneous disorder with strong neurobiological basis that afflicts millions of individuals of all ages worldwide. Although the stimulants remain the mainstay of treatment for this disorder, a new generation of non-stimulant drugs is emerging that provides viable alternatives for patients and families. It is essential to apply a careful differential diagnosis in the assessment of the ADHD patient that considers psychiatric, social, cognitive, educational, and medical/neurological factors that may contribute to the subject's clinical presentation. Realistic expectations of interventions, careful definition of target symptoms, and careful assessment of the potential risks and benefits of each type of intervention for such patients are major ingredients for success.

REFERENCES

Abramowicz, M. (1990). Sudden death in children treated with a tricyclic antidepressant. *Medical Letter on Drugs and Therapeutics*, **32**, 53.

Adler, L., Resnick, S., Kunz, M., and Devinsky, O. (1995). *Open-Label Trial of Venlafaxine in Attention Deficit Disorder*. Orlando, FL: New Clinical Drug Evaluation Unit Program.

Barkley, R. A. (1977). A review of stimulant drug research with hyperactive children. *Journal of Child Psychology and Psychiatry*, **18**, 137–65.

Barrickman, L., Noyes, R., Kuperman, S., Schumacher, E., and Verda, M. (1991). Treatment of ADHD with fluoxetine: a preliminary trial. *Journal of the American Academy of Child and Adolescent Psychiatry*, **30**, 762–7.

Barrickman, L., Perry, P., Allen, A., *et al.* (1995). Bupropion versus methylphenidate in the treatment of attention-deficit hyperactivity disorder. *Journal of the American Academy of Child and Adolescent Psychiatry*, **34**, 649–57.

Bergman, A., Winters, L., and Cornblatt, B. (1991). Methylphenidate: effects on sustained attention. In: *Ritalin: Theory and Patient Management*, ed. L. Greenhill and B. Osman. New York: Mary Ann Liebert, pp. 223–31.

Biederman, J., Gastfriend, D. R., and Jellinek, M. S. (1986). Desipramine in the treatment of children with attention deficit disorder. *Journal of Clinical Psychopharmacology*, **6**, 359–63.

Biederman, J., Baldessarini, R. J., Wright, V., Knee, D., and Harmatz, J. (1989). A double-blind placebo controlled study of desipramine in the treatment of attention deficit disorder: I. Efficacy. *Journal of the American Academy of Child and Adolescent Psychiatry*, **28**, 777–84.

Biederman, J., Faraone, S. V., Keenan, K., *et al.* (1992). Further evidence for family-genetic risk factors in attention deficit hyperactivity disorder. Patterns of comorbidity in probands and relatives in psychiatrically and pediatrically referred samples. *Archives of General Psychiatry*, **49**, 728–38.

Biederman, J., Baldessarini, R. J., Wright, V., Keenan, K., and Faraone, S. (1993). A double-blind placebo controlled study of desipramine in the treatment of attention deficit disorder: III. Lack of impact of comorbidity and family history factors on clinical response. *Journal of the American Academy of Child and Adolescent Psychiatry*, **32**, 199–204.

Biederman, J., Milberger, S., Faraone, S., *et al.* (1994). Family environmental risk factors for attention deficit hyperactivity disorder: a test of Rutter's indicators of adversity. In: *Scientific Proceedings of the Annual Meeting of the American Academy of Child and Adolescent Psychiatry*, ed. N. Alessi and S. Porter. Washington, DC: American Academy of Child and Adolescent Psychiatry.

Biederman, J., Thisted, R., Greenhill, L., and Ryan, N. (1995a). Estimation of the association between desipramine and the risk for sudden death in 5- to 14-year-old children. *Journal of Clinical Psychiatry*, **56**, 87–93.

Biederman, J., Wilens, T., Mick, E., *et al.* (1995b). Psychoactive substance use disorder in adults with attention deficit hyperactivity disorder: effects of ADHD and psychiatric comorbidity. *American Journal of Psychiatry*, **152**, 1652–8.

Biederman, J., Wilens, T., Mick, E., Spencer, T., and Faraone, S. V. (1999). Pharmacotherapy of attention-deficit/hyperactivity disorder reduces risk for substance use disorder. *Pediatrics*, **104**, e20.

Biederman, J., Lopez, F., Boellner, S., and Chandler, M. (2002a). A randomized, double-blind placebo-controlled, parallel-group study of SLI381 in children with ADHD. *Pediatrics*, **110**, 258–66.

Biederman, J., Quinn, D., Wigal, S., *et al.* (2002b). Methylphenidate hydrochloride extended release capsules: once-daily therapy for ADHD. In: *Annual Meeting of the American Psychiatric Association*. Philadelphia, PA: American Psychiatric Association, p. 29.

Brown, R. T., Wynne, M. E., and Slimmer, L. W. (1984). Attention deficit disorder and the effect of methylphenidate on attention, behavioral, and cardiovascular functioning. *Journal of Clinical Psychiatry*, **45**, 473–6.

Buitelaar, J., van de Gaag, R., Swaab-Barneveld, H., and Kuiper, M. (1996). Pindolol and methylphenidate in children with attention deficit hyperactivity disorder. *Journal of Child and Adolescent Psychiatry*, **36**, 587–95.

Casat, C. D., Pleasants, D. Z., and Van Wyck Fleet, J. (1987). A double-blind trial of bupropion in children with attention deficit disorder. *Psychopharmacology Bulletin*, **23**, 120–2.

Casat, C. D., Pleasants, D. Z., Schroeder, D. H., and Parler, D. W. (1989). Bupropion in children with attention deficit disorder. *Psychopharmacology Bulletin*, **25**, 198–201.

Castellanos, F., Giedd, J., Marsh, W., *et al.* (1996). Quantitative brain magnetic resonance imaging in attention deficit hyperactivity disorder. *Archives of General Psychiatry*, **53**, 607–16.

Chandler, M. C., Lopez, F. A., and Biederman, J. (2002). Long-term safety and efficacy of Adderall extended release in children with ADHD. In: *Annual Meeting of the American Psychiatric Association*. Philadelphia, PA: American Psychiatric Association, p. 19.

Chappell, P., Riddle, M., Scahill, L., *et al.* (1995). Guanfacine treatment of comorbid attention-deficit hyperactivity disorder and Tourette's syndrome. *Journal of the American Academy of Child and Adolescent Psychiatry*, **34**, 1140–6.

Comings, D. E. and Comings, B. G. (1988). Tourette's syndrome and attention deficit disorder. In: *Tourette's Syndrome and Tic Disorders: Clinical Understanding and Treatment*, ed. D. J. Cohen, R. D. Bruun, and J. F. Leckman. New York: John Wiley, pp. 119–36.

Connor, D., Ozbayrak, K., Benjamin, S., Ma, Y., and Fletcher, K. (1997). A pilot study of nadolol for overt aggression in developmentally delayed individuals. *Journal of the American Academy of Child and Adolescent Psychiatry*, **36**, 826–34.

Conners, K., Casat, C., Gualtieri, T., *et al.* (1996). Bupropion hydrochloride in attention deficit disorder with hyperactivity. *Journal of the American Academy of Child and Adolescent Psychiatry*, **35**, 1314–21.

Conners, C. K., Casat, C., Coury, D., *et al.* (2001). Randomized trial of dex-methylphenidate (*d*-MPH) and *d,l*- MPH in children with ADHD. In: *48th Annual Meeting of the American Academy of Child and Adolescent Psychiatry*. Honolulu, HW: AACAP.

Cox, W. (1982). An indication for the use of imipramine in attention deficit disorder. *American Journal of Psychiatry*, **139**, 1059–60.

DeVane, C. (1998). Differential pharmacology of newer antidepressants. *Journal of Clinical Psychiatry*, **59**, 85–93.

Dillon, D. C., Salzman, I. J., and Schulsinger, D. A. (1985). The use of imipramine in Tourette's syndrome and attention deficit disorder: case report. *Journal of Clinical Psychiatry*, **46**, 348–9.

Ding, Y. S., Fowler, J. S., Volkow, N. D., *et al.* (1995). Carbon-11-*d*-threo-methylphenidate binding to dopamine transporter in baboon brain. *Journal of Nuclear Medicine*, **36**, 2298–305.

Donnelly, M., Zametkin, A. J., Rapoport, J. L., *et al.* (1986). Treatment of childhood hyperactivity with desipramine: plasma drug concentration, cardiovascular effects, plasma and urinary catecholamine levels, and clinical response. *Clinical Pharmacological and Therapeutics*, **39**, 72–81.

Donnelly, M., Rapoport, J. L., Potter, W. Z., *et al.* (1989). Fenfluramine and dextroamphetamine treatment of childhood hyperactivity. *Archives of General Psychiatry*, **46**, 205–12.

Douglas, V., Barr, R., Amin, K., O'Neill, M., and Britton, B. (1988). Dosage effects and individual responsivity to methylphenidate in attention deficit disorder. *Journal of Child Psychology and Psychiatry*, **29**, 453–75.

Famularo, R. and Fenton, T. (1987). The effect of methylphenidate on school grades in children with attention deficit disorder without hyperactivity: a preliminary report. *Journal of Clinical Psychiatry*, **48**, 112–14.

Faraone, S. V. (2000). Genetics of childhood disorders: XX. ADHD, Part 4: is ADHD genetically heterogeneous? *Journal of the American Academy of Child and Adolescent Psychiatry*, **39**, 1455–7.

Faraone, S. V. and Biederman, J. (1999). The neurobiology of attention deficit hyperactivity disorder. In: *Neurobiology of Mental Illness*, ed. D. S. Charney, E. J. Nestler, and B. S. Bunney. New York: Oxford University Press, pp. 788–801.

Faraone, S. V., Biederman, J., Krifcher Lehman, B., *et al.* (1993). Intellectual performance and school failure in children with attention deficit hyperactivity disorder and in their siblings. *Journal of Abnormal Psychology*, **102**, 616–23.

Findling, R., Schwartz, M., Flannery, D., and Manos, M. (1996). Venlafaxine in adults with ADHD: an open trial. *Journal of Clinical Psychiatry*, **57**, 184–9.

Fung, Y. K. (1988). Postnatal behavioural effects of maternal nicotine exposure in rats. *Journal of Pharmacy and Pharmacology*, **40**, 870–2.

Fung, Y. K. and Lau, Y. S. (1989). Effects of prenatal nicotine exposure on rat striatal dopaminergic and nicotinic systems. *Pharmacology, Biochemistry and Behavior*, **33**, 1–6.

Gadow, K. D., Nolan, E. E., and Sverd, J. (1992). Methylphenidate in hyperactive boys with comorbid tic disorder: II. Short-term behavioral effects in school settings. *Journal of the American Academy of Child and Adolescent Psychiatry*, **31**, 462–71.

Gadow, K., Sverd, J., Sprafkin, J., Nolan, E., and Ezor, S. (1995). Efficacy of methylphenidate for attention-deficit hyperactivity disorder in children with tic disorder [published erratum appears in *Archives of General Psychiatry* (1995) **52**, 836]. *Archives of General Psychiatry*, **52**, 444–55.

Garfinkel, B. D., Wender, P. H., Sloman, L., and O'Neill, I. (1983). Tricyclic antidepressant and methylphenidate treatment of attention deficit disorder in children. *Journal of the American Academy of Child and Adolescent Psychiatry*, **22**, 343–8.

Gastfriend, D. R., Biederman, J., and Jellinek, M. S. (1985). Desipramine in the treatment of attention deficit disorder in adolescents. *Psychopharmacology Bulletin*, **21**, 144–5.

Gittelman-Klein, R. (1974). Pilot clinical trial of imipramine in hyperkinetic children. In: *Clinical Use of Stimulant Drugs in Children*, ed. C. Conners. The Hague, Netherlands: Excerpta Medica, pp. 192–201.

Gittelman-Klein, R. (1987). Pharmacotherapy of childhood hyperactivity: an update. In: *Psychopharmacology: The Third Generation of Progress*, ed. H. Y. Meltzer. New York: Raven Press, pp. 1215–24.

Gittelman, R. (1980). Childhood disorders. In: *Drug Treatment of Adult and Child Psychiatric Disorders*, ed. D. Klein, F. Quitkin, A. Rifkin and R. Gittelman. Baltimore, MD: Williams and Wilkins, pp. 576–756.

Gittelman, R. and Mannuzza, S. (1988). Hyperactive boys almost grown up: III. Methylphenidate effects on ultimate height. *Archives of General Psychiatry*, **45**, 1131–4.

Goldman, L., Genel, M., Bezman, R., and Slanetz, P. (1998). Diagnosis and treatment of attention-deficit/hyperactivity disorder in children and adolescents. *Journal of the American Medical Association*, **279**, 100–7.

Greenberg, L., Yellin, A., Spring, C., and Metcalf, M. (1975). Clinical effects of imipramine and methylphenidate in hyperactive children. *International Journal of Mental Health*, **4**, 144–56.

Greenblatt, D., Moltke, L., Harmatz, J., and Shader, R. (1998). Drug interactions with newer antidepressants: role of human cytochromes P450. *Journal of Clinical Psychiatry*, **59**, 19–27.

Greenhill, L., Halperin, J., Abikoff, H. (1998). Stimulant medications. *Journal of the American Academy of Child and Adolescent Psychiatry*, **38**, 503–12.

Greenhill, L. L., Findling, R. L., and Swanson, J. M. (2002). A double-blind, placebo-controlled study of modified-release methylphenidate in children with attention-deficit/hyperactivity disorder. *Pediatrics*, **109**, E39–9.

Gross, M. (1973). Imipramine in the treatment of minimal brain dysfunction in children. *Psychosomatics*, **14**, 283–5.

Gross, M. (1976). Growth of hyperkinetic children taking methylphenidate, dextroamphetamine, or imipramine/desipramine. *Journal of Pediatrics*, **58**, 423–31.

Gualtieri, C. T. and Evans, R. W. (1988). Motor performance in hyperactive children treated with imipramine. *Perceptual and Motor Skills*, **66**, 763–9.

Gunning, B. (1992). *A Controlled Trial of Clonidine in Hyperkinetic Children, in Department of Child and Adolescent Psychiatry*. Rotterdam, the Netherlands: Academic Hospital Rotterdam – Sophia Children's Hospital.

Hoge, S. K. and Biederman, J. (1986). A case of Tourette's syndrome with symptoms of attention deficit disorder treated with desipramine. *Journal of Clinical Psychiatry*, **47**, 478–9.

Hornig-Rohan, M. and Amsterdam, J. (1995). *Venlafaxine vs. Stimulant Therapy in Patients with Dual Diagnoses of ADHD and Depression*. Orlando, FL: New Clinical Drug Evaluation Unit Program.

Horrigan, J. P. and Barnhill, L. J. (1995). Guanfacine for treatment of attention-deficit hyperactivity disorder in boys. *Journal of Child and Adolescent Psychopharmacology*, **5**, 215–23.

Huessy, H. and Wright, A. (1970). The use of imipramine in children's behavior disorders. *Acta Paedopsychiatrie*, **37**, 194–9.

Hunt, R. D. (1987). Treatment effects of oral and transdermal clonidine in relation to methylphenidate: an open pilot study in ADD-H. *Psychopharmacology Bulletin*, **23**, 111–14.

Hunt, R. D., Minderaa, R. B., and Cohen, D. J. (1985). Clonidine benefits children with attention deficit disorder and hyperactivity: report of a double-blind placebo-crossover therapeutic trial. *Journal of the American Academy of Child Psychiatry*, **24**, 617–29.

Hunt, R. D., Capper, L., and O'Connell, P. (1990). Clonidine in child and adolescent psychiatry. *Journal of Child and Adolescent Psychopharmacology*, **1**, 87–102.

Hunt, R., Arnsten, A., and Asbell, M. (1995). An open trial of guanfacine in the treatment of attention-deficit hyperactivity disorder. *Journal of the American Academy of Child and Adolescent Psychiatry*, **34**, 50–4.

Hunt, R., Sachs, D. P., Glover, E. D., *et al.* (1997). A comparison of sustained-release bupropion and placebo for smoking cessation. *New England Journal of Medicine*, **337**, 1195–202.

Johns, J. M., Louis, T. M., Becker, R. F., and Means, L. W. (1982). Behavioral effects of prenatal exposure to nicotine in guinea pigs. *Neurobehavioral Toxicology and Teratology*, **4**, 365–9.

Jones, G., Sahakian, B., Levy, R., Warburton, D., and Gray, J. (1992). Effects of acute subcutaneous nicotine on attention, information and short-term memory in Alzheimer's disease. *Psychopharmacology*, **108**, 485–94.

Klein, R. G. (1987). Pharmacotherapy of childhood hyperactivity: an update. In: *Psychophar-macology: The Third Generation of Progress*, ed. H. Y. Meltzer. New York: Raven Press, pp. 1215–25.

Kratochvil, C. J., Bohac, D., Harrington, M., *et al.* (2001). An open-label trial of tomoxetine in pediatric attention deficit hyperactivity disorder. *Journal of Child and Adolescent Psychophar-macology*, **11**, 167–70.

Kupietz, S. S. and Balka, E. B. (1976). Alterations in the vigilance performance of children receiving amitriptyline and methylphenidate pharmacotherapy. *Psychopharmacology*, **50**, 29–33.

Kupietz, S. S., Winsberg, B. G., Richardson, E., Maitinsky, S., and Mendell, N. (1988). Effects of methylphenidate dosage in hyperactive reading-disabled children: I. Behavior and cognitive performance effects. *Journal of the American Academy of Child Adolescent Psychiatry*, **27**, 70–7.

Kurlan, R. (2002). Treatment of ADHD in children with tics: a randomized controlled trial. *Neurology*, **58**, 527–36.

Landgraf, J. (1995). *Child Health Questionnaire – Parent Form CHQ-PF 50*. Boston, MA: Health Institute of New England Medical Center, 1995.

Leckman, J. F., Hardin, M. T., Riddle, M. A., *et al.* (1991). Clonidine treatment of Gilles de la Tourette's syndrome. *Archives of General Psychiatry*, **48**, 324–8.

Levin, E., Conners, C., Sparrow, E., *et al.* (1996). Nicotine effects on adults with attention-deficit/hyperactivity disorder. *Psychopharmacology*, **123**, 55–63.

Lowe, T. L., Cohen, D. J., and Detlor, J. (1982). Stimulant medications precipitate Tourette's syndrome. *Journal of the American Medical Association*, **247**, 1168–9.

Luh, J., Pliszka, S., Olvers, R., and Tatum, R. (1996). *An Open Trial of Venlafaxine in the Treatment of Attention Deficit Hyperactivity Disorder: A Pilot Study*. San Antonio, TX: University of Texas Health Science Center at San Antonio.

Malhotra, S. and Santosh, P. J. (1998). An open clinical trial of buspirone in children with attention deficit/hyperactivity disorder. *Journal of the American Academy of Child and Adolescent Psychiatry*, **37**, 364–71.

Mattes, J. A. (1986). Propranolol for adults with temper outbursts and residual attention deficit disorder. *Journal of Clinical Psychopharmacology*, **6**, 299–302.

Mattes, J. A. and Gittelman, R. (1983). Growth of hyperactive children on maintenance regimen of methylphenidate. *Archives of General Psychiatry*, **40**, 317–21.

McCracken, J. T., Biederman, J., Greenhill, L. L., *et al.* (2000). Analog classroom assessment of SLI381 for treatment of ADHD. In: *The 47th Annual Meeting of the American Academy of Child and Adolescent Psychiatry*. New York, NY: AACAP, p. 104.

Meck, W. and Church, R. (1987). Cholinergic modulation of the content of temporal memory. *Behavioral Neuroscience*, **101**, 457–64.

Mereu, G., Yoon, K., Gessa, G., Naes, L., and Westfall, T. (1987). Preferential stimulation of ventral tegmental area dopaminergic neurons by nicotine. *European Journal of Pharmacology*, **141**, 395–9.

Michelson, D., Faries, D., Wernicke, J., *et al.* (2001). Atomoxetine in the treatment of children and adolescents with attention-deficit/hyperactivity disorder: a randomized, placebo-controlled, dose–response study. *Pediatrics*, **108**, E83.

Milberger, S., Biederman, J., Faraone, S. V., Chen, L., and Jones, J. (1996). Is maternal smoking during pregnancy a risk factor for attention deficit hyperactivity disorder in children? *American Journal of Psychiatry*, **153**, 1138–42.

Milberger, S., Biederman, J., Faraone, S., Chen, L., and Jones, J. (1997a). ADHD is associated with early initiation of cigarette smoking in children and adolescents. *Journal of the American Academy of Child and Adolescent Psychiatry*, **36**, 37–43.

Milberger, S., Biederman, J., Faraone, S., Guite, J. and Tsuang, M. (1997b). Pregnancy delivery and infancy complications and ADHD: issues of gene–environment interactions. *Biological Psychiatry*, **41**, 65–75.

MTA Cooperative Group (1999). A 14-month randomized clinical trial of treatment strategies for attention-deficit/hyperactivity disorder. Multimodal treatment study of children with ADHD [see comments]. *Archives of General Psychiatry*, **56**, 1073–86.

Nemeroff, C., DeVane, L., and Pollock, B. (1996). Newer antidepressants and the cytochrome P450 system. *American Journal of Psychiatry*, **153**, 311–20.

NIMH (1996). *Alternative Pharmacology of ADHD*. National Institute of Mental Health.

Palumbo, D. (2002). Impact of ADHD treatment once-daily OROS formulation of MPH on tics. In: *Annual Meeting of the American Psychiatric Association*. Philadelphia, PA: American Psychiatric Association, p. 30.

Parrott, A. C. and Winder, G. (1989). Nicotine chewing gum (2 mg, 4 mg) and cigarette smoking: comparative effects upon vigilance and heart rate. *Psychopharmacology*, **97**, 257–61.

Peeke, S. and Peeke, H. (1984). Attention, memory, and cigarette smoking. *Psychopharmacology*, **84**, 205–16.

Pelham, W. E., Bender, M. E., Caddell, J., Booth, S., and Moorer, S. H. (1985). Methylphenidate and children with attention deficit disorder. *Archives of General Psychiatry*, **42**, 948–52.

Pelham, W. E., Gnagy, E. M., Burrows-Maclean, L., *et al.* (2001). Once-a-day Concerta methylphenidate versus three-times-daily methylphenidate in laboratory and natural settings. *Pediatrics*, **107**, E105.

Pentikis, H. S., Simmons, R. D., Benedict, M. F., and Hatch, S. J. (2002). Methylphenidate bioavailability in adults when an extended-release multiparticulate formulation is administered sprinkled on food or as an intact capsule. *Journal of the American Academy of Child and Adolescent Psychiatry*, **41**, 443–9.

Pomerleau, O., Downey, K., Stelson, F., and Pomerleau, C. (1996). Cigarette smoking in adult patients diagnosed with ADHD. *Journal of Substance Abuse*, **7**, 373–8.

Prince, J., Wilens, T., Biederman, J., Spencer, T., and Wozniak, J. (1996). Clonidine for ADHD related sleep disturbances: a systematic chart review of 62 cases. *Journal of the American Academy of Child and Adolescent Psychiatry*, **35**, 599–605.

Prince, J., Wilens, T., Biederman, J., *et al.* (1999). A controlled study of nortriptyline in children and adolescents with attention deficit hyperactivity disorder. *Scientific Proceedings of the American Academy of Child and Adolescent Psychiatrists*, Chicago, IL: AACAP.

Quinn, P. O. and Rapoport, J. L. (1975). One-year follow-up of hyperactive boys treated with imipramine or methylphenidate. *American Journal of Psychiatry*, **132**, 241–5.

Quitkin, F. M., Harrison, W., Stewart, J. W., *et al.* (1991). Response to phenelzine and imipramine in placebo nonresponders with atypical depression. *Archives of General Psychiatry*, **48**, 319–23.

Rapoport, J. L., Quinn, P., Bradbard, G., Riddle, D., Brooks, E. (1974). Imipramine and methylphenidate treatment of hyperactive boys: a double-blind comparison. *Archives of General Psychiatry*, **30**, 789–93.

Rapport, M. D., Jones, J. T., DuPaul, G. J., *et al.* (1987). Attention deficit disorder and methylphenidate: group and single-subject analyses of dose effects on attention in clinic and classroom settings. *Journal of Clinical Child Psychology*, **16**, 329–38.

Rapport, M. D., Stoner, G., DuPaul, G. J., *et al.* (1988). Attention deficit disorder and methylphenidate: a multilevel analysis of dose–response effects on children's impulsivity across settings. *Journal of the American Academy of Child and Adolescent Psychiatry*, **27**, 60–9.

Rapport, M. D., DuPaul, G. J., and Kelly, K. L. (1989a). Attention deficit hyperactivity disorder and methylphenidate: the relationship between gross body weight and drug response in children. *Psychopharmacology Bulletin*, **25**, 285–90.

Rapport, M. D., Quinn, S. O., DuPaul, G. J., Quinn, E. P., and Kelly, K. L. (1989b). Attention deficit disorder with hyperactivity and methylphenidate: the effects of dose and mastery level on children's learning performance. *Journal of Abnormal Child Psychology*, **17**, 669–89.

Rapport, M., Carlson, G., Kelly, K., and Pataki, C. (1993). Methylphenidate and desipramine in hospitalized children: I. Separate and combined effects on cognitive function. *Journal of the American Academy of Child and Adolescent Psychiatry*, **32**, 333–42.

Ratey, J., Greenberg, M., and Lindem, K. (1991). Combination of treatments for attention deficit disorders in adults. *Journal of Nervous and Mental Disorders*, **176**, 699–701.

Reimherr, F. W., Wender, P. H., Wood, D. R., and Ward, M. (1987). An open trial of L-tyrosine in the treatment of attention deficit disorder, residual type. *American Journal of Psychiatry*, **144**, 1071–3.

Reimherr, F., Hedges, D., Strong, R., and Wender, P. (1995). *An Open-Trial of Venlaxine in Adult Patients with Attention Deficit Hyperactivity Disorder*. Orlando, FL: New Clinical Drug Evaluation Unit Program.

Riddle, M. A., Hardin, M. T., Cho, S. C., Woolston, J. L., and Leckman, J. F. (1988). Desipramine treatment of boys with attention-deficit hyperactivity disorder and tics: preliminary clinical experience. *Journal of the American Academy of Child and Adolescent Psychiatry*, **27**, 811–14.

Riddle, M. A., Nelson, J. C., Kleinman, C. S., *et al.* (1991). Sudden death in children receiving norpramin: a review of three reported cases and commentary. *Journal of the American Academy of Child and Adolescent Psychiatry*, **30**, 104–8.

Safer, D. J., Allen, R. P., and Barr, E. (1972). Depression of growth in hyperactive children on stimulant drugs. *New England Journal of Medicine*, **287**, 217–20.

Satterfield, J. H., Cantwell, D. P., Schell, A., and Blaschke, T. (1979). Growth of hyperactive children treated with methylphenidate. *Archives of General Psychiatry*, **36**, 212–17.

Scahill, L., Chappell, P. B., Kim, Y. S., *et al.* (2001). A placebo-controlled study of guanfacine in the treatment of children with tic disorders and attention deficit hyperactivity disorder. *American Journal of Psychiatry*, **158**, 1067–74.

Silva, R., Munoz, D., and Alpert, M. (1996). Carbamazepine use in children and adolescents with features of attention-deficit hyperactivity disorder: a meta-analysis. *Journal of the American Academy of Child and Adolescent Psychiatry*, **35**, 352–8.

Singer, S., Brown, J., Quaskey, S., *et al.* (1994). The treatment of attention-deficit hyperactivity disorder in Tourette's syndrome: a double-blind placebo-controlled study with clonidine and desipramine. *Pediatrics*, **95**, 74–81.

Spencer, T. (2002). ADHD treatment with once-daily OROS formulation of MPH: effect on growth. In: *Annual Meeting of the American Psychiatric Association.* Philadelphia, PA: American Psychiatric Association, p. 30.

Spencer, T., Biederman, J., Wilens, T., Steingard, R., and Geist, D. (1993a). Nortriptyline in the treatment of children with attention deficit hyperactivity disorder and tic disorder or Tourette's syndrome. *Journal of the American Academy of Child and Adolescent Psychiatry*, **32**, 205–10.

Spencer, T., Biederman, J., Kerman, K., Steingard, R., and Wilens, T. (1993b). Desipramine in the treatment of children with tic disorder or Tourette's syndrome and attention deficit hyperactivity disorder. *Journal of the American Academy of Child and Adolescent Psychiatry*, **32**, 354–60.

Spencer, T., Wilens, T., Biederman, J., *et al.* (1995). A double-blind, crossover comparison of methylphenidate and placebo in adults with childhood-onset attention-deficit hyperactivity disorder. *Archives of General Psychiatry*, **52**, 434–43.

Spencer, T. J., Biederman, J., Wilens, T., *et al.* (1996). Pharmacotherapy of attention deficit hyperactivity disorder across the lifecycle: a literature review. *Journal of the American Academy of Child and Adolescent Psychiatry*, **35**, 409–32.

Spencer, T., Biederman, J., and Wilens, T. (1997). Pharmacotherapy of ADHD: a life span perspective. In: *American Psychiatric Press Review of Psychiatry*, ed. J. Oldham and M. Riba. Washington, DC: APA, pp. 87–128.

Spencer, T., Biederman, J., and Wilens, T. (1998a). Growth deficits in children with attention deficit hyperactivity disorder. *Pediatrics*, **102**, 501–6.

Spencer, T., Biederman, J., Wilens, T. E., and Faraone, S. V. (1998b). Adults with attention-deficit/hyperactivity disorder: a controversial diagnosis. *Journal of Clinical Psychiatry*, **59**, 59–68.

Spencer, T., Biederman, J., Wilens, T., *et al.* (1998c). Effectiveness and tolerability of tomoxetine in adults with attention deficit hyperactivity disorder. *American Journal of Psychiatry*, **155**, 693–5.

Spencer, T., Biederman, J., Coffey, B., *et al.* (1999). The 4-year course of tic disorders in boys with attention-deficit/hyperactivity disorder. *Archives of General Psychiatry*, **56**, 842–7.

Spencer, T., Swanson, J., Weidenman, M., *et al.* (2000). Pharmacodynamic profile of Ritalin LA, a new extended-release dosage form of Ritalin, in children with ADHD. In: *The 47th Annual Meeting of the American Academy of Child and Adolescent Psychiatry.* New York, NY: AACAP.

Spencer, T., Biederman, J., Heiligenstein, J., *et al.* (2001). An open-label, dose-ranging study of atomoxetine in children with attention deficit hyperactivity disorder. *Journal of Child and Adolescent Psychopharmacology*, **11**, 251–65.

Spencer, T., Biederman, J., Coffey, B., *et al.* (2002a). A double-blind comparison of desipramine and placebo in children and adolescents with chronic tic disorder and comorbid attention-deficit/hyperactivity disorder. *Archives of General Psychiatry*, **59**, 649–56.

Spencer, T., Heiligenstein, J., Biederman, J., *et al.* (2002b). Results from two proof-of-concept, placebo-controlled studies of atomoxetine in children with ADHD. *Journal of Clinical Psychiatry*, **63**, 1140–7.

Steingard, R., Biederman, J., Spencer, T., Wilens, T., and Gonzalez, A. (1993). Comparison of clonidine response in the treatment of attention deficit hyperactivity disorder with and without comorbid tic disorders. *Journal of the American Academy of Child and Adolescent Psychiatry*, **32**, 350–3.

Swanson, J., Agler, D., Fineberg, E., *et al.* (2000). University of California, Irvine, laboratory school protocol for pharmacokinetic and pharmacodynamic studies. In: *Ritalin: Theory and Practice*, 2nd edn, ed. L. Greenhill and B. Osman. Larchmont, New York: Mary Ann Liebert, pp. 405–30.

Tannock, R., Schachar, R. J., Carr, R. P., and Logan, G. D. (1989). Dose–response effects of methylphenidate on academic performance and overt behavior in hyperactive children. *Pediatrics*, **84**, 648–57.

Taylor, F. B. (2000). Comparing guanfacine and dextroamphetamine for adult ADHD: Efficacy and implications. In: *153rd Annual Meeting of the American Psychiatric Association*. Chicago, IL: American Psychiatric Association.

Watter, N. and Dreyfuss, F. E. (1973). Modifications of hyperkinetic behavior by nortriptyline. *Virginia Medical Monthly*, **100**, 123–6.

Wender, P. H. and Reimherr, F. W. (1990). Bupropion treatment of attention-deficit hyperactivity disorder in adults. *American Journal of Psychiatry*, **147**, 1018–20.

Werry, J. (1980). Imipramine and methylphenidate in hyperactive children. *Journal of Child Psychology and Psychiatry*, **21**, 27–35.

Wesnes, K. and Warburton, D. (1984). The effects of cigarettes of varying yield on rapid information processing performance. *Psychopharmacology*, **82**, 338–42.

West, S., Johnson, D. E., Wigal, S., and Zeldis, J. (2002). Withdrawal trial of dex-methylphenidate (Focalin) in children with ADHD. In: *Annual Meeting of the American Psychiatric Association*. Philadelphia, PA: American Psychiatric Association, p. 30.

Westfall, T., Grant, H., and Perry, H. (1983). Release of dopamine and 5-hydroxytryptamine from rat striatal slices following activation of nicotinic cholinergic receptors. *General Pharmacology*, **14**, 321–5.

Wilens, T. and Biederman, J. (1992). The stimulants. In: *Psychiatric Clinics of North America*, ed. D. Schaffer. Philadelphia, PA: W. B. Saunders, pp. 191–222.

Wilens, T. E. and Spencer, T. J. (1999). Combining methylphenidate and clonidine: a clinically sound medication option. *Journal of the American Academy of Child and Adolescent Psychiatry*, **38**, 614–22.

Wilens, T. E., Biederman, J., Geist, D. E., Steingard, R., and Spencer, T. (1993). Nortriptyline in the treatment of attention deficit hyperactivity disorder: a chart review of 58 cases. *Journal of the American Academy of Child and Adolescent Psychiatry*, **32**, 343–9.

Wilens, T. E., Biederman, J. B., Mick, E., and Spencer, T. (1995). A systematic assessment of tricyclic antidepressants in the treatment of adult attention-deficit hyperactivity disorder. *Journal of Nervous and Mental Diseases*, **183**, 48–50.

Wilens, T. E., Biederman, J., Abrantes, A. M., and Spencer, T. J. (1996a). A naturalistic assessment of protriptyline for attention-deficit hyperactivity disorder. *Journal of the American Academy of Child and Adolescent Psychiatry*, **35**, 1485–90.

Wilens, T. E., Biederman, J., Prince, J., et al. (1996b). Six-week, double-blind, placebo-controlled study of desipramine for adult attention deficit hyperactivity disorder. *American Journal of Psychiatry*, **153**, 1147–53.

Wilens, T., Spencer, T., Biederman, J., et al. (1999a). *A Controlled Trial of Bupropion SR for Attention Deficit Hyperactivity Disorder in Adults*. Boca Raton, FL: New Clinical Drug Evaluation Unit Program.

Wilens, T., Biederman, J., Spencer, T., et al. (1999b). A pilot controlled clinical trial of ABT-418, a cholinergic agonist, in the treatment of adults with attention deficit hyperactivity disorder. *American Journal of Psychiatry*, **156**, 1931–7.

Wilens, T. E., Biederman, J., Spencer, T. J., et al. (1999c). Controlled trial of high doses of pemoline for adults with attention-deficit/hyperactivity disorder. *Journal of Clinical Psychopharmacology*, **19**, 257–64.

Wilens, T., Pelham, W. E., Stein, M., and Conners, C. K. (2002). ADHD treatment with a once-daily formulation of methylphenidate: a two-year study. In: *Annual Meeting of the American Psychiatric Association*. Philadelphia, PA: American Psychiatric Association, p. 19.

Winsberg, B. G., Bialer, I., Kupietz, S., and Tobias, J. (1972). Effects of imipramine and dextroamphetamine on behavior of neuropsychiatrically impaired children. *American Journal of Psychiatry*, **128**, 1425–31.

Wolraich, M. L., Greenhill, L. L., Pelham, W., et al. (2001). Randomized, controlled trial of oros methylphenidate once a day in children with attention-deficit/hyperactivity disorder. *Pediatrics*, **108**, 883–92.

Yepes, L. E., Balka, E. B., Winsberg, B. G., and Bialer, I. (1977). Amitriptyline and methylphenidate treatment of behaviorally disordered children. *Journal of Child Psychology and Psychiatry*, **18**, 39–52.

Zametkin, A. J. and Rapoport, J. L. (1987). Noradrenergic hypothesis of attention deficit disorder with hyperactivity: a critical review. In: *Psychopharmacology: The Third Generation of Progress*, ed. H. Y. Meltzer. New York: Raven Press, pp. 837–42.

Zametkin, A., Rapoport, J. L., Murphy, D. L., Linnoila, M., and Ismond, D. (1985). Treatment of hyperactive children with monoamine oxidase inhibitors: I. Clinical efficacy. *Archives of General Psychiatry*, **42**, 962–6.

Zametkin, A. J., Nordahl, T. E., Gross, M., et al. (1990). Cerebral glucose metabolism in adults with hyperactivity of childhood onset. *New England Journal of Medicine*, **323**, 1361–6.

11

Evidence-based pharmacotherapy of Alzheimer's disease

John Grimley Evans,[1] Gordon Wilcock,[2] and Jacqueline Birks[1]

[1] University of Oxford, UK
[2] University of Bristol, UK

In broad terms, dementia is conceptualized as an acquired global impairment of cognitive capacities – such as memory, reasoning, language, and performance of effective executive action – of sufficient severity to interfere with normal functioning. Most forms are progressive and with an onset after the age of 65. So-called presenile dementias appear at earlier ages and some have a single-gene cause. Approximately 5% of people aged over 65 are affected by dementia and the prevalence doubles with each 5 years of age, to reach 20% of people aged over 80. Some 70% of cases of dementia are thought to be due primarily to Alzheimer's disease.

The term "Alzheimer's disease" is loosely used in a variety of ways. At present it is most usefully restricted to specifying a disease of the brain associated with a characteristic pathology of intracellular argyrophilic "tangles" and extracellular "plaques" of amyloid material surrounded by swollen neurites. Dementia is a clinical syndrome, of which Alzheimer's disease is one common cause. Although there is a quantitative link between the degree and distribution of Alzheimer's-type changes in the brain and the clinical severity of dementia, not everyone with the brain changes of Alzheimer's disease will show dementia.

Alzheimer's disease was originally described as a cause of "presenile dementia," that is to say, dementia with onset before the age of 65. In the 1960s it was observed that at autopsy most cases of later-onset "senile dementia," widely supposed up to that time to be a manifestation of "normal aging," were associated with the same pathological features as Alzheimer's disease. It was also shown that there was a significant correlation between the degree of dementia exhibited by affected old people before death and quantitative measures of the Alzheimer-type changes in their brains at autopsy (Blessed et al., 1968; Wilcock and Esiri, 1982; Wilcock et al., 1982). This supported a causal relationship between brain pathology and function. "Senile dementia" is now obsolete as a diagnostic term.

Accuracy of diagnosis

Although descriptions of the clinical manifestations of Alzheimer's disease have been increasingly refined in the last decade there is no diagnostic test for what remains fundamentally a pathologically defined condition. There is a wide range of other causes of dementia in later life, but numerically the most prevalent, after Alzheimer's disease, are brain ischemia secondary to cerebrovascular disease, and dementia with Lewy bodies. The former may take the form of infarcts in the brain due to thromboembolic events that may be clinically manifest as strokes, but cognitive impairment and dementia may more frequently be due to microvascular disease causing leukoaraiosis in the periventricular white matter visible on computed tomography or magnetic resonance imaging brain scanning. Dementia with Lewy bodies shares some features with Alzheimer's disease, but often has a different clinical presentation and differs histologically. There are fewer cortical neurofibrillary tangles, but, as the name suggests, Lewy bodies similar to those seen in the basal ganglia in Parkinson's disease are found in the cerebral cortex.

Alzheimer's disease and brain ischemia may coexist. There is a long-recognized epidemiological phenomenon, known as Berkson's bias, that results in people with two diseases being more likely to come to medical notice than people with only one. This form of bias must be expected to be especially powerful where the two diseases produce the same cardinal effect. People with mixed forms of dementia due to a combination of Alzheimer's and cerebrovascular disease will be identified sooner on average than people with either disease alone. Since the causes and mechanisms of dementia are likely to differ between Alzheimer's disease and cerebrovascular disease, for both research and management purposes, attempts are made to distinguish the two clinically. The accuracy of the diagnosis of Alzheimer's disease is partly dependent on the sensitivity and specificity of methods for identifying cerebrovascular disease, and patients thought to have cerebrovascular dementia may well have Alzheimer's disease as well and vice versa. Neuropathological study confirms that most older people showing cognitive decline have mixed vascular and Alzheimer's disease (Neuropathology Group, 2001).

Problems with clinical trials in Alzheimer's disease

The fact that Alzheimer's disease as diagnosed at autopsy may or may not correspond with Alzheimer's disease diagnosed clinically needs to be borne in mind in interpreting the results of clinical trials of treatment. This is particularly true in comparing trials performed at periods when diagnostic criteria differed and sensitive radiological techniques for identifying cerebrovascular disease varied in their availability.

Many people with dementia do not come to medical notice; those who do are selected in ways dependent on their social situation and the workings of the local medical and social systems of care. Patients enrolled into clinical trials in one country may not be representative of those presenting for medical care in another. A new medical treatment needs to undergo three levels of appraisal: for (1) efficacy; (2) effectiveness; and (3) efficiency. In broad terms, efficacy implies that a drug does something that might be desirable, while effectiveness implies that some patients at least experience benefit if given the drug. Efficiency relates to the cost-effectiveness of the drug in comparison with alternatives that may be other drugs or treatments, or simply letting a disease run its natural course. It is important, when evaluating efficiency in particular, that investigators are sensitive to issues in the selection of the patients who entered the trials showing a drug's effectiveness.

Mode of action

Interventions relevant to Alzheimer's disease fall broadly into three groups: (1) those that interfere with its etiology; (2) those that interrupt the mechanisms of the pathogenesis of the disease; and (3) those that modify its manifestations. The first will reduce or postpone the incidence of the disease, the second will modify its natural history, and the third will be essentially palliative. These distinctions need to be held in mind when assessing the clinical significance of the results of a trial. A drug that improves the natural history of the disease by retarding deterioration is potentially of greater value than one that merely produces a short-lived improvement in function. A commonly overlooked problem in research on the treatment of Alzheimer's disease is that sufferers may be depressed, and drugs with an antidepressant action may, by improving cognition and daily functioning, be presentable as "antidementia."

Much prescribing for people with Alzheimer's disease is directed not at the disease itself but at its manifestations and consequences, particularly depression and challenging behaviors. These aspects of treatment, which often have to be prescribed as part of an integrated management strategy linked with medical, nursing, and social care of both patient and carer, are outside the scope of this chapter. They do, however, raise some general concerns, in particular the problems of adverse effects and drug interactions. Many of the antidepressants and neuroleptics have central anticholinergic actions that can exacerbate the cognitive problems of someone with Alzheimer's disease. Hypotensive reactions are a potential risk with both the cholinesterase inhibitors (ChEIs) and many other drugs commonly prescribed for people with Alzheimer's disease. Drug prescriptions should be kept to a minimum and regularly reviewed. Abrupt deterioration in a patient with Alzheimer's disease should lead first to a search for intercurrent illness rather than a prescription pad.

Assessing the evidence

As a consequence of professional and lay interest in treatments for Alzheimer's disease, the performance of the drugs is an area of intense study. A complicating factor is the commercial competition between the pharmaceutical companies involved and some published reviews must be viewed as possibly partisan. The Cochrane Collaboration is an international organization dedicated to producing strictly dispassionate systematic reviews of evidence relating to drugs or other treatments. A systematic review has to start by identifying all available evidence, published or unpublished, and assessing its methodological quality. This initial stage of identifying all the evidence is crucial since bias can arise if only positive trials are published or if drug companies conceal negative data. (Obviously an annotation in a Cochrane review that a drug company has refused to make data from one or more of its trials available should raise questions in a reader's mind.) From this overview, the results from all randomized controlled trials of reliable quality may be included in a statistical process of meta-analysis. This process aims at combining the results from separate trials to provide more precise and reliable estimates of the size of treatment effects. It also, however, involves an assessment of whether the results of the different trials are compatible in the sense of the trials having involved sufficiently similar patients and methods for a combination of their results to be clinically meaningful.

What is the first-line pharmacotherapy of Alzheimer's disease?

All clinicians and certainly all patients would consider cholinergic drugs to be first-line pharmacotherapy for Alzheimer's disease. The rationale for the use of cholinergic drugs for people with Alzheimer's disease lies in enhancing the secretion or prolonging the half-life of acetylcholine in the synaptic clefts in relevant areas of the brain. It has been known for many years that degeneration in the cholinergic neural pathways in the brain underlies some of the manifestations of advanced Alzheimer's disease, and in particular contributes to the characteristic deficits in cognition. Several cholinergic approaches, such as muscarinic and nicotinic receptor agonists, and compounds to enhance acetylcholine release, have been tried as treatment for Alzheimer's disease, but without clinically useful effects. Some compounds have been too ephemeral in their pharmacological effects, and a common and predictable problem has been a high incidence of adverse effects due to peripheral cholinergic actions.

Nicotine

Some observational studies have suggested a negative association between tobacco smoking and Alzheimer's disease, raising the possibility of a beneficial effect of nicotine. However, epidemiological studies may be biased by the diagnostic problems mentioned earlier; people with Alzheimer's disease plus any of the cardiovascular diseases associated with smoking may be presumed to have vascular dementia. A review of four prospective studies (Doll *et al.*, 2000) found no evidence of any association between smoking and Alzheimer's disease.

Most of the receptors in the parts of the brain affected by Alzheimer's disease are muscarinic rather than nicotinic, but nicotine does have a presynaptic effect in releasing acetylcholine in addition to its postsynaptic agonist effects. There is also some evidence from animal model studies that nicotine might reduce the accumulation of beta-amyloid in brain tissue (Nordberg *et al.*, 2002), and in some animal models nicotine has been found to enhance memory or awareness. A Cochrane review concluded that at present there is no useful evidence on the effect of nicotine as a treatment for Alzheimer's disease (López-Arrieta *et al.*, 2004). There was only one randomized, double-blind, placebo-controlled trial of nicotine for Alzheimer's disease that could be included in the review. This small, 10-week, crossover trial testing a nicotine patch in eight people who had been non-smokers for at least a year provided no interpretable results.

The cholinesterase inhibitors

ChEIs that delay the breakdown of naturally secreted acetylcholine have provided the most significant advance. To be useful such drugs must cross the blood–brain barrier and, to minimize adverse effects, inhibit the breakdown of acetylcholine to a lesser degree in the rest of the body than in the brain.

The first of the ChEIs to be marketed for the treatment of Alzheimer's disease was tacrine, which, although shown to be effective in clinical trials (Qizilbash *et al.*, 1998), had a high incidence of potentially serious adverse effects and has now been overtaken by new drugs. The three currently on the market are donepezil (Aricept), rivastigmine (Exelon), and galantamine (Reminyl). They differ to some extent in their pharmacological properties. Unlike donepezil, rivastigmine inhibits butyrylcholinesterase as well as acetylcholinesterase. In addition to its inhibition of acetylcholinesterase, galantamine has nicotinic agonist activity. The clinical significance of these differences is not yet established. Donepezil has a long half-life that makes once-daily dosage logical.

Do the cholinesterase inhibitors work?

If the rationale underlying the development of the drugs is the whole story, it is not to be expected that ChEIs will change the natural course of deterioration in Alzheimer's disease. That would require drugs that interfere in the pathogenetic process, rather than merely mitigating some of its consequences. The trials have therefore focused on detecting differences between treatment and placebo groups of patients in their rates of deterioration of cognitive function over quite small time intervals, typically 3–6 months.

Tables 11.1–11.4 summarize the details of included trials and results from systematic reviews carried out by the Cochrane Dementia and Cognitive Improvement Group (Birks and Harvey, 2004; Birks et al., 2004a; Olin and Schneider, 2004). The Group is happy to acknowledge the cooperation of the relevant pharmaceutical companies in obtaining access to trial results for the reviews. In the trials various different drug dosages were used, but for simplicity the tables show data relating to dosages recommended by the manufacturers for clinical use. The doses reported on are total daily doses of 10 mg for donepezil, 24 mg for galantamine, and 6–12 mg for rivastigmine. Donepezil was taken once a day, while galantamine and rivastigmine were distributed over twice-daily dosage. For all three drugs titration up to this dose is recommended in order to minimize the incidence and severity of adverse effects. The results summarized in the tables are as observed after 6 months of treatment, pooled across all relevant studies. It should be noted that Cochrane reviews are updated regularly, with new studies included as the results become available.

Although it might be technically feasible to standardize the drug dosages pharmacologically in terms of, say, their percentage inhibition of brain acetylcholinesterase in some laboratory preparation, this has not been done. Rather, the manufacturers have chosen dosages to strike a balance between beneficial and adverse effects. Most of the ill effects of the drugs, as with the beneficial effects, will be due to cholinergic actions and dose-dependent. Differences between the drugs in their performance in trials may reflect physiological non-equivalence of dosages rather than different intrinsic virtues. If this is so, there will be a direct relationship, other things being equal, between the efficacy of a drug and the incidence of its pharmacologically predictable adverse effects.

Which patients?

Defects in the cholinergic system may contribute to cognitive impairment in conditions other than Alzheimer's disease. The Cochrane review of cholinesterase inhibitors for dementia with Lewy bodies (Wild et al., 2004) included only one randomized, double-blind trial (McKeith et al., 2000), in which rivastigmine was compared with placebo in 120 patients over 20 weeks. There was no evidence of benefit for rivastigmine compared with placebo for behavior as assessed by the Neuropsychiatric Inventory (NPI, Cummings et al., 1994), cognitive function, and global assessment for the intent-to-treat (ITT) analysis, but limited evidence of benefit for rivastigmine for behavior in the completers' analysis. There is increasing evidence of the efficacy of the cholinesterase inhibitors in vascular dementia. The Cochrane review of donepezil for vascular cognitive impairment (Maloof and Birks, 2004) included two 24-week randomized, double-blind, placebo-controlled

Table 11.1 Summary of double-blind, randomized, placebo-controlled, parallel-group trials of cholinesterase inhibitors for Alzheimer's disease

Drug	Author	Sample size	Duration (weeks)	Dose (mg/day)	Outcomes
Donepezil	Homma *et al.* (1998)	190	12	1,3	Cognition, global, ADL
Donepezil	Homma *et al.* (2000)	268	24	5	Cognition, global, ADL
Donepezil	Rogers (1996)	161	12	1,3,5	Cognition, global, ADL, QoL
Donepezil	Tune *et al.* (1998)	28	24	10	Cognition, behavior
Donepezil	Unpublished	67	24	10	Cognition
Donepezil	Unpublished	12	12	10	Cognition, ADL, QoL
Donepezil	Rogers *et al.* (1998a)	468	12	5,10	Cognition, global, QoL
Donepezil	Rogers *et al.* (1998b)	473	24	5,10	Cognition, global, QoL
Donepezil	Burns *et al.* (1999)	818	24	5,10	Cognition, global, ADL, QoL
Donepezil	Unpublished	39	12	10	Cognition
Donepezil	Tariot *et al.* (2001)	208	24	10	Cognition, behavior
Donepezil	Mohs *et al.* (2001)	431	54	10	Cognition, ADL
Donepezil	Bentham *et al.* (2002)	566	60	5,10	Cognition, ADL, behavior, QoL
Donepezil	Robert *et al.* (2000)	318	12	10	Cognition, ADL, behavior
Donepezil	Feldman *et al.* (2001)	473	24	10	Cognition, global, ADL, behavior
Donepezil	Meadows *et al.* (2000)	60	12	5	Cognition, global
Donepezil	Winblad *et al.* (2001)	286	52	10	Cognition, global, ADL
Galantamine	Wilkinson and Murray (2001)	285	12	18, 24, 36	Cognition, global, ADL
Galantamine	Unpublished	554	29	32	Cognition, global, ADL
Galantamine	Wilcock *et al.* (2000)	653	26	24, 32	Cognition, ADL
Galantamine	Rockwood *et al.* (2001)	386	12	24–32	Cognition, ADL, behavior
Galantamine	Raskind *et al.* (2000)	636	26	24, 32	Cognition, global, ADL
Galantamine	Tariot *et al.* (2000)	978	22	8, 16, 24	Cognition, global, behavior, ADL
Galantamine	Kewitz *et al.* (1994)	95	13	20–50	Cognition, global, ADL
Rivastigmine	Anand *et al.* (1996)	402	13	4, 6	Cognition, global, ADL
Rivastigmine	Anand *et al.* (1996)	114	18	6–12	Cognition, global
Rivastigmine	Anand *et al.* (1996)	50	9	6–12	Cognition, global, ADL
Rivastigmine	Rösler *et al.* (1999)	725	26	1–4, 6–12	Cognition, global, ADL
Rivastigmine	Unpublished	677	26	2–12	Cognition, global, ADL
Rivastigmine	Unpublished	702	26	3,6,9	Cognition, global, ADL
Rivastigmine	Corey-Bloom *et al.* (1998)	699	26	1–4, 6–12	Cognition, global, ADL
Rivastigmine	Tai *et al.* (2000)	80	26	Maximum tolerated	Cognition, global, ADL

ADL, activities of daily living; QoL, quality of life.

Table 11.2 Efficacy of donepezil, rivastigmine, and galantamine in patients with Alzheimer's disease: mean changes in scores from baseline at 6 months

	Favors	Treatment effect (mean difference)	95% confidence limits	Test for effect P-value	Number on treatment	Number on placebo	Number of studies pooled
Observed cases							
Cognition: ADAS-Cog (score 0–70, improvement is associated with a decrease in score)							
Donepezil	Treatment	−2.92	−3.64 to −1.61	<0.00001	346	390	4
Galantamine	Treatment	−3.52	−4.26 to −2.79	<0.00001	498	553	3
Rivastigmine	Treatment	−2.62	−3.29 to −1.94	<0.00001	670	709	4
Cognition: MMSE (score 0–30, improvement is associated with an increase in score)							
Donepezil	Treatment	1.50	0.97 to 2.04	<0.00001	342	377	3
Activities of daily living: DAD (score 0–100, improvement is associated with an increase in score)							
Donepezil	Treatment	8.00	3.61 to 12.39	0.0004	121	126	1
Galantamine	–	2.5	−0.80 to 5.80	0.14	159	177	1
Behavioral disturbance: NPI (score 0–144, improvement is associated with a decrease in score)							
Donepezil	Treatment	−4.42	−7.93 to −0.91	0.01	119	125	1
Behavioral disturbance: NPI (score 0–120, improvement is associated with a decrease in score)							
Galantamine	Treatment	−2.40	−4.63 to −0.17	0.04	212	234	1
Intent-to-treat							
Cognition: ADAS-Cog (score 0–70, improvement is associated with a decrease in score)							
Donepezil	Treatment	−2.91	−3.65 to −2.16	<0.00001	404	417	4
Galantamine	Treatment	−3.29	−3.92 to −2.65	<0.00001	675	677	3
Rivastigmine	Treatment	−2.09	−2.65 to −1.54	<0.00001	1054	863	4
Cognition: MMSE (score 0–30, improvement is associated with an increase in score)							
Donepezil	Treatment	1.35	0.84 to 1.85	<0.00001	385	396	4
Rivastigmine	Treatment	0.83	0.53 to 1.12	<0.00001	1054	867	4
Activities of daily living: DAD (score 0–100, improvement is associated with an increase in score)							
Donepezil	Treatment	8.24	4.46 to 12.02	<0.0001	134	140	1
Galantamine	–	1.4	−0.69 to 3.49	0.19	398	406	2
Activities of daily living: PDS (score 0–100, improvement is associated with a decrease in score)							
Rivastigmine	Treatment	−2.15	−3.16 to −1.13	<0.0001	1048	864	4
Behavioral disturbance: NPI (score 0–144, improvement is associated with a decrease in score)							
Donepezil	Treatment	−5.6	−8.95 to −2.25	0.001	138	144	1
Behavioral disturbance: NPI (score 0–120, improvement is associated with a decrease in score)							
Galantamine	–	−2.00	−4.08 to 0.08	0.06	253	262	1

ADAS-Cog, cognitive scale of the Alzheimer Disease and Associated Disorders scale; MMSE, Mini-Mental State Examination; DAD, Disability Assessment for Dementia; PDS, Progressive Deterioration Scale; NPI, Neuropsychiatric Inventory.

Table 11.3 Benefit and risk of donepezil, galantamine, and rivastigmine in Alzheimer's disease: intent-to-treat analyses

	Treatment events (%)	Placebo events (%)	Odds ratio	95% confidence interval	Test for effect *P*-value	Number of studies
CIBIC-plus	Global assessment with carer input, no change or worse at 6 months					
Donepezil	293/390 (75)	356/409 (87)	0.46	0.32–0.66	<0.0001	2
Galantamine	319/392 (81)	338/398 (85)	0.78	0.53–1.12	0.18	2
Rivastigmine	468/660 (71)	551/693 (80)	0.63	0.49–0.81	0.0004	4
CIBIC-plus	Global assessment with carer input, no change or improved at 6 months					
Galantamine	263/392 (67)	212/399 (53)	1.82	1.36–2.43	<0.0001	2
Rivastigmine	505/759 (67)	350/615 (57)	1.47	1.18–1.84	0.0007	3
Withdrawals before the end of treatment						
Donepezil	171/725 (24)	146/735 (20)	1.25	0.97–1.60	0.08	5
Galantamine	173/705 (25)	116/714 (16)	1.67	1.29–2.17	<0.0001	3
Rivastigmine	367/1052 (35)	145/868 (17)	2.40	1.95–2.96	<0.00001	4
Withdrawals due to adverse events before the end of treatment						
Donepezil	99/711 (14)	67/721 (9)	1.58	1.14–2.19	0.006	5
Galantamine	107/705 (15)	45/714 (6)	2.09	1.51–2.91	<0.0001	3
Rivastigmine	257/1052 (24)	74/868 (9)	2.97	2.33–3.79	<0.00001	4

CIBIC-plus, Clinician Interview-Based Impression of Charge-plus.

trials of donepezil in 1219 patients with cognitive decline probably caused by vascular dementia. The donepezil (10 mg/day) group showed statistically significant benefit compared with placebo for cognitive function and activities of daily living. There is one published trial (Erkinjuntti *et al.*, 2002) on the use of galantamine in Alzheimer's disease and vascular dementia. There was no difference between galantamine and placebo for cognition, global assessment, activities of daily living, or behavioral symptoms in the vascular dementia subgroup of 188 patients.

There are no completed trials in acute delirium, although these are in progress. The majority of trials with patients suffering from Alzheimer's disease included only subjects with mild to moderate disease represented by Mini-Mental State Examination (MMSE) scores (out of 30) of 10 or 11 to 24 or 26 (Folstein *et al.*, 1975). This group of patients was targeted partly because they are at the stage of disease at which there seems most to gain from interventions, but also because of ethical difficulties in involving people too demented to give informed consent in trials of drugs with yet uncertain risks of adverse effects. Two studies of donepezil (Feldman *et al.*, 2001; Tariot *et al.*, 2001) included severely demented patients (MMSE 5–17) and there is no evidence to suggest that the effects of donepezil for such people differ

Table 11.4 Risk of donepezil, galantamine, and rivastigmine in Alzheimer's disease: adverse effects

	Treatment events (%)	Placebo events (%)	Odds ratio	95% confidence interval	Test for effect P-value	Number of studies
At least one adverse event of nausea at 6 months						
Donepezil	111/653 (17)	35/658 (5)	3.31	2.34–4.68	<0.00001	4
Galantamine	206/705 (29)	67/714 (9)	3.69	2.82–4.82	<0.00001	3
Rivastigmine	490/1052 (47)	105/868 (12)	5.40	4.44–6.58	<0.00001	4
At least one adverse event of vomiting at 6 months						
Donepezil	84/677 (12)	32/687 (5)	2.73	1.86–4.00	<0.00001	4
Galantamine	116/705 (16)	41/714 (6)	3.01	2.15–4.21	<0.00001	3
Rivastigmine	321/1052 (31)	49/868 (6)	5.28	4.19–6.65	<0.00001	4
At least one adverse event of diarrhea at 6 months						
Donepezil	105/677(16)	39/687 (6)	2.83	2.01–4.00	<0.00001	4
Galantamine	57/705 (8)	43/714 (6)	1.37	0.91–2.05	0.13	3
Rivastigmine	195/1052 (19)	99/868 (11)	1.77	1.38–2.28	<0.00001	4
At least one adverse event of anorexia at 6 months						
Donepezil	41/533 (8)	10/541 (2)	3.64	2.07–6.38	<0.00001	3
Galantamine	69/711 (10)	29/714 (4)	1.84	1.24–2.73	0.002	3
Rivastigmine	171/1052 (16)	27/868 (3)	4.46	3.31–6.01	<0.00001	4
At least one adverse event of headache at 6 months						
Donepezil	71/520 (14)	57/525 (11)	1.30	0.90–1.88	0.07	3
Galantamine	21/220 (10)	7/215 (3)	2.83	1.32–6.09	0.008	1
Rivastigmine	177/1052 (17)	97/868 (11)	1.61	1.24–2.10	<0.00001	4
At least one adverse event of abdominal pain at 6 months						
Donepezil	19/247 (8)	15/251 (6)	1.31	0.65–2.62	0.45	2
Galantamine	14/212 (7)	9/213 (4)	1.59	0.69–3.68	0.28	1
Rivastigmine	137/1052 (13)	51/868 (6)	2.24	1.65–3.05	<0.00001	4
At least one adverse event of dizziness at 6 months						
Donepezil	55/677 (8)	35/687 (5)	1.63	1.07–2.50	0.02	4
Galantamine	53/432 (12)	34/420 (8)	1.62	1.04–2.52	0.03	2
Rivastigmine	230/1052 (22)	114/868 (13)	1.29	1.00–1.67	0.05	4
At least one adverse event of tremor at 6 months						
Donepezil	8/103 (8)	2/105 (2)	3.58	1.01–12.71	0.05	1
Galantamine	11/212 (5)	1/213 (<1)	5.56	1.77–17.50	0.003	1
Rivastigmine	–	–	–	–	–	–
At least one adverse event of weight loss at 6 months						
Donepezil	30/247 (12)	16/251 (6)	2.02	1.09–3.73	0.02	2
Galantamine	43/432 (10)	11/428 (3)	3.55	2.04–6.17	<0.00001	2
Rivastigmine	–	–	–	–	–	–

from those for mildly to moderately demented patients. The data summarized in the tables relate only to subjects diagnosed as having Alzheimer's disease according to standardized criteria of National Institute of Neurologic, Communicative Disorders and Stroke and Alzheimer's Disease and Related Disorders Association (NINCDS-ADRDA) (McKhann *et al.*, 1984) and *Diagnostic and Statistical Manual, 3rd edition* (DSM-III-R) (American Psychiatric Association, 1987). These clinical criteria perform only moderately well against autopsy diagnosis of Alzheimer's disease, and variable individual responses may reflect differences in underlying pathological processes. There were minor differences between the trials in other inclusion and exclusion criteria.

In the summary tables presented, Tables 11.2–11.4, differences are noted as statistically significant where the 95% confidence intervals on the odds ratios do not embrace 1.0, and on the mean difference do not embrace zero. In Table 11.2 the results are presented on an intent-to-treat basis (which includes all patients who were randomized to treatment, received at least one dose of the study drug, and had at least one postbaseline assessment), and on an observed-case basis (which includes all randomized patients who had an evaluation on treatment at the designated endpoint). Despite the greater number of patients who did not complete treatment in the therapy group, the results are similar. The ADAS-Cog – the cognitive scale of the Alzheimer Disease and Associated Disorders scale (Rosen *et al.*, 1984) – and the MMSE are composite scores representing a range of different cognitive functions. For ADAS-Cog these include memory, orientation, spoken-language ability and comprehension, recall of test instructions, word-finding, following commands, naming objects, construction drawing, ideational praxis, orientation, word recall, and word recognition. There was a significant benefit in favor of the active treatment for donepezil, galantamine, and rivastigmine (−2.9, −3.5, and −2.6 points out of a total score of 70). With the ADAS-Cog a fall in score indicates functional improvement.

MMSE includes tests of orientation, immediate recall, attention and calculation, delayed recall, and language. The MMSE was originally devised as a screening instrument for cognitive impairment and its use in clinical trials to measure changes in function is common but not strictly appropriate, particularly as it is rather insensitive to change. Improvement is associated with an increase of score. There was a significant benefit in favor of the active treatment for donepezil and rivastigmine (1.4 and 0.8 points out of a total score of 30); MMSE was not assessed in the galantamine trials. The Clinician Interview-Based Impression of Change-plus (CIBIC-plus) (Schneider *et al.*, 1997) in Table 11.3 reflects the clinician's overall impression, also making use of carers' observations, of the degree to which a patient is better or worse than when seen initially. At first attendance the patient is allocated a score of 4 and the next score is noted in the range 1 (marked improvement) to 7 (marked deterioration). For the analyses reported in the trials, CIBIC-plus is dichotomized in one of two ways, either counting those patients assessed as worse or unchanged against those assessed as improved, or counting those assessed as unchanged or improved against those assessed as worse. For the first method, for donepezil and rivastigmine, treatment is significantly better than placebo, but there is no difference between galantamine and placebo. For the second method, for galantamine and rivastigmine, treatment is significantly better than placebo, but there are no data for donepezil.

Over the period that the drugs have been undergoing evaluation there have been important developments in the methodology of trials of antidementia interventions. This has included efforts to measure outcomes more directly related than cognitive function to the functional and behavioral manifestations of dementia and to the sense of well-being of patients and carers. The importance of such measures is reflected in the requirements of some regulatory bodies. The European Medicines Evaluation Agency, for example, requires assessment in at least two of the three domains of cognition, global assessment, and function. Outcomes other than cognition assessed in some of the studies were: activities of daily living as judged by a carer; neuropsychiatric features; quality of life; and severity of disease. Information on activities of daily living is assessed using several rating scales. The Disability Assessment for Dementia (DAD) scale (Gelinas *et al.*, 1999; Wilcock *et al.*, 2000) was used in trials of galantamine and donepezil. There was a significant difference in favor of treatment for donepezil; the magnitude was 8.0 points (total range 100 points) but not for the galantamine study. The rivastigmine studies all included an assessment of the activities of daily living using the Progressive Deterioration Scale (PDS) (DeJong *et al.*, 1989) and there was a significant benefit for treatment of 2.2 points (total range 100).

One study of galantamine and one of donepezil used the NPI (Cummings *et al.*, 1994) and found no difference between treatment and placebo for galantamine and a significant difference in favor of donepezil (5.6 points on a scale of 0–120). No rivastigmine studies assessed psychiatric features. A patient-rated measure of quality of life (Blau, 1977) was included in both the relevant studies of donepezil; there was no significant difference between treatment and placebo. The burden on carers was assessed in the four rivastigmine studies using the Caregiver Activity Survey (CAS), in which the carer estimates the time spent per 24 h helping the patient with the activities of daily living. The results are not mentioned in reports of the studies.

Adverse effects

As to be expected, adverse effects were quite common. Table 11.3 summarizes the data on withdrawals from treatment and placebo groups according to whether the withdrawal was due to an adverse event or for any reason. For all three drugs, withdrawals for any reason and withdrawals due to adverse events were significantly higher for treatment than for placebo groups. Fifteen percent of patients on treatment and 9% of those on placebo withdrew from the trials on account of adverse events but overall only 70% of patients on treatment completed the study, compared with 82% on placebo. Table 11.4 lists those specific adverse effects noted for one of more of the drugs to be significantly more common in the treatment than in the placebo groups. Not all types of adverse effects were reported in all trials, but as expected most are explicable in terms of the drugs' cholinergic actions. It is to be expected that rarer and idiosyncratic drug reactions will be seen in clinical practice, as will any long-term or delayed adverse effects not observable in short-term trials. Overall, specific adverse effects were more frequent in the treatment groups of the rivastigmine trials than in the trials of the other drugs but the same was true of the placebo groups, and the risk ratios between treatment and placebo groups were not consistently higher for rivastigmine. The titration schemes now recommended by the pharmaceutical companies for donepezil, galantamine, and rivastigmine, are more gradual than those used in these trials in order to decrease the risk of an adverse event.

There are two short-term randomized, single-blind, head-to-head studies comparing donepezil, galantamine, and rivastigmine. They were both of 12 weeks, duration and the drugs were administered according to the recommended regimens on the product labels. From a head-to-head study, Bullock *et al.* (2001) reported statistically significant benefit for donepezil compared with rivastigmine for the numbers that did not complete the 12 weeks of treatment (6/57 compared with 17/55, odds ratio (OR) (0.30 95% confidence intervals (CIs) 0.12–0.74, $P = 0.009$)), for the numbers who reported at least one adverse event of nausea (6/57 compared with 13/55, OR (0.28 95% CIs 0.10–0.79, $P = 0.0002$)), and vomiting (4/57 compared with 17/55, OR (0.30 95% CIs 0.12–0.74, $P = 0.02$)). Bullock *et al.* also reported that the carers and physicians rated satisfaction and ease of use as significantly better with donepezil than with rivastigmine, but did not present the relevant data.

The head-to-head study reported by Passmore *et al.* (2002) showed statistically significant benefit for donepezil compared with galantamine for the numbers who remained on the maximum dose during the 12 weeks' treatment (59/64 compared with 40/56, OR (0.24 95% CIs 0.09–0.62, $P = 0.003$)). Passmore *et al.* also reported, but without data, that the carers and physicians rated satisfaction and ease of use as significantly better with donepezil than with galantamine.

More recently, a 12-month head-to head-study of galantamine against donepezil has been reported (Wilcock *et al.*, 2003), in which there were no statistically significant differences in an activities of daily living scale as the primary outcome measure. However there were minor differences in favor of galantamine in some of the secondary outcome measures assessing cognition.

So which drug?

All three drugs show similar effects, and in the data from the trials there is no justification for concluding that any one is preferable. The trials were not designed to produce comparative evidence that could only emerge from direct "head-to-head" randomized trials of one drug against another. The two small head-to-head trials reported benefit for donepezil compared with galantamine and rivastigmine for ease of use and adverse gastrointestinal effects, but not for cognitive function and activities of daily living.

Important evidence about the utility of drugs often emerges from clinical experience. In clinical practice doctors often develop different dosage regimes, and particularly more gradual titration from starting to maintenance doses, that reduce the incidence of adverse effects. Conversely, a low incidence of adverse effects in trials, such as those reported here, where subjects were required to have a carer to help with dosages may be increased, or decreased, when the drug is prescribed in the real world of old people living alone. A simple once-a-day dosage regime, as possible with the long half-life of donepezil, may prove easier to manage in such circumstances. On the other hand, against the benefits of fewer errors in simpler dosage, there was evidence in the Cochrane review of rivastigmine that distributed dosage was associated with a lower incidence of withdrawals than less frequent regimens. In the one study that reported comparable data on twice-daily and thrice-daily dosage, the latter was associated with significantly fewer withdrawals due to adverse events at 26 weeks (24/227 compared with 39/228).

Clinical experience will also be necessary to extend knowledge about the benefits and risks of the drugs for patients not represented in the trials. In particular, frailer patients and those with significant comorbidity or taking other drugs were excluded, but are likely to present in the real world of clinical practice. Current evidence for benefit from the drugs is restricted to patients with mild to moderate cognitive impairment in all but two trials, but it is doubtful whether trials in earlier or more severe disease will be mounted before public pressure extends the use of the drugs to such areas. It is unfortunate that there are not more adequate formal arrangements in place to collect systematic data on how new drugs perform in clinical use. While more serious adverse effects are likely to emerge from ordinary postmarketing surveillance, even if rare, minor problems may be difficult to discern, even if common. More important is the absence of systematic monitoring of the natural history of illness in treated patients that might provide insight into the best strategy for prescribing the drugs.

Drug interactions can be anticipated, and some can be predicted from what is already known about the pharmacology of the ChEIs. It would not normally be logical to prescribe drugs that cross the blood–brain barrier and have anticholinergic actions. These will include some antiparkinsonian drugs, phenothiazines, antihistamines, and cimetidine. The drugs may interfere with the actions of muscle relaxants used in anesthesia. Care will also be needed in the use of medications that are likely to reinforce the peripheral cholinergic actions of the drugs. Of specific concern will be drugs that induce bradycardia such as beta-blockers, and the drugs will be best avoided for patients with sick sinus syndrome or cardiac conduction block. Care may also be needed with patients with urinary retention due to prostatic disease, with obstructive pulmonary disease or gastrointestinal complaints. The manufacturers of rivastigmine claim that the cytochrome P450 complex is less involved in the metabolism of rivastigmine than with donepezil or galantamine, but whether this leads to a lower risk of drug interactions will emerge in clinical practice.

Cost-effectiveness

Other things being equal, doctors and patient have an interest in choosing the cheapest drug or the one easiest to administer, for example, a once-daily dosage may be important for some people. But the drug that is cheapest at the point of delivery to the direct purchaser may not be the cheapest from the perspective of the health economist concerned with cost-effectiveness. Into the cost-effectiveness equation go the cost of the drug, its prescription and supervision, and the impact of any adverse effects, all set off against the direct benefits of the drug and any savings from other interventions avoided. With dementia treatments the discounted savings from delayed institutionalization are of particular significance, and the burden of care falling on relatives should be included in the equation. There have been several attempts at estimating the cost-effectiveness of the cholinergic drugs, but most have been vitiated by insufficient appropriate data (Fenn and Gray, 1999; Neumann *et al.*, 1999). A review of the three cholinergic drugs, commissioned for the National Institute of Clinical Excellence in the UK (Clegg *et al.*, 2002), reported that there are five economic evaluations of donepezil published, and four of rivastigmine, though none of galantamine. These studies were carried out in Europe or North America. The donepezil studies produced conflicting results, that cast doubt on the robustness of the estimates, and the rivastigmine studies were difficult to interpret owing to inadequate reporting of cost-effectiveness ratios. The review concluded that the main issue remains not the cost of the drugs but the impact across other aspects of care.

A recent study (Garfield *et al.*, 2002) estimated the economic impact on public health costs in Sweden of galantamine. As with several of the economic studies, the cost estimates are based on extrapolation of the results of cognitive tests from randomized controlled trials of patients with mild to moderate dementia to predict the time until full-time care in an institution is needed. The study reported that galantamine could increase the time before patients needed full-time care, and thus could prove to be a cost-effective treatment. The weakness of this study, as in several others, lies in the lack of robust data describing the progression of patients to full-time care and death with and without ChEI treatment. This same weakness applies to an economic evaluation of donepezil treatment for Alzheimer's disease in Japan (Ikeda *et al.*, 2002), which also concluded that there are small cost advantages of using donepezil.

Cholinesterase inhibitors in clinical practice

As there is no clear winner among the cholinesterase inhibitors, each physician will make an empirical choice and become familiar with a particular therapeutic regime. In some patients the slower titration that is possible with galantamine may be preferable, whilst in others a once-daily dosage may be essential for practical reasons. Whichever drug is given, the principles of prescribing thereafter are similar. A careful watch must be kept for adverse effects, and if they occur, a decision must be made about their management. In some people it will be necessary to discontinue the treatment, but in many cases the temporary use (2–3 days) of an antiemetic will help overcome nausea and vomiting, which often only occur for a short while during dose adjustment.

When adverse effects are due, as is usually the case, to the expected mode of action of the ChEIs, there is no scientific rationale for switching from one of the drugs to another. However, there may be clinical situations, for example where titration has proved difficult, a patient has developed an antipathy to a drug, or the carer expresses a strong preference where changing drugs may be required. It is important to bear in mind the half-life of the different drugs in this situation. Substituting a short-acting for a long-acting drug without allowing for a washout period could result in acute overdosage (Taylor *et al.*, 2002).

Responders and non-responders?

The efficiency of a drug may be improved by appropriate targeting – only prescribing it for those patients who benefit and only for as long as they continue to do so. An important proportion of the patients enrolled in the trials showed no improvement with the drugs, but no reliable indicators are yet available to identify which patients with Alzheimer's disease are likely to benefit. Many prescribing guidelines, including those in the UK from the National Institute for Clinical Excellence (2001), recommend an objectively monitored clinical trial for each patient. Formal diagnosis and assessment using accepted rating scales should be employed, and prescription should not be continued if there is no benefit. Defining absence of benefit is controversial. At what interval should it be assessed, given that Alzheimer's disease is progressive? Should a patient whose cognitive function shows no change over the assessment period be regarded as a responder or a non-responder? Clinical practice will undoubtedly evolve, but at present a trial period of 3 months, as endorsed in the UK by the National Institute of Clinical Excellence (2001), is commonly regarded as appropriate. Stabilization or improvement in score on the ADAS-Cog, MMSE, some form of global impression assessment, and activities of daily living performance over that period would normally indicate response, and deterioration non-response. For some patients, rating scales chosen more individually to reflect particular problems, for example challenging behavior, sleep disturbance, or incontinence, may be more relevant.

Ethical issues may arise; guidelines from bodies such as the National Institute of Clinical Excellence are aimed primarily at controlling drug costs, on a basis of overall cost-effectiveness, and should not be invoked to prevent optimal or humane care of individual patients. Changes in scores over an observation period need to be interpreted in the light of the background trend that can be expected from the "natural history" of a progressive disorder such as Alzheimer's disease. In clinical trials this is, on average, in the range of 2 points per year for the MMSE and 4.5 points per year for ADAS-Cog for the placebo groups. In other groups of patients faster decrements may be observed. There is also within-subject variation to consider. Over a period of time as short as 1 month, patients in the placebo group can show variation of as much as 5 points for the MMSE and 10 points for the ADAS-Cog. This will partly reflect fluctuation in a patient's condition and partly measurement error. Whether it is justifiable to extrapolate these data to the general population of patients with Alzheimer's disease is, of course, uncertain. Making individual patient decisions on the basis of average scores is even more questionable.

How should pharmacotherapy of Alzheimer's disorder continue?

The most difficult decision is when to stop treatment. If a problem such as the onset of agitation arises after the patient has been treated for some while on a stable dose, and this is suspected to be a late adverse event of treatment, the decision is relatively simple. In many instances, however, there will only be a suspicion that the treatment effect is wearing off, based either on a global impression, or deterioration on a scale if one is being used. In these circumstances it has been suggested that a "drug holiday" – discontinuation of treatment for a short period followed by reassessment – might be informative. Discontinuation is probably best initiated by gradually reducing the dose if there is scope for this, although the long half-life of donepezil may obviate this need. It is clinically unjustifiable, although it has been suggested (National Institute for Clinical Excellence, 2001), to specify a point on a scale, such as the MMSE, below which the drug is stopped automatically. Such a score should rather remind the physician to make a careful assessment of the situation when this stage is reached.

An important issue is whether temporarily stopping a ChEI might cause irreversible harm to a patient with Alzheimer's disease. There is no *a priori* pathophysiological reason why this should be so. A phase III, open-label extension study (Doody *et al.*, 2001) evaluated treatment with donepezil for up to 144 weeks. All patients entering the extension had completed a previous trial of donepezil, for either 12 weeks of treatment followed by 3 weeks' placebo washout, or 24 weeks' treatment followed by 6 weeks' washout. Doody *et al.* evaluated the progress of the patients who were classified by their previous treatment group by making comparisons between the groups within trials and concluded that after the 6-week washout the benefits of the previous 24 weeks of donepezil were completely lost, but for patients who had experienced a 3-week washout after 12 weeks of treatment some of the benefits were retained. However, this is not a randomized or blind trial and no standard errors are reported for any values and no statistical tests are reported. The report raises an important question but does not answer it.

Many clinicians will feel that if there is doubt about whether a drug is doing more harm – clinical or financial – than good, a trial of withdrawal is appropriate. If no obvious deterioration occurs and there is no significant change in performance scores after a washout period of around 6 weeks, restarting the drug is unlikely to produce benefit.

There are philosophical, and even political, dimensions to policy choices in this situation. Doctors remunerated on a fee-for-service basis, and pharmaceutical companies, will wish to believe that drugs, once started, should be continued under regular review. Salaried doctors, and insurers or governments who pay the bills, will be more interested in there being demonstrable benefit from treatment for each individual patient. It will not be surprising if different health care systems generate different patterns of clinical practice.

Treatment with drugs other than cholinesterase inhibitors

Memantine

A rational approach to the development of antidementia drugs based on the neurochemical pathology of these conditions has suggested another potentially useful drug, memantine, which modulates the glutamatergic system by blocking the (*N*-methyl-D-aspartate) (NDMA) type of glutamate receptor. L-glutamate is the main excitatory neurotransmitter in the central nervous system, implicated in the neural transmission of learning and memory processes and in neuronal plasticity (Sucher *et al.*, 1996). There is evidence that enhancement of the excitatory action of this amino acid plays a role in the pathogenesis of the damage due to an ischemic stroke and possibly in Alzheimer's disease (Cacabelos *et al.*, 1999). However, physiological glutamate activity is required for normal brain activity and cannot be abolished completely (Kornhuber and Weller, 1997). Low-affinity NMDA receptor antagonists, such as memantine, might prevent excitatory amino acid neurotoxicity without interfering with the physiological actions of glutamate that are required for learning and memory function.

Memantine was first synthesized as an agent to lower elevated blood sugar level, but was ineffective. Subsequently the drug was tested in animal models of cognition and found to reverse deficits in learning and synaptic plasticity. In the last 15 years it has been tested in trials involving people with Alzheimer's, vascular, and mixed dementia at different stages. In all studies the reported incidence and severity of adverse effects have been low. Memantine was approved in February 2002 by the European Agency for the Evaluation of Medicinal Products (2002) for the treatment of "moderately severe to severe Alzheimer's disease."

A systematic review (Areosa Sastre and Sherriff, 2004) included seven trials involving different types of dementia. The number of participants ranged from 60 to 579. The diagnosis of dementia was established using editions of the DSM. Only one study was restricted to people with Alzheimer's disease diagnosed according to NINCDS-ADRDA criteria. Three studies included Alzheimer's disease and vascular dementia in various proportions, with the Hachinski score used to differentiate the two.

Overall, the reviewers concluded that, at daily dosages of 20 or 30 mg, memantine was associated with a small improvement in cognitive function for at least 28 weeks in people with mild to moderate Alzheimer's disease, vascular, or mixed dementia. At the higher dose there was an early beneficial effect on mood and behavior. A significant improvement in global ratings in three trials suggested that the functional improvements were large enough to be of clinical relevance. The overall incidence of adverse events and dropouts did not differ significantly between treatment and placebo groups, but in three trials the incidence of restlessness or agitation was greater in the memantine than in the placebo group.

The data were not sufficient to permit analysis of results for people with Alzheimer's disease alone. It would now be regarded as ethically unacceptable to conduct placebo-controlled trials of drugs for Alzheimer's disease, and direct comparisons of memantine with ChEIs are required. Since the mechanism of action of memantine differs from that of the ChEIs, a factorial design trial of memantine versus ChEI versus both together would be valuable. There is also a need for longer-term studies.

Selegiline

Selegiline is an inhibitor of monoamine oxidase. It was originally developed as an antihypertensive agent but found to be ineffective for that purpose. It later found a place as ancillary treatment for Parkinson's disease, in which it prolongs the time over which patients function well enough to be able to continue working. In low doses it selectively inhibits monoamine oxidase B (MAO-B), an enzyme that accounts for 80% of monoamine oxidase activity in the brain, and is increased in the brains of people with Alzheimer's disease, possibly as a result of gliosis. Inhibition of MAO-B reduces the breakdown of dopamine and selegiline also inhibits presynaptic uptake of dopamine, so stimulating its synthesis. In high doses, selegiline also inhibits MAO-A, which breaks down norepinephrine (noradrenaline) and serotonin. Inhibition of oxidative deamination is thought to reduce oxidative damage to neurons.

The highest concentration of MAO-B is found in the hippocampus, a brain region with a crucial role in the memory function disturbed early and radically in Alzheimer's disease. By inhibiting MAO-B, selegiline may enhance catecholamine neurotransmission in this region. It has also been suggested that inhibition of MAO-B may reduce the production of free radicals and oxidative stress, thought to contribute to neuronal damage in Alzheimer's as in Parkinson's disease.

A systematic review using individual patient data from 14 trials that met specified quality criteria was reported on behalf of the trialists by Wilcock *et al.* (2002). This concluded that, although there was some evidence of improvement in cognition and activities of daily living associated with selegiline in the short term, the magnitude of the effect was not of clinical importance, and there was no evidence of long-term benefit.

Vitamin E

Vitamin E is a collective name for a group of naturally occurring lipid-soluble chemicals derived from tocopherol and tocotrienol. Alpha-tocopherol is the standard form for medical uses. The compounds are found in vegetable oils and nuts and are antioxidants that neutralize free radicals. Vitamin E supplements are widely available "over the counter" and have been claimed to prevent a wide range of age-associated diseases. A systematic review (Tabet *et al.*, 2004) found only one acceptable trial of vitamin E as treatment for Alzheimer's disease. In that trial, Sano *et al.* (1997) included vitamin E with selegiline in a 2 by 2 factorial study of people with moderately severe Alzheimer's disease. The outcome measures were based on time to reach prespecified endpoints indicative of increase in severity, including death and institutionalization. Preliminary analysis revealed no apparent benefit from vitamin E but unfortunately the placebo and treatment groups had not been comparable at baseline. When allowance was made for the significantly higher baseline MMSE scores in the placebo group, a benefit from vitamin E emerged. The appropriateness of the statistical methods used to derive this result was subsequently a topic of considerable and unresolved controversy.

Tabet *et al.* (2004) reanalyzed the published summary data of the trial by simply comparing the group receiving vitamin E alone with that receiving placebo. This analysis also found evidence of benefit from vitamin E; fewer patients reached the endpoints on vitamin E than on placebo (45/77 compared with 58/78, OR 0.49, 95% CI 0.49–0.96), associated with a significant but unexplained increase in the risk of falls. The reviewers concluded that, although the results were sufficiently promising to justify further research, the evidence for clinical efficacy of vitamin E in Alzheimer's disease was insufficient. Further trials are in progress.

Ginkgo biloba

Extracts of the leaves of ginkgo biloba, the maidenhair tree, have been a component of traditional Chinese medicine for centuries. The active components of ginkgo biloba consist of flavonoids and terpenoids, found extensively in plants, and terpene lactones (ginkgolides and bilobalide) that are unique to ginkgo biloba. A well-defined extract, EGb 761, is marketed as Tanakan, Tebonin, or Rökan. The extract is widely prescribed in Germany and France for cerebral insufficiency, a diagnosis that can cover a range of conditions, including memory and concentration problems, confusion, depression, anxiety, dizziness, tinnitus, and headache. It is not licenced as a drug in the UK, Canada, and the USA but is available as a food supplement.

The extract has been claimed to have a wide range of actions, including increasing blood supply by dilating arterioles, and reducing the density of free radicals. It has a low incidence of adverse effects, mostly gastrointestinal, but there have been isolated case reports of subdural hematoma associated with high doses and of hyphema (spontaneous bleeding into the anterior chamber of the eye) following combined therapy with ginkgo extract and aspirin. However, there is no consistent experimental evidence of an effect of ginkgo extract on blood clotting.

A systematic review (Birks *et al.*, 2004b) identified 33 trials, involving 3106 participants, of methodological quality sufficient for inclusion. The trials included participants with a range of possible diagnoses and the reviewers did not consider it feasible to analyze separately trials relating to people with Alzheimer's disease alone. Many of the trials were of small size and carried out in Germany under the sponsorship of the manufacturing company. These were early trials and tended to have more positive results than four more modern trials, but the methodology, the analyses, and reporting of results was open to criticism, and publication bias could not be excluded. The more recent trials were of larger size and the methodology has improved. Two of these showed no statistically significant benefit for ginkgo, one has not published sufficient information for interpretation, and another, that claimed benefit, used unsound methods. In a meta-analysis, there was evidence linking ginkgo extract with short-term benefits in cognition and activities of daily living and also in mood. It is possible that at least part of the benefits associated with ginkgo arose from an antidepressant action. There were no significant differences between treatment and placebo groups in the incidence or severity of adverse effects. The available evidence does not establish the efficacy of ginkgo biloba for dementia. A large trial using modern methods is now underway in the UK.

Piracetam

Piracetam (2-oxo-1-pyrrolidine-acetamide) is chemically related to the inhibitory neurotransmitter gamma-aminobutyric acid (GABA). It has been classed as a "nootropic," a group of drugs conceptualized as enhancing cognitive function without sedation or psychostimulation. It is marketed for the treatment of a wide range of "organic psychosyndromes" in countries where such diagnoses are still recognized, and for the treatment of cerebrovascular accidents. In the UK it is prescribed for the adjunctive treatment of cortical myoclonus.

A systematic review and meta-analysis by Waegemans et al. (2002) included 19 published and unpublished studies of piracetam for cognitive impairment. The outcome common to the studies was a measure of clinical global impression of change. Meta-analysis revealed significant benefits associated with piracetam. A test for heterogeneity between the studies was statistically highly significant ($P < 0.001$). Seventeen of the included studies enrolled participants with broad diagnoses implying cognitive impairment – "psycho-organic syndromes," "dementia syndromes," "disorders of senescence," "cerebral sclerosis," and "mild primary dementia." One recruited participants with age-associated memory impairment diagnosed according to Age-Associated Memory Impairment–National Institute of Mental Health criteria. Only one small study (Croisile et al., 1993) specifically involved people with Alzheimer's disease (NINCDS-ADRDA criteria) and produced non-significant results. The evidence at present therefore would justify further research rather than prescription for Alzheimer's disease.

Evidence from observational studies

Observational studies, case-control or cohort, can be valuable in generating hypotheses about factors in lifestyles or environment that might be protective against cognitive impairment or dementia. However, it is impossible reliably to exclude the influence of confounding factors in observational studies by statistical means, and only interventive studies can prove causation. It is unfortunate that the differing epistemological standing of observational and interventive studies is not better understood in the lay, and, all too often, the scientific press. In some cases it is clear that the inappropriate credence given to observational evidence is weighted by a degree of wishful thinking.

In studies of dementia, education and premorbid intelligence are particularly powerful influences. Higher education and intelligence are associated with lower risks for dementia and Alzheimer's disease but are also linked to wealth and healthy lifestyles, factors particularly linked in developed societies to cardiovascular disease. However education and intelligence may also equip a person to preserve mental function by deploying compensatory mechanisms against brain damage from Alzheimer's disease or other pathology.

Hormone replacement therapy

Extensive observational data suggested that hormone replacement therapy might reduce the incidence of coronary heart disease in postmenopausal women (Grady *et al.*, 1992), although Barrett-Connor (1991) had warned of the impact of bias arising from the social and behavioral patterns linked with use or non-use of hormone replacement therapy. Observational data had also suggested that hormone replacement therapy might benefit the cognitive function of postmenopausal women and reduce the incidence of dementia (Zandi *et al.*, 2002). A systematic review (Hogervorst *et al.*, 2004a) found little evidence of benefit from estrogen, with or without progestogen, on cognitive function of postmenopausal women. What evidence there is would be compatible with a short-term benefit secondary to relief of severe postmenopausal symptoms. A systematic review of hormone replacement therapy to maintain cognitive function in women with dementia (Hogervorst *et al.*, 2004b) identified five trials involving 210 women with Alzheimer's disease and found no evidence of clinically significant benefit.

A long-term randomized controlled trial of estrogen and progestogen was halted prematurely as treatment was found to be associated with an increased risk of coronary heart disease as well as breast cancer, stroke, and pulmonary embolism (Writing Group for the Women's Health Initiative Investigators, 2002). A further report of this study found that estrogen plus progestogen increased rather than decreased the risk of dementia (Schumaker *et al.*, 2003). Whether this effect was mediated through an impact on Alzheimer's disease or cerebrovascular disease is speculative. The estrogen-only branch of the study is continuing, and it may yet emerge that the progestogen rather than hormone replacement therapy *per se* is responsible for the ill effects so far reported.

Anti-inflammatory drugs

It has been suggested that inflammatory processes may be involved in the brain damage produced by Alzheimer's disease and observational studies have found an association between the use of anti-inflammatory drugs and a lower risk of Alzheimer's disease (Etminan *et al.*, 2003). There is a paucity of evidence from clinical trials. Tabet and Feldman (2004) were able to find only one trial of indometacin for people with Alzheimer's disease. Treatment was not associated with benefit in terms of cognitive function, and, as to be expected, there was a higher incidence of adverse effects in the treatment than in the placebo group. Trials with ibuprofen, and other non-steroidal anti-inflammatory drugs, are under way.

Statins

Observational studies have also identified the statin group of drugs, used for treating certain types of hyperlipidemia, as having a possible protective effect against dementia (Jick *et al.*, 2000; Wolozin *et al.*, 2000). This may not be a class effect, as not all statins are associated with a lower risk of dementia. Trials are needed to ascertain whether this is truly an effect of these compounds, or results from inclusion or other biases in the cohort studies (Scott and Laake, 2004).

Folate deficiency and hyperhomocysteinemia

Low blood folate level is a further factor linked to dementia and Alzheimer's disease in observational studies (Snowdon *et al.*, 2000). Here the problem is whether the folate deficiency is a cause of the dementia or a consequence of the poor diet taken by many demented people. One consequence of folate deficiency is accumulation of homocysteine in the blood stream and within cells. Hyperhomocysteinemia is a risk factor for cardiovascular disease so low folate might contribute to a vascular component of dementia. High intracellular levels of homocysteine might also have a directly toxic effect on neurons. It is also possible that folate deficiency may affect central neuronal function by other mechanisms. There is no good evidence from trials of folic acid in the treatment or prevention of Alzheimer's disease, but good clinical care should ensure that patients are not deficient in folate or any other vitamin.

What is the best pharmacotherapy approach to resistant Alzheimer's disorder?

Clearly much is now happening and clinical practice will change rapidly. At present, people with mild to moderate Alzheimer's disease merit a trial of a ChEI for at least 3 months. If there is no response, or initial benefit is lost, memantine can be substituted or added. Memantine is specifically licenced in Europe for patients presenting with severe Alzheimer's disease, but many clinicians will also try ChEIs in this situation on the grounds that there is no evidence that they will not work with severe as with mild to moderate disease.

At present the evidential base for prescribing other drugs is less well established. Whether doctors feel able to endorse the use of ginkgo biloba will depend partly on the cost to their patients in countries where it is not reimbursable by the health services. While it has been recognized since the work of Sigmund Freud that patients value a treatment in proportion to how much it has cost them, most patients with Alzheimer's disease are not only old but poor.

The dementing disorders such as Alzheimer's disease are among the cruellest afflictions with which nature plagues the human race. Patients and their carers will want treatment to be prescribed, and will want to believe that it works. The only drugs without adverse effects are those that do not work at all. In dealing with dementia, doctors face in particularly stark form the need to balance human realities against the costs and risk of adverse effects from pharmacologically powerful drugs.

REFERENCES

American Psychiatric Association (1987). *Diagnostic and Statistical Manual of Mental Disorders*, 3rd edn. Washington, DC: American Psychiatric Association.

Anand, R., Gharabawi, G., and Enz, A. (1996). Efficacy and safety results of the early phase studies with Exelon (ENA-713) in Alzheimer's disease: an overview. *Journal of Drug Development and Clinical Practice*, **8**, 109–16.

Areosa Sastre, M. A. and Sherriff, F. (2004). Memantine for dementia (Cochrane Review). In: *The Cochrane Library*, issue 1, 2004. Chichester, UK: John Wiley.

Barrett-Connor, E. (1991). Postmenopausal estrogen and prevention bias. *Annals of Internal Medicine*, **115**, 455–6.

Bentham, P., Gray, R., Hill, R., Sellwood, E., and Courtney, C. (2002). Twelve week response to cholinesterase inhibitors does not predict future benefit, the AD2000 trial experience. In: *The 8th Conference on Alzheimer's Disease and Related Disorders*. Stockholm, Sweden, 337.

Birks, J. and Harvey, R. (2004).The efficacy of donepezil for mild and moderate Alzheimer's disease (Cochrane Review). In: *The Cochrane Library*, issue 1, 2004. Chichester, UK: John Wiley.

Birks, J., Grimley Evans, J., Iakovidou, V., and Tsolaki, M. (2004a). Rivastigmine for Alzheimer's disease (Cochrane Review). In: *The Cochrane Library*, issue 1, 2004. Chichester, UK: John Wiley.

Birks, J., Grimley Evans, J., and Van Dongen, M. (2004b). Ginkgo biloba for dementia and cognitive impairment (Cochrane Review). In: *The Cochrane Library*, issue 1, 2004. Chichester, UK: John Wiley.

Blau, T. H. (1977). Quality of life, social indicators and criteria of change. *Professional Psychologist*, **8**, 464–73.

Blessed, G., Tomlinson, B. E., and Roth, M. (1968). The association between quantitative measures of dementia and of senile change in the cerebral grey matter of elderly subjects. *British Journal of Psychiatry*, **114**, 797–811.

Bullock, R., Passmore, P., Potocnik, F., and Hock, C. (2001). The tolerability, ease of use and efficacy of donepezil and rivastigmine in Alzheimer's disease patients: a 12-week, multinational, comparative study. *Journal of the American Geriatrics Society*, **49**, S19.

Burns, A., Rossor, M., Hecker, J., *et al.* (1999). The effects of donepezil in Alzheimer's disease – results from a multinational trial. *Dementia and Geriatric Cognitive Disorders*, **10**, 237–44.

Cacabelos, R., Takeda, M., and Winblad, B. (1999). The glutamatergic system and neurodegeneration in dementia: preventive strategies in Alzheimer's disease. *International Journal of Geriatric Psychiatry*, **14**, 3–47.

Clegg, A., Bryant, J., Nicholson, T., *et al.* (2002). Clinical and cost-effectiveness of donepezil, rivastigmine, and galantamine for Alzheimer's disease: a systematic review. *International Journal of Technology Assessment in Health Care*, **18**, 497–507.

Corey-Bloom, J., Anand, R., and Veach, J. for ENA 713 B352 Study Group. (1998). A randomized trial evaluating the efficacy and safety of ENA 713 (rivastigmine tartrate), a new acetylcholinesterase inhibitor, in patients with mild to moderately severe Alzheimer's disease. *International Journal of Geriatric Psychopharmacology*, **1**, 55–65.

Croisile, B., Trillet, M., Fonderai, J., *et al.* (1993). Long-term and high-dose piracetam treatment of Alzheimer's disease. *Neurology*, **43**, 301–5.

Cummings, J. L., Mega, M., Gray, K., *et al.* (1994). The neuropsychiatric inventory: comprehensive assessment of psychopathology in dementia. *Neurology*, **44**, 2308–14.

DeJong, R., Osterlund, O. W., and Roy, G. W. (1989). Measurement of quality-of-life changes in patients with Alzheimer's disease. *Clinical Therapeutics*, **11**, 545–54.

Doll, R., Peto, R., Boreham, J., and Sutherland, I. (2000). Smoking and dementia in male British doctors: prospective study. *British Medical Journal*, **320**, 1097–102.

Doody, R. S., Geldmacher, D. S., Gordon B., *et al.* (2001). Open-label, multicenter, phase 3 extension study of the safety and efficacy of donepezil in patients with Alzheimer's disease. *Archives of Neurology*, **58**, 427–33.

Erkinjuntti, T., Kurz, A., Gauthier, S., *et al.* (2002). Efficacy of galantamine in probable vascular dementia and Alzheimer's disease combined with cerebrovascular disease: a randomised trial. *Lancet*, **359**, 1283–90.

Etminan, M., Gill, S., and Samii, A. (2003). Effect of non-steroidal anti-inflammatory drugs on risk of Alzheimer's disease: systematic review and meta-analysis of observational studies. *British Medical Journal*, **327**, 128–31.

European Agency for the Evaluation of Medicinal Products (2002). Committee for Proprietary Products European Public Assessment Report (EPAR). Ebixa, international nonproprietary name (INN) Memantine. CPMP/1604/02. Available online at: www.eudra.org/humandocs/PDFs/EPAR/ebixa/160402en1.pdf.

Feldman, H., Gauthier, S., Hecker, J., *et al.* (2001). A 24-week, randomized, double-blind study of donepezil in moderate to severe Alzheimer's disease. *Neurology*, **57**, 613–20.

Fenn, P. and Gray, A. (1999). Estimating long term cost savings from treatment of Alzheimer's disease. *Pharmacoeconomics*, **16**, 165–74.

Folstein, M. F., Folstein, S. E., and McHugh, P. R. (1975). 'Mini-Mental State': a practical method for grading the cognitive state of patients for the clinician. *Journal of Psychiatric Research*,

12, 189–98.

Garfield, F. B., Getsios, D., Caro, J. J., Wimo, A., and Winblad, B. (2002). Assessment of health economics in Alzheimer's disease (AHEAD). *Pharmacoeconomics*, **20**, 629–37.

Gelinas, I., Gauthier, L., McIntyre, M., and Gauthier, S. (1999). Development of a functional measure for persons with Alzheimer's disease: the disability assessment for dementia. *American Journal of Occupational Therapy*, **53**, 471–81.

Grady, D., Rubin, S. M., Petitti, D. B., *et al.* (1992). Hormone therapy to prevent disease and prolong life in postmenopausal women. *Annals of Internal Medicine*, **117**, 1016–37.

Hogervorst, E., Yaffe, K., Richards, M., and Huppert, F. (2004a). Hormone replacement therapy for cognitive function in postmenopausal women (Cochrane Review). In: *The Cochrane Library*, issue 1, 2004. Chichester, UK: John Wiley.

Hogervorst, E., Yaffe, K., Richards, M., and Huppert, F. (2004b). Hormone replacement therapy to maintain cognitive function in women with dementia (Cochrane Review). In: *The Cochrane Library*, issue 1, 2004. Chichester, UK: John Wiley.

Homma, A., Imai, Y., Hagiguchi, S., *et al.* (1998). Late phase II clinical study of acetyl cholinesterase inhibitor E2020 in patients with Alzheimer-type dementia. *Clinical Evaluation*, **26**, 251–84.

Homma, A., Takeda, M., Imai, Y., *et al.* (2000). Clinical efficacy and safety of donepezil on cognitive and global function in patients with Alzheimer's disease: a 24-week, multicenter, double-blind, placebo-controlled study in Japan. *Dementia and Geriatric Cognitive Disorders*, **11**, 299–313.

Ikeda, S., Yamada, Y., and Ikegami, N. (2002). Economic evaluation of donepezil treatment for Alzheimer's disease in Japan. *Dementia and Geriatric Cognitive Disorders*, **13**, 33–9.

Jick, H., Zornberg, G. L., Jick, S. S., Seshadri, S., and Drachman, D. A. (2000). Statins and the risk of dementia. *Lancet*, **356**, 1627–31.

Kewitz, H., Berzewski, H., Rainer, M., *et al.* (1994). Galantamine, a selective non-toxic acetyl-cholinesterase inhibitor is significantly superior over placebo in treatment of SDAT. *Neuropsychopharmacology*, **10**, 130S.

Kornhuber, J. and Weller, M. (1997). Psychotogenicity and N-methyl-D-aspartate receptor antagonism: implications for neuroprotective pharmacotherapy. *Biological Psychiatry*, **41**, 135–44.

López-Arrieta, J. M., Rodriguez, J. L., and Sanz, F. (2004). Efficacy and safety of nicotine on Alzheimer's disease patients (Cochrane Review). In: *The Cochrane Library*, issue 1, 2004. Chichester, UK: John Wiley.

Maloof, R. and Birks, J. (2004). Donepezil for cognitive vascular impairment (Cochrane Review). In: *The Cochrane Library*, issue 1, 2004. Chichester, UK: John Wiley.

McKeith, I., Del Ser, T., Spano, P., *et al.* (2000). Efficacy of rivastigmine in dementia with Lewy bodies: a randomised, double-blind, placebo-controlled international study. *Lancet*, **356**, 2031–6.

McKhann, G., Dracman, D., Folstein, M., *et al.* (1984). Clinical diagnosis of Alzheimer's disease: report of the NINCDS-ADRDA work group under the auspices of Department of Health and Human Services Task Force on Alzheimer's disease. *Neurology*, **4**, 939–44.

Meadows, M. E., Sperling, R. A., Growdon, J. H., *et al.* (2000). Donepezil therapy in clinical practice: a randomized crossover study. *Archives of Neurology*, **5**, 94–9.

Mohs, R. C., Doody, R. S., Morris, J. C., *et al.* (2001). A 1-year, placebo-controlled preservation of function survival study of donepezil in AD patients. *Neurology*, **57**, 481–8.

National Institute for Clinical Excellence (2001). Guidance on the use of donepezil, rivastigmine and galantamine for the treatment of Alzheimer's disease. Available online at: www.nice.org.uk/pdf/ALZHEIMER_full_guidance.pdf.

Neumann, P. J., Hermann, R. C., Kuntz, K. M., *et al.* (1999). Cost-effectiveness of donepezil in the treatment of mild or moderate Alzheimer's disease. *Neurology*, **52**, 1138–45.

Neuropathology Group of the Medical Research Council Cognitive Function and Ageing Study (MRC CFAS) (2001). Pathological correlates of late-onset dementia in a multicentre, community-based population in England and Wales. *Lancet*, **357**, 169–75.

Nordberg, A., Hellstrom-Lindahl, E., Lee, M., *et al.* (2002). Chronic nicotine treatment reduces beta-amyloidosis in the brain of a mouse model of Alzheimer's disease (APPsw). *Journal of Neurochemistry*, **81**, 655–8.

Olin, J. and Schneider, L. (2004). Galantamine for Alzheimer's disease (Cochrane Review). In: *The Cochrane Library*, issue 1, 2004. Chichester, UK: John Wiley.

Passmore, P., Wetterberg, P., Alder, G., *et al.* (2002). First head to head study comparing the tolerability, ease of use and efficacy of donepezil and galantamine in Alzheimer's disease. In: *The 8th Conference on Alzheimer's Disease and Related Disorders*. Stockholm, Sweden.

Qizilbash, N., Whitehead, A., Higgins, J., *et al.* (1998). Cholinesterase inhibition for Alzheimer's disease: a meta-analysis of the tacrine trials. Dementia Trialists' Collaboration. *Journal of the American Medical Association*, **280**, 1777–82.

Raskind, M. A., Peskind, E. R., Wessel, T., *et al.* (2000). Galantamine in AD: a 6-month randomized placebo-controlled trial with a 6-month extension. *Neurology*, **54**, 2261–8.

Robert, P., Lebert, F., Goni, S., *et al.* (2000). The impact on caregiver distress of donepezil treatment of patients with mild Alzheimer's disease. In: *Proceedings of the Quality Research in Dementia*. London.

Rockwood, K., Mintzer, J., Truyen, L., *et al.* (2001). Effects of a flexible galantamine dose in Alzheimer's disease: a randomized, controlled trial. *Journal of Neurology, Neurosurgery and Psychiatry*, **71**, 589–95.

Rogers, S. L., Friedhoff, L. T. and the Donepezil Study Group (1996). The efficacy and safety of donepezil in patients with Alzheimer's disease: results of a US multicentre, randomised, double-blind, placebo-controlled trial. *Dementia*, **7**, 293–303.

Rogers, S. L., Doody, R. S., Mohs, R. C., *et al.* (1998a). Donepezil improves cognition and global function in Alzheimer disease. *Archives of Internal Medicine*, **158**, 1021–31.

Rogers, S. L., Farlow, M. R., Doody, R. S., *et al.* (1998b). A 24-week, double-blind, placebo-controlled trial of donepezil in patients with Alzheimer's disease. *Neurology*, **50**, 136–45.

Rosen, W. G., Mohs, R. C., and Davis, K. L. (1984). A new rating scale for Alzheimer's disease. *American Journal of Psychiatry*, **41**, 356–64.

Rösler, M., Anand, R., Cicin-Sain, A., *et al.* (1999). Efficacy and safety of rivastigmine in patients with Alzheimer's disease: international randomised controlled trial. *British Medical Journal*, **319**, 633–8.

Sano, M., Ernesto, C., Thomas, R. G., *et al.* (1997). A controlled trial of selegiline, alpha tocopherol, or both as treatment for Alzheimer's disease. *New England Journal of Medicine*, **336**, 1216–22.

Schneider, L. S., Olin, J. T., Doody, R. S., *et al.* (1997). Validity and reliability of the Alzheimer's disease cooperative study-clinical global impression of change. *Alzheimer Disease and Asso-*

ciated Disorders, **11** (suppl. 2), 22–32.

Schumaker, S. A., Legault, C., Rapp, S. R., *et al.* (2003). Estrogen plus progestin and the incidence of dementia and mild cognitive impairment in postmenopausal women. The Women's Health Initiative Memory Study: a randomized controlled trial. *Journal of the American Medical Association*, **289**, 2651–62.

Scott, H. D. and Laake, K. (2004). Statins for the prevention of Alzheimer's disease (Cochrane Review). In: *The Cochrane Library*, issue 1. 2004. Chichester, UK: John Wiley.

Snowdon, D. A., Tully, C. L., Smith, C. D., Riley, K. P., and Markesbery, W. R. (2000). Serum folate and the severity of atrophy of the neocortex in Alzheimer disease: findings from the Nun study. *American Journal of Clinical Nutrition*, **71**, 993–8.

Sucher, N. J., Awobuluyi, M., Choi, Y. B., and Lipton, S. A. (1996). NMDA receptors: from genes to channels. *Trends in Pharmacological Science*, **17**, 348–55.

Tabet, N. and Feldman, H. (2004). Indomethacin for the treatment of Alzheimer's disease patients (Cochrane Review). In: *The Cochrane Library*, issue 1, 2004. Chichester, UK: John Wiley.

Tabet, N., Birks, J., Grimley Evans, J., Orrel, M., and Spector, A. (2004). Vitamin E for Alzheimer's disease (Cochrane Review). In: *The Cochrane Library*, issue 1, 2004. Chichester, UK: John Wiley.

Tai, C. T., Liu, C. K., Sung, S. M., Pai, M. C., and Hsu, C. Y. (2000). The safety and efficacy of Exelon in Alzheimer's patients: a multicentre, randomized, 26-week study in Taiwan. *International Journal of Neuropsychopharmacology*, **3** (suppl. 1), S356.

Tariot, P. N., Solomon, P. R., Morris, J. C., *et al.* (2000). A 5-month, randomized, placebo-controlled trial of galantamine in AD. *Neurology*, **54**, 2269–76.

Tariot, P. N., Cummings, J. L., Katz, I. R., *et al.* (2001). A randomised, double-blind, placebo-controlled study of the efficacy and safety of Donepezil in patients with Alzheimer's disease in the nursing home setting. *Journal of the American Geriatrics Society*, **49**, 1590–99.

Taylor, A. M., Hoehns, J. D., Anderson, D. M., and Tobert, D. G. (2002). Fatal aspiration pneumonia during transition from donepezil to rivastigmine. *Annals of Pharmacotherapy*, **36**, 1550–3.

Tune, L. E., Tiseo, P. J., Hoffman, J. M., *et al.* (1998). Functional brain activity in Alzheimer's disease. In: *Proceedings of the 151st Annual Meeting of the American Psychiatric Association*. Toronto: NR345.

Waegemans, T., Wilsher, C. R., Danniau, A., *et al.* (2002). Clinical efficacy of piracetam in cognitive impairment: a meta-analysis. *Dementia and Geriatric Cognitive Disorders*, **13**, 217–24.

Wilcock, G. K. and Esiri, M. M. (1982). Plaques, tangles and dementia: a quantitative study. *Journal of Neurological Science*, **56**, 343–56.

Wilcock, G. K., Esiri, M. M., Bowen, D. M., and Smith, C. C. T. (1982). Alzheimer's disease: correlation of cortical choline acetyltransferase activity with the severity of the dementia and histological abnormalities. *Journal of Neurological Science*, **57**, 407–17.

Wilcock, G. K., Lilienfeld, S., and Gaens, E. (2000). Efficacy and safety of galantamine in patients with mild to moderate Alzheimer's disease: multicentre randomised controlled trial. Galantamine International-1 Study Group. *British Medical Journal*, **321**, 1445–9.

Wilcock, G. K., Birks, J., Whitehead, A., and Grimley Evans, J. (2002). The effect of selegiline in the treatment of people with Alzheimer's disease: a meta-analysis of published trials.

International Journal of Geriatric Psychiatry, **17**, 175–83.

Wilcock, G., Howe, I., Coles, H., *et al.* (2003). A long-term comparison of galantamine and donepezil in the treatment of Alzheimer's disease. *Drugs and Aging*, **20**, 777–89.

Wild, R., Pettit, T., and Burns, A. (2004). Cholinesterase inhibitors for dementia with Lewy bodies (Cochrane Review). In: *The Cochrane Library*, issue 1, 2004. Chichester, UK: John Wiley.

Wilkinson, D. and Murray, J. (2001). Galantamine: a randomized, double-blind, dose comparison in patients with Alzheimer's disease. *International Journal of Geriatric Psychiatry*, **16**, 852–7.

Winblad, B., Engedal, K., Soininen, H., *et al.* (2001). A 1-year, randomized, placebo-controlled study of donepezil in patients with mild to moderate AD. *Neurology*, **57**, 489–95.

Wolozin, B., Kellman, W., Rousseau, P., Celesia, C. G., and Siegel, G. (2000). Decreased prevalence of Alzheimer disease associated with 3-hydroxy-3-methylglutaryl coenzyme A reductase inhibitors. *Archives of Neurology*, **57**, 1439–43.

Writing Group for the Women's Health Initiative Investigators (2002). Risk and benefits of estrogen plus progestin in healthy postmenopausal women. Principal results from the Women's Health Initiative randomized controlled trial. *Journal of the American Medical Association*, **288**, 321–33.

Zandi, P. P., Carlson, M. C., Plassman, B. L., *et al.* (2002). Hormone replacement therapy and incidence of Alzheimer disease in older women. The Cache County study. *Journal of the American Medical Association*, **288**, 2123–9.

12

Drug interactions

C. Lindsay DeVane

Medical University of South Carolina, Charleston, SC, USA

Introduction

Daily exposure to multiple drugs has become a fact of life for an increasing proportion of the population. Reasons for this situation include the appearance of chronic disease with advancing age, the development of drugs with highly specific pharmacologic effects, and evidence that health benefits accrue from prophylaxis of an increasingly recognized number of preventable illnesses. Also, the popularity of herbal preparations is increasing, and unanticipated short-term illness, especially infections and transient painful conditions, frequently require intervention with brief, but potent, drug treatment. As the number of drugs taken on a daily basis increases, concern also rises about the occurrence of harmful drug interactions. Among the elderly, many hospitalizations for drug toxicity (Juurlink *et al.*, 2003) occur after avoidable administration of a drug known to cause drug interactions. The frequency and cost of serious adverse drug reactions are high (Azaz-Livshits *et al.*, 1998; Moore *et al.*, 1998) and drug-related morbidity and death occur in both hospital and ambulatory settings (Juntti-Patinen and Neuvonen, 2002; Gandhi *et al.*, 2003). Meta-analyses of deaths occurring in hospital implicate drugs as a contributing factor in many cases. Many of these serious adverse drug events are presumed to result from drug interactions.

Numerous drug interactions involving psychoactive drugs have been reported in the literature and the theoretical numbers of interactions are much higher. These predictions are supported by recognition that many drugs are metabolized by identical enzymatic pathways and that competitive inhibition can occur between drugs with high affinity for the same enzyme when given in sufficiently high doses. Additionally, some psychoactive drugs have the capacity independently to inhibit or induce the activity of drug-metabolizing enzymes (Fang and Gorrod, 1999). This situation creates concern for patient safety as the stability of many psychiatric patients is often fragile, even brittle, and poor drug tolerability as a result of adverse drug events from a drug interaction can have a pronounced effect on well-being. The reality that drug interactions can contribute to morbidity has sensitized clinicians to the need to anticipate and avoid drugs in combination that may interact.

The number of potential drug interactions is too high for a practical memorization of all drug combinations that produce potentially significant interactions. In addition, the literature on drug interactions is expanding at such a rapid pace that the interpretation of the clinical significance of combining specific drugs is frequently unclear. An evidence-based approach to classifying all the reported drug interactions in psychiatry is beyond the scope of this chapter. However, an alternative to memorization of drug combinations is to develop an understanding of the principles underlying drug interactions. This should serve to increase confidence that individualizing pharmacotherapy with previously unencountered drug combinations may be advantageous and can be accomplished in a safe and effective manner without producing untoward consequences.

This chapter will explain some fundamental principles of pharmacokinetics as they apply to drug interactions. The mechanism most often documented in investigations of pharmacokinetic interactions is an inhibition or induction of metabolic clearance of one drug by another (Markowitz and DeVane, 1999, 2000). The degree of alteration in clearance is a primary determinant of the magnitude of a change in systemic drug concentration. This change, in turn, influences the magnitude of change in pharmacologic effect from an interaction. By understanding some basic concepts of pharmacokinetic interactions, the clinician should be better able to foresee the consequences of many drug combinations and avoid untoward events. An intuitive prediction of an alteration in clearance can be made with as little data as a knowledge of the individual drug's elimination pathways. A more quantitative prediction can be made using inhibitory constants of drugs obtained *in vitro*. Complementary data includes knowledge of previous patients who have received the drug combination in question and the results of formal drug interaction studies conducted in humans. Most often, complete information is unavailable to guide the clinician. The discussion below, preceded by comments on the history of drug interactions in psychiatry, focuses on key pharmacokinetic principles that serve as a background for the use of data in subsequent tables that allow potential interactions to be identified.

Historical perspective of drug interactions in psychiatry

Some drug interactions in psychiatry have been documented to result in severe clinical consequences. Most of these interactions are mediated by a pharmacokinetic mechanism while some result from pharmacodynamic consequences at sites of action. However, pharmacokinetic interactions may ultimately lead to adverse or toxic reactions of a pharmacodynamic nature (Bhatara *et al.*, 1998). Particularly notable are drug interactions with lithium and the monoamine oxidase inhibitors. Lithium toxicity as a result of fluid and electrolyte imbalance secondary to changes in hydration status and/or co-administration of specific diuretics is one of the most predictable drug interactions in psychopharmacology. The combination of a monoamine oxidase inhibitor with a tricyclic antidepressant or sympathomimetic amine can result in an unbridled catecholamine stimulation with a consequent hypertensive response. These severe, but relatively rare, outcomes of drug interactions have served to emphasize a need early in the modern history of psychopharmacology to collect systematic evidence of drug interactions during the initial phases of a drug's development. Regulatory agencies now routinely require specific studies for documentation of safety regarding drug interactions. Specific sections on drug interactions are routinely incorporated into product prescribing information and package labeling.

In the 1980s, relatively few new antipsychotics or antidepressants became available for clinical use that differed substantially in their pharmacologic effects from the existing phenothiazines and other conventional antipsychotics and from the tricyclic antidepressants. There was a clear need during this period for alternative drugs, as mirrored by the popularity of combining drugs from these two classes to improve therapeutic outcomes. A few commercial products were available that consisted of fixed combinations of a phenothiazine and tricyclic. One widely prescribed product combined perhenazine with amitriptyline. In retrospect, these combination products were irrational and contributed to underdosing of depression along with the development of tardive dyskinesia. Ironically, they combined drugs that interacted with each other.

A few investigations were reported in the 1980s of drug interactions between antidepressants and antipsychotics. Notable were the studies demonstrating that tricyclics and antipsychotics could cause an apparent mutual metabolic inhibition that raised the plasma concentration of both drugs compared to their administration separately. Loga *et al.* (1981) showed that this practice led to increased side-effects in some patients (Kudo and Ishizaki, 1999; Shin *et al.*, 1999). About the same time as the above reports were appearing, there was increasing recognition of the role of specific P450 isozymes in the metabolism of psychoactive drugs. This advancement in pharmacology stimulated a decade of intense research activity into drug interactions that continues today.

With the introduction of the selective serotonin reuptake inhibitors (SSRIs) in the late 1980s and early 1990s, it was natural to combine fluoxetine and other members of this new drug class with the tricyclics in order to improve treatment response in recalcitrant depressed patients. This practice produced a few reports of increased tricyclic plasma concentration secondary to the addition of an SSRI. Subsequent investigations revealed that drug interactions were occurring with fluoxetine through inhibition of the metabolism of the tricyclic causing an increase in the tricyclic plasma concentration. Given the lack of specific studies at that time of the various SSRIs combined with drugs commonly used in medical practice, the field had to rely upon *in vitro* studies to determine the affinity and inhibitory constants of the various antidepressants for P450 enzymes. These data were eventually supplemented with data from healthy volunteer pharmacokinetic studies investigating interactions of specific SSRIs with drugs selected as representative of all substrates for a particular P450 enzyme. From these data, extrapolations could be made that a specific SSRI would inhibit the metabolism of various substrates metabolized by the same enzymatic pathway. One result of these studies has been the prediction of numerous potential drug–drug interactions, but confirmatory data have been slow to emerge. Most drug–drug interactions are only problematic under certain circumstances.

Classification of drug interactions

Drug interactions can be classified into one or more of three different categories. Pharmaceutic interactions occur through physical interactions of drugs *ex vivo*. Interactions of this type are less likely to occur in the practice of psychiatry than in other medical specialties where drugs are more often mixed for intravenous administration (oncology, infectious disease, parenteral nutrition).

A second category of interactions are pharmacodynamic. These occur when drugs interact in the body to produce alterations of pharmacologic effects at a site of action (Sternbach, 1991; Demers and Malone, 2001). Such sites are commonly thought to involve receptors but can also occur at membrane ion channels, enzymes, or other sites. An alteration of effect occurs in the absence of a change in drug concentration; however, a drug concentration change may be independent of the change in pharmacodynamic effect. Pharmacodynamic interactions are commonly referred to as additive, synergistic, or antagonistic, depending upon the specific change in pharmacologic effect. Pharmacodynamic interactions are not necessarily undesirable as some drugs are commonly administered for their intended effects with other drugs. Examples include drug combinations in the treatment of infectious disease, in neurology, and in oncology. The overall effect of administering selected drug combinations in these areas of medicine is to produce a greater and more beneficial effect than either of the drugs given alone. Often, the sum of the combined effects appears greater than each of the drug's individual contributions. In psychiatry, unplanned pharmacodynamic interactions between drugs can be difficult to detect as they may be subtle and the measurement instruments are not always available to quantify their magnitude. Obviously, as these interactions by definition occur at sites of action, they are difficult to assess in psychiatry as the sites of action are generally located in the central nervous system.

Pharmacokinetic interactions are the third and often most easily studied category of drug interactions. However, the clinical significance of a pharmacokinetic interaction is not always so easily determined. The threshold for producing a measurable and clinically meaningful change in pharmacologic effect may be above the threshold for producing a change in drug concentration. This situation, where drug concentration changes without a change in pharmacologic effect, can be viewed as clinically insignificant and so such interactions in routine clinical care may go undetected unless prospectively studied. The significance of drug interactions could be easily determined if the following information were available with each psychoactive drug interaction: a measurement of the plasma concentration time course of all interacting drugs, definition of the applicable clinical circumstances, and a quantitative measure of the patient's pharmacologic effects. As the clinical effects of psychoactive drugs are often not immediately apparent, investigation of their interactions is hindered by an inability to determine when there is an unfavorable effect on the patient.

Of the several means by which one drug may have its concentration altered by another, the most common are interactions that result in a change in drug clearance. With chronic dosing, clearance is the pharmacokinetic parameter that determines the steady-state concentration of a drug in the body. Clearance may either be increased or decreased, resulting in a decrease or increase in drug concentration, respectively. In recent years, the effect of cytochrome P450 induction or inhibition on clearance has been extensively studied. An understanding of the concept of drug clearance and its relationship to steady-state drug concentration improves the ability to predict the consequences of pharmacokinetic interactions.

Pharmacokinetic principles

Role of drug clearance

A drug's clearance, often estimated following data collected in a single-dose study, is the major determinant of the steady-state concentration when the drug is chronically administered. A single-dose study often suffices for estimating clearance as this parameter remains relatively constant across the range of clinically useful doses for most drugs. The utility of knowing a drug's clearance is different from knowing its elimination half-life ($t^{1/2}$), the most commonly quoted pharmacokinetic parameter. Knowledge of a drug's elimination half-life enables a prediction of the time required for drug to be completely eliminated from the body upon cessation of dosing and also the time to achieve a steady-state drug concentration in the body with constant dosing. This period of time is equal to a multiple of 4 to 5 times the value of the elimination half-life. Half-life determinations do not enable a prediction of the magnitude of steady-state drug concentration, or the change in concentration

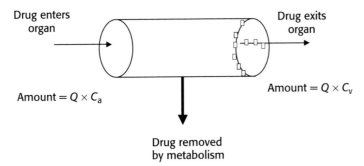

Figure 12.1 Organ clearance model for drug elimination. Drug entering the organ is the product of blood flow (Q) and arterial drug concentration (C_a) and the amount leaving is the product of blood flow (Q) and venous concentration (C_v).

that may occur following a drug interaction, although half-life may be altered by an interaction (DeVane, 1998).

Drugs that circulate in the blood are cleared from the body by being extracted by an eliminating organ, mostly the kidneys or liver. For drugs that undergo renal clearance, drug molecules are subject to glomerular filtration followed by elimination in the urine. Depending upon the specific drug, some renal tubular reabsorption or tubular secretion may occur. This process of clearing a drug from the body by the kidney is analogous to creatinine clearance. Drug clearance is defined as the volume of blood from which drug is irreversibly removed per unit of time. Thus, like renal clearance of creatinine, drug clearance has units of volume/time. Nearly all drugs undergo some degree of renal clearance, although most psychoactive drugs are highly metabolized and may be excreted in the urine as a small percentage ($<5\%$) of the unchanged form of the administered drug.

Hepatic clearance of drugs can be viewed in much the same manner as renal clearance. To illustrate this concept, a simple organ clearance model for drug elimination can be considered, as shown in Figure 12.1. Assume that the liver does not accumulate drug, so that all drug that enters via the arterial circulation (C_a) either exits the organ in the venous circulation (C_v) or is removed during passage through the liver by metabolism. The amount of drug that is removed by the organ is the amount that is extracted over time. To quantify this process, an extraction ratio, E, can be calculated as follows:

$$E = (C_a - C_v)/C_a \qquad \text{(equation 1)}$$

The amount entering the organ is controlled by the hepatic blood flow, Q. Thus, clearance can be expressed as:

$$Cl = Q(C_a - C_v)/C_a \qquad \text{(equation 2)}$$

and simplified to:

$$Cl = Q \times E \qquad \text{(equation 3)}$$

Physiologically, clearance of drug by an organ is equal to the blood flow to the organ times the extraction ratio of the organ. Its numerical value reflects how much of a drug delivered to an organ is irreversibly removed over time.

The ability of hepatocytes to extract and then metabolize drugs as they pass through the liver is influenced by several factors. The degree of plasma protein binding of drugs, the amount and activity of metabolizing enzymes, and the affinity between drug and enzyme will all contribute to how efficiently drugs are extracted. As many hepatic enzymes can exist in a polymorphic form, genetic heritability plays a role in drug extraction by the liver (Otani and Aoshima, 2000). Many enzymes can be induced or inhibited, so their activity is an important determinant of the extraction ratio. As can be seen from equation 3, clearance is proportional to the extraction ratio, E. How a change in hepatic enzyme activity can influence the extraction ratio and, in turn, influence a change in steady-state drug concentration, can be conceptualized by the following equation relating steady-state drug concentration in plasma (C_{pss}) with clearance:

$$C_{pss} = F \times \text{dose}/Cl \times \tau \qquad \text{(equation 4)}$$

This equation states that the steady-state plasma drug concentration is determined by a drug's bioavailability, F, the size of the dose, Dose, divided by the value of clearance adjusted for the dosage interval, τ. Thus, any influence on clearance will cause the drug concentration to change in the opposite direction. Well-recognized influences on clearance include age, diet, and the concomitant administration of some drugs.

The difference in utility of knowing clearance and half-life may be usefully illustrated with an example. Two drugs with a similar elimination half-life (mean of 12–16 h) are valproate and clozapine. They are also typically given in a similar dosage, 600 mg/day, but chronic dosing results in widely different steady-state plasma concentrations. For example, 100 μg/ml for valproate is regarded as a therapeutic concentration while 350 ng/ml is usual and appropriate for clozapine. Thus, valproate circulates at a therapeutic concentration nearly 300-fold higher than clozapine, yet the drugs have similar half-lives. The explanation is due to the much higher hepatic extraction and clearance for clozapine, 11–105 l/h, compared to an average clearance for valproate of 0.5–1.1 l/h (Eiermann et al., 1997). Differences in bioavailability and distribution may contribute to fluctuations of drug concentration over a dosage interval, but it is the value of clearance as shown in equation 4 that is the major determinant of the average steady-state plasma drug concentration. Any change in clearance produced by a drug interaction results in a change in steady-state drug concentration that may influence pharmacologic effects.

Role of protein binding

The role of drug protein binding is often mentioned in conjunction with drug interactions. Psychoactive drugs, with few exceptions such as lithium and gabapentin, circulate in the blood bound to various plasma proteins. For most drugs, the percentage of total circulating concentration bound to proteins is quite high, frequently greater than 90%. A widely accepted principle is that it is the free, non-protein-bound drug that is available to distribute to target sites outside the circulation. Thus, drug interactions that result in displacement of drug from their plasma protein-binding sites could theoretically increase the amount of free drug available to produce pharmacologic effects. In reality, the displacement of one drug from its protein-binding sites by another drug frequently results in only a transient change in free drug concentration that is buffered by a compensatory change in clearance or a change in bioavailability. This restores the free drug concentration to its pre-interaction value, although total drug concentration in plasma may be reduced. For this reason, the clinical significance of protein-binding drug interactions has likely been overemphasized in the literature (DeVane, 2002).

Mechanisms of pharmacokinetic drug interactions

Various opportunities exist for one drug to influence another drug's concentration or time course of passage through the body. Each of the elements of a drug's disposition, including absorption, protein binding and distribution, hepatic metabolism, and renal elimination, offer opportunities for one drug to interfere with the usual transit of another drug through the body.

Altered bioavailability

Most psychoactive drugs are administered orally, with the expectation that they will produce a high enough concentration at the target sites of action to be clinically effective. The movement of an orally administered drug through the body occurs with interactions of numerous membranes, carrier proteins, and enzymes. Specific physiological mechanisms exist either to impede a drug's progress or hasten its elimination. In evolutionary terms, these processes appear to have developed in response to the need to protect critical organs from insult by chemicals in the environment. They are first encountered by a drug in the gastrointestinal tract and can be influenced by concomitant drug administration.

For drugs to be absorbed orally, they must solubilize from a solid dosage form shortly after administration. Drug complexation, decreased peristaltic

Table 12.1 Selected substrates, inhibitors, and inducers of P-glycoprotein and the major human P450 (CYP) and uridine glucuronyltransferase (UGT) enzymes involved in drug metabolism. Drugs used in psychiatry that are CYP substrates are shown in Table 12.2

Enzyme or transporter	Substrates	Inhibitors	Inducers
P-glycoprotein	Amitriptyline, olanzapine, risperidone, quetiapine, methadone, digoxin, verapamil, rifampin	Verapamil, quinidine	St. John's wort
CYP1A2	Caffeine, theophylline, verapamil, warfarin	Fluoroquinolones (ciprofloxacin, norfloxacin, fluvosamine, cimetidine)	Charcoal-broiled beef, cigarette smoke, cruciferous vegetables, marijuana smoke, omeprazole
CYP2A6	Coumarin, nicotine	Tranylcypromine	Barbiturates
CYP2B6	Nicotine, tamoxifen, cyclophosphamide		Phenobarbital, cyclophosphamide
CYP2C9	Metoclopramide, diclofenac, phenytoin, propranolol, tetrahydrocannabinol, tolbutamide, warfarin	Fluvoxamine, D-propoxyphene, disulfiram, fluconazole, sulfaphenazole	Rifampin, phenytoin, secobarbital
CYP2C19	Ibuprofen, S-mephenytoin, moclobemide, naproxen, omeprazole, piroxicam, tenoxicam	Omeprazole	Rifampin
CYP2D6	Codeine, debrisoquin, dextromethorphan, metoclopramide, metoprolol, mexiletine, ondansetron, orphenadrine, pindolol, propafenone, propranolol, timolol	Fluoxetine, paroxetine, quinidine, sertraline	None identified *in vivo*
CYP2E1	Ethanol, caffeine, dapsone	Disulfiram	Ethanol
CYP3A4	Amiodarone, caffeine, clarithromycin, codeine, cortisol ciclosporin, erythromycin, estradiol, ethinylestradiol, lidocaine, lovastatin, nicardipine, nifedipine, omeprazole, ondansetron, orphenadrine, quinidine, rifampin, tamoxifen, verapamil	Fluoxetine, fluvoxamine, detoconazole, naringenin, cimetidine, erythromycin, indinavir, ritonavir, saquinavir	Barbiturates, dexamethasone, phenytoin, rifampin, St. John's wort
UGT1A3	Amitriptyline, chlorpromazine, clozapine, doxepin, ibuprofen, imipramine, ketoprofen, morphine, naloxone, naproxen, valproate		
UGT1A4	Amitriptyline, chlorpromazine, clozapine, imipramine, lamotrigine, olanzapine		
UGT1A9	Acetaminophen (paracetamol), dapsone, ethinylestradiol, furosemide, ibuprofen, ketoprofen, labetalol, naproxen, propranolol		
UGT2B7	Chloramphenicol, codeine, fenoprofen, ibuprofen, ketoprofen, morphine, nalorphine, naloxone, naltrexone, oxazepam, propranolol, valproate, temazepam		

movements, and alteration in gastric pH favoring an ionized species are all mechanisms whereby one drug may interfere with the absorption of another. It should be noted that the process of drug absorption implies both the rate at which drugs move across the gastrointestinal membranes as well as the completeness of the absorbed dose.

While not usually considered a drug interaction, the effect of food on drug absorption is a practical consideration in drug administration. There are rare examples of food increasing the amount of drug absorbed (propranolol, theophylline), but the presence of food usually serves to diminish the rate of drug absorption, prolonging the time to reach maximum plasma concentration following a dose, and/or diminishing the maximum concentration obtained in plasma following a single dose. Food effects on drug absorption tend to be less significant when drugs are taken in regard to meals in a consistent daily manner.

A major determinant of oral drug bioavailability is the activity of P-glycoprotein (P-gp) (Carson *et al.*, 2002). P-gp is a transmembrane transport pump that causes the efflux of various drugs from cells. It is one of a family of transporter proteins that serve a protective function of critical organs by excluding small molecules from passing membranes. For drugs that are substrates of P-gp, some portion of an oral dose will be excluded from absorption by affinity for P-gp which deposits the drug back into the gastrointestinal tract. The distribution of P-gp in the body includes the epithelial cells lining the luminal surface of enterocytes in the small intestine as well as the endothelial cells making up the blood–brain barrier. The now well-recognized effects of flavonoids (or other constituents) in grapefruit juice, increasing the bioavailability of various drugs, is believed to be in part due to an inhibitory effect on intestinal P-gp (Markowitz *et al.*, 2000).

The significance of P-gp for drug interactions in psychiatry is that several psychoactive drugs are substrates for P-gp. These are listed in Table 12.1. The activity of P-gp can be both inhibited and induced and inducers and inhibitors of P-gp may alter the amount of a substrate that is absorbed following oral administration. An example of an interaction involving P-gp is the effect that the herbal preparation St. John's wort produces to reduce the plasma concentration of digoxin and other drugs. Constituents in St. John's wort induce the activity of intestinal P-gp, which in turn increases the effectiveness of this protein transporter in limiting access of drugs to the systemic circulation.

Altered protein binding

Most drugs circulate in the blood bound to some extent to plasma proteins. The fraction of the total drug circulating in plasma that is bound to proteins depends upon several factors. These include the drug concentration, its affinity for the binding protein, and the protein concentration and number of available binding sites.

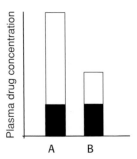

Figure 12.2 The influence of a displacement interaction on the total and free-drug concentration of a low-extraction restrictively cleared drug. A, bound + free drug during monotherapy; B, bound + free drug following displacement interaction. Filled columns, drug circulating as unbound; open columns, drug bound to protein.

Drug–protein binding is normally a reversible process and occurs so rapidly that a disturbance in the amount bound is quickly countered by a reequilibration. The potential consequences of changes in drug binding from a displacement interaction are best understood by examining the effects on clearance.

The effects of a protein-binding displacement interaction differ for drugs according to whether their extraction ratio as they pass through the liver is high or low relative to the hepatic blood flow. For all drugs, a protein-binding displacement interaction will immediately increase the free fraction of drug in plasma. This situation allows more free drug to distribute to sites of action outside the circulation. It also means more free drug is exposed to organs of elimination. For drugs that have a low extraction ratio by the liver, an increase in free fraction from a binding interaction results in a greater drug clearance. An increased clearance causes the total drug concentration in plasma to fall. Consequently, this fall in total concentration results in a return of free drug to its pre-interaction level. The transient increase in free drug concentration may or may not be clinically significant. The results of this binding interaction are shown in Figure 12.2.

For drugs that are highly extracted by the liver, a binding displacement interaction also transiently increases the free fraction in plasma. However, this increase will be offset by a decrease in oral bioavailability. The binding interaction results in a small but meaningful increase in the extraction ratio which diminishes the amount of drug absorbed. The consequences of this displacement interaction are a lower bioavailability that decreases the total concentration resulting in little or no change in free concentration compared with the pre-interaction situation. The consequence of these interactions, for drugs that have either a low or high hepatic extraction, is that total concentration of drug in plasma has decreased while the free concentration, although not the free fraction, has remained the same.

Theoretically, no change in pharmacologic effect should occur after reequilibration. With no change in free concentration, then no reason exists to increase the daily dose, even though a measurement of total drug in plasma suggests an interaction has decreased the plasma concentration. Examples of this type of interaction can be found with the anticonvulsant/mood-stabilizer drugs. Displacement of phenytoin from its albumin-binding sites can result in a lower total drug concentration in plasma but no need to increase the dose to maintain therapeutic effects as the free concentration has not changed.

Enzyme induction

Drug metabolism in the liver is accomplished by phase I and phase II enzymes as the principal means by which the body eliminates drugs and xenobiotics ingested from the environment. Although many foreign compounds undergo some degree of renal elimination, these processes are complementary and form a substantial physiological barrier to the organism being overcome by ingested chemicals in food and the environment. The general effect of drug metabolism is to render foreign compounds more water-soluble so that they may be excreted more easily in the urine. Given the extraordinary diversity of chemicals to which humans are exposed, the body has developed numerous enzymes to cope with their presence and accomplish biotransformation.

Phase I enzymes oxidize drugs to more elemental forms. Of the phase I reactions, the cytochrome P450 family of enzymes has stimulated the most recent research. Phase II enzymes biotransform drugs by conjugating them with another molecule, such as glucuronide, sulfate, glycine, and glutathione (Liston *et al.*, 2001). The most prominent of the phase II enzymes are the family of uridine glucuronyl-transferases (UGTs). Phase I and II enzymes are complementary in the sense that, following oxidation by a cytochrome P450 enzyme, many drugs then undergo glucuronidation before excretion. Psychoactive drugs are substrates for phase I and II enzymes, although the precise enzymes for metabolizing many drugs have not been determined. The principal pathways for psychoactive drug disposition are listed in Table 12.2.

Most enzymes can be inhibited and/or induced. The term enzyme induction generally refers to a process whereby an increased amount of enzyme is available in an eliminating organ to extract substrate drugs. The result is an increased ability to perform metabolism which increases the extraction ratio and clearance (equations 1 through 3) and reduced steady-state plasma drug concentration (equation 4).

An increased amount of enzyme can occur through two broad mechanisms. Either the rate of synthesis of new enzyme can be increased or the rate of degradation of enzyme can be slowed. Most induction phenomena occur by increased synthesis (Sogawa and Fujii-Kuriyama, 1997; Bertilsson *et al.*, 1998; Lehmann *et al.*, 1998). Of

Table 12.2 Pharmacokinetic drug interaction pharmacology of selected psychoactive drugs

Drug	Pathways of elimination	Inhibitory (inductive) potential	Effects on other drugs[a]	Effects by other drugs[a]
Anxiolytics				
Alprazolam	Renal <2%; CYP3A4			Common CYP3A4 inhibitors (ketoconazole, itraconazole, erythromycin, nefazodone, fluoxetine, fluvoxamine, cimetidine) and inducers (St. John's wort, carbamazepine)
Buspirone	CYP3A4			
Clonazepam	Renal <2%; non-P450 reduction			Phenytoin, carbamazepine, phenobarbital decrease plasma concentration by 30%
Diazepam	CYP2C19; CYP3A4			
Lorazepam	UGTs			
Oxazepam	UGTs			
Sedative/hypnotics				
Flurazepam	CYP?, UGTs			Expected effects from non-selective inhibitors (cimetidine, disulfiram)
Temazepam	UGTs			Lacks well-documented interactions
Triazolam	CYP3A4, UGTs			Ketoconazole, erythromycin, diltiazem, nefazodone, ritonavir, grapefruit juice; reduced by rifampicin
Zaleplon	Aldehyde oxidase (major), CYP3A4 (minor)			Cimetidine
Zolpidem	CYP3A4, CYP1A2, CYP2D6, UGTs			Inhibited by ritonavir, induced by rifampicin; no change by cimetidine
Tricyclic/older antidepressants				
Amoxapine				
Amitriptyline	CYP1A2; CYP2C9/19; CYP2D6			
Clomipramine	CYP1A2; CYP2C19			
Desipramine	CYP2D6			

Table 12.2 (*cont.*)

Drug	Pathways of elimination	Inhibitory (inductive) potential	Effects on other drugs[a]	Effects by other drugs[a]
Imipramine	CYP2D6; CYP2C19	CYP2C19		
Nortriptyline	CYP2D6			
Trazodone	CYP3A4; CYP2D6	CYP3A4		
Newer antidepressants				
Bupropion	CYP2B6	CYP2D6	Desipramine; other CYP2D6 substrates	No effect by cimetidine
Citalopram	CYP2C19; CYP3A4			
Duloxetine	CYP1A2; CYP2D6			
Escitalopram				
Fluoxetine	Renal 2–5%; CYP2D6; multiple isozymes	CYP2D6 inhibitor Inhibitory constant <1 μmol/l; weak effects norfluoxetine on CYP3A4		
Fluvoxamine	CYP1A2; CYP2D6	CYP1A2; CYP2C19; CYP2C9; CYP3A4		
Mirtazapine	CYP2D6; CYP3A4			
Nefazodone	CYP3A4	CYP3A4		
Paroxetine	Renal 2%; CYP2D6	CYP2D6	Desipramine; other CYP2D6 substrates	
Sertraline	Renal <5% Multiple CYP isoforms: 2D6; 2C9; 2B6; 2C19; 3A4 glucuronidation of metabolites	Weak inhibitor of CYP2D6; 3A4; 2C19		
Venlafaxine	CYP2D6			
Traditional antipsychotics				
Chlorpromazine	CYP2D6; CYP3A4	CYP2D6		
Haloperidol	CYP1A2; CYP2D6; CYP3A4	CYP2D6		
Fluphenazine	CYP2D6	CYP2D6		
Perphenazine	CYP2D6	CYP2D6		
Thioridazine	CYP2D6	CYP2D6		

(*cont.*)

Table 12.2 (*cont.*)

Drug	Pathways of elimination	Inhibitory (inductive) potential	Effects on other drugs[a]	Effects by other drugs[a]
Trifluperazine				
Atypical antisychotics				
Aripiprazole	CYP2D6; CYP3A4			
Clozapine	CYP1A2; CYP3A4			
Olanzapine	CYP1A2; CYP2D6; UGTs			
Risperidone	CYP2D6; CYP3A4			
Quetiapine				
Ziprasidone	CYP3A4			
Mood stabilizers				
Carbamazepine	CYP3A4	(CYP2C19); (CYP3A4); UGTs		
Gabapentin	Renal Cl = 100%			
Lamotrigine				
Lithium	Renal Cl = 100%			
Topiramate				
Valproate	UTGs (50%); P450 oxidation (10%)	CYP2C9; UGTs	Plasma concentration including: clozapine, lamotrigine, lorazepam, zidovudine; binding interactions with phenytoin	Aspirin (binding); lamotrigine (NS); UGT inducers
Psychostimulants				
Atamoxetine	CYP2D6			
Amfetamine	CYP2D6			
Methylphenidate				
Modafinil				
Cognition promoters				
Donepezil	Renal Cl = 17%; CYP3A4; CYP2D6; UGTs			Ketoconazole and quinidine; no effect of cimetidine

Table 12.2 (*cont.*)

Drug	Pathways of elimination	Inhibitory (inductive) potential	Effects on other drugs[a]	Effects by other drugs[a]
Galantamine	Renal Cl = 20%; CYP2D6; CYP3A4; UGTs	No effects *in vitro*		CYP2D6 and CYP3A4 inhibitors; ketoconazole and paroxedine, cimetidine
Rivastigmine	Hydrolysis by esterases (non-P450)	No P450 effects	Not expected	
Tacrine	CYP1A2	CYP1A2	Theophylline (competitive inhibition of CYP1A2)	Cimetidine including AUC 64%; fluvoxamine

[a] CYP, cytochrome P450; UGTs, uridine diphosphate glucuronyltransferases; NS, rarely or non-significant; AUC, area under the drug concentration versus time-curve. UGT inducers: phenytoin, carbamazepine, phenobarbital; rifampin.

the major P450 enzymes, CYP1A2, CYP2E1, and CYP3A4 are subject to induction. Some known inducers are listed in Table 12.1. While CYP enzymes show broad variability in their inherent activity, induction of CYP1A2 is controversial and induction of CYP2D6 is generally acknowledged not to occur.

Enzyme induction takes a variable amount of time to occur. Once an inducer is introduced in the body, the effects on enzyme activity may not peak until days or weeks later. In a similar manner, once an inducer is withdrawn, a period of days or weeks may be required for the enzyme activity to return to the pre-induction state. Common enzyme inducers include several of the mood stabilizers/anticonvulsants (phenobarbital, phenytoin, carbamazepine), cigarette smoking, and alcohol. Unfortunately, the precise increase in extraction efficiency by enzyme induction has been difficult to predict, but is generally a graded phenomenon dependent upon the dose of inducer.

Enzyme inhibition

Inhibition of drug-metabolizing enzymes is a more common mechanism of drug interactions in psychiatry than enzyme induction. Inhibition can occur as a reversible effect where the normal function of the enzyme returns as the inhibitor is eliminated from the body. The basis for this type of interaction is a competitive inhibition as the inhibitor prevents further binding of the substrate to its metabolizing enzyme. Theoretically, any two drugs metabolized by the same enzyme, if administered in sufficiently high doses, could compete for binding sites, resulting in an inhibition of metabolism of one or both compounds. Other types of inhibition are characterized as non-competitive and mechanism-based. These interactions occur with more irreversible characteristics. Typically, an inhibitor binds to an enzyme and prevents it from metabolizing normal substrates or forms an inactive complex which requires the synthesis of new enzyme for the metabolic activity to be restored to normal. For all types of enzyme inhibition, the outcome is a reduced clearance and increased plasma drug concentration of the affected substrate. The inhibitor itself may or may not be a substrate of the inhibited enzyme.

In contrast to the delayed effects of an inducer, administration of an inhibitor can have a more immediate effect on the clearance of other drugs. While the time required for an inhibited drug to reach a new steady-state plasma concentration will depend upon the change in clearance and elimination half-life, the full inhibitory effects may not be apparent until the inhibitor has also reached a steady-state concentration upon its chronic dosing. The clinical significance of enzyme inhibition will partly depend upon how important that specific enzyme is to the overall elimination of a particular substrate. In Table 12.2, many psychoactive drugs can be noted to be metabolized by several CYP enzymes. If an inhibited enzyme is the primary means of elimination of the drug of interest, then the interaction will be more prominent than if the inhibited enzyme is of only minor importance in the drug's overall elimination.

Prediction of *in vivo* drug interactions

Given the theoretically large numbers of psychoactive drug-co-medication combinations that could be administered, an efficient approach to predict the occurrence and clinical significance of drug interactions is unavailable. However, a rudimentary approach can be used by knowing the pathways of elimination of drug combinations selected for use. Table 12.1 lists common drugs that are substrates for P-gp and the most common CYP and UGT enzymes involved in drug metabolism. Table 12.2 lists major drugs used in psychiatry, their elimination pathways, and a notation of whether they have been implicated as having the potential to interfere with the clearance of other drugs and documented effects from other drugs. When drugs are eliminated by the same pathways, then a potential for interaction exists. Unfortunately, for many marketed drugs this information is incomplete. The development of new drugs is now accompanied by identification of the specific enzymes involved in their elimination along with an assessment of their potential to cause enzyme induction and inhibition. When drugs are combined with any of the specific inhibitors or inducers, then a pharmacokinetic interaction can be anticipated. Unfortunately, these predictions do not allow for an estimate of the magnitude or clinical significance of an interaction. The clinical significance of a psychoactive drug interaction depends upon multiple factors, including the clinical state of the patient, the order in which drugs were administered to the patient, the doses used, length of dosing, and other patient-specific factors.

Some newer antidepressants have shown a potent ability to inhibit some CYP enzymes. Fluoxetine and paroxetine have *in vitro* determined inhibitory constants in the micromolar range for the CYP2D6 enzyme. This implies that a potent inhibitory effect should occur for all co-administered CYP2D6 substrates. However, even in well-controlled pharmacokinetic studies, these drugs do not reliably convert extensive metabolizers of CYP2D6 to the poor metabolizer status. In a prospective, postmarketing surveillance program of over 200 patients, we were unable to confirm that the newer antidepressants inhibited concomitant pharmacotherapy in all but a few individuals (DeVane *et al.*, 2001). Part of the explanation for this lack of documented interaction may lie in how clinicians dose antidepressants and other psychoactive drugs. The usual routine is to start with low doses and proceed according to patient response and tolerability. This approach to pharmacotherapy may ameliorate the expression of drug interactions in some patients by allowing a tolerance to any increased drug concentration to occur. Also, as most drugs are metabolized by multiple enzymes, then compensatory pathways may play a proportionally larger role in overall clearance as one enzymatic pathway is blocked. Nevertheless, drug interactions do occur and by applying fundamental knowledge of drug metabolism and pharmacokinetic principles, they can be predicted and appropriate precautions taken to avoid untoward effects.

REFERENCES

Azaz-Livshits, T., Levy, M., Sadan, B., *et al.* (1998). Computerized surveillance of adverse drug reactions in hospital: pilot study. *British Journal of Clinical Pharmacology*, **45**, 309–14.

Bertilsson, G., Heidrich, J., Svensson, K., *et al.* (1998). Identification of a human nuclear receptor defines a new signaling pathway for CYP3A induction. *Proceedings of the National Academy of Science of the USA*, **95**, 12208–13.

Bhatara, V. S., Magnus, R. D., Paul, K. L., and Preskorn, S. H. (1998). Serotonin syndrome induced by venlafaxine and fluoxetine: a case study in polypharmacy and potential pharmacodynamic and pharmacokinetic mechanisms. *Annals of Pharmacotherapy*, **32**, 432–6.

Carson, S. W., Ousmanou, A. D., and Hoyler, S. L. (2002). Emerging significance of P-glycoprotein in understanding drug disposition and drug interactions in psychopharmacology. *Psychopharmacology Bulletin*, **36**, 67–81.

Demers, J. C. and Malone, M. (2001). Serotonin syndrome induced by fluvoxamine and mirtazapine. *Annals of Pharmacotherapy*, **35**, 1217–20.

DeVane, C. L. (1998). Clinical implications of dose-dependent cytochrome P-450 drug interactions with antidepressants. *Human Psychopharmacology*, **13**, 329–36.

   (2002). Clinical significance of drug plasma protein binding and binding displacement drug interactions. *Psychopharmacology Bulletin*, **36**, 5–21.

DeVane, C. L., Markowitz, J. S., Liston, H. L., and Risch, S. C. (2001). Charleston Antidepressant Drug Interactions Surveillance Program (CADISP). *Psychopharmacology Bulletin*, **35**, 50–61.

Eiermann, B., Engel, G., Johansson, I., *et al.* (1997). The involvement of CYP1A2 and CYP3A4 in the metabolism of clozapine. *British Journal of Clinical Pharmacology*, **44**, 439–46.

Fang, J. and Gorrod, J. W. (1999). Metabolism, pharmacogenetics, and metabolic drug–drug interactions of antipsychotic drugs. *Cell and Molecular Neurobiology*, **19**, 491–510.

Gandhi, T. K., Weingart, S. N., Borus, J., *et al.* (2003). Adverse drug events in ambulatory care. *New England Journal of Medicine*, **348**, 1556–64.

Juntti-Patinen, L. and Neuvonen, P. J. (2002). Drug-related deaths in a university central hospital. *European Journal of Clinical Pharmacology*, **58**, 479–82.

Juurlink, D. N., Mamdani, M., Kopp, A., Laupacis, A., and Redelmeier, D. A. (2003). Drug–drug interactions among elderly patients hospitalized for drug toxicity. *Journal of the American Medical Association*, **289**, 1652–8.

Kudo, S. and Ishizaki, T. (1999). Pharmacokinetics of haloperidol: an update. *Clinical Pharmacokinetics*, **37**, 435–56.

Lehmann, J. M., McKee, D. D., Watson, M. A., *et al.* (1998). The human orphan nuclear receptor PXR is activated by compounds that regulate CYP3A4 gene expression and cause drug interactions. *Journal of Clinical Investigation*, **102**, 1016–23.

Liston, H. L., Markowitz, J. S., and DeVane, C. L. (2001). Drug glucuronidation in clinical psychopharmacology. *Journal of Clinical Psychopharmacology*, **21**, 500–15.

Loga, S., Curry, S., and Lader, M. (1981). Interaction of chlorpromazine and nortriptyline in patients with schizophrenia. *Clinical Pharmacokinetics*, **6**, 454–62.

Markowitz, J. S. and DeVane, C. L. (1999). Suspected ciprofloxacin-related increase in olanzapine plasma concentration. *Journal of Clinical Psychopharmacology*, **19**, 289–90.

Markowitz, J. S. and DeVane, C. L. (2000). Rifampin induced selective serotonin reuptake inhibitor withdrawal syndrome in a patient treated with sertraline. *Journal of Clinical Psychopharmacology*, **20**, 109–10.

Markowitz, J. S., DeVane, C. L., Boulton, D. W., *et al.* (2000). Effect of St. John's wort (*Hypericum perforatum*) on cytochrome P-450 2D6 and 3A4 activity in healthy volunteers. *Life Sciences*, **66**, 133–9.

Moore, N., Lecointre, D., Noblet, C., and Mabille, M. (1998). Frequency and cost of serious adverse drug reactions in a department of general medicine. *British Journal of Clinical Pharmacology*, **45**, 301–8.

Otani, K. and Aoshima, T. (2000). Pharmacogenetics of classical and new antipsychotic drugs. *Therapy and Drug Monitoring*, **22**, 118–21.

Shin, J. G., Soukhova, N., and Flockhart, D. A. (1999). Effect of antipsychotic drugs on human liver cytochrome P-450 (CYP) isoforms *in vitro*: preferential inhibition of CYP2D6. *Drug Metabolism and Disposal*, **27**, 1078–84.

Sogawa, K. and Fujii-Kuriyama, Y. (1997). Ah receptor, a novel ligand activated transcription factor. *Journal of Biochemistry*, **122**, 1075–9.

Sternbach, H. (1991). The serotonin syndrome. *American Journal of Psychiatry*, **148**, 705–13.

Index